The Neuro-ophthalmology
Survival Guide

THIRD EDITION

The Neuro-ophthalmology Survival Guide

ANTHONY PANE, MBBS, MMedSc, FRANZCO, PhD
Neuro-ophthalmologist
Queensland Eye Institute
Brisbane, Australia

NEIL R. MILLER, MD, FACS
Professor Emeritus of Ophthalmology, Neurology and Neurosurgery
Wilmer Eye Institute
Johns Hopkins Hospital
Baltimore, Maryland, United States of America

MICHAEL BURDON, BSc, MB, BS, MRCP, FRCOphth
Consultant Neuro-ophthalmologist
County Durham and Darlington NHS Foundation Trust
United Kingdom

For additional online content visit eBooks+.com.

ELSEVIER

ISBN: 978-0-443-11598-1

Content Strategist: Trinity Hutton
Content Project Manager: Tapajyoti Chaudhuri
Design: Miles Hitchen
Marketing Manager: Deborah J. Watkins

Printed in India.

Last digit is the print number: 9 8 7 6 5 4 3 2 1

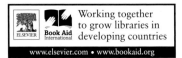

Working together to grow libraries in developing countries

www.elsevier.com • www.bookaid.org

CONTENTS

8. Abnormal movement or orientation of the visual world

Whether you are a busy optometrist who primarily performs refractions, an ophthalmologist who sees patients with cataracts or glaucoma, or a neurologist who sees a lot of patients with headache, you never know when a patient with a potentially vision- or life-threatening disorder will come to your clinic with a visual problem. Over the many years that we have practiced neuro-ophthalmology, we have encountered many patients who became permanently blind or neurologically impaired or who died because their otherwise skilled and well-meaning ophthalmologists, optometrists, or neurologists failed to **recognize** that they had a potentially devastating but treatable neuro-ophthalmic condition. This, despite the existence of many excellent and detailed neuro-ophthalmology texts. The problem is that none of these texts are written for the vast majority of practitioners who have no particular interest or expertise in neuro-ophthalmology. In addition, most of these texts are diagnosis based and therefore only helpful once the diagnosis had been made. However, in our opinion, the three most difficult challenges for most practitioners are to recognize that their patient has a "neuro-ophth" problem in the first place, then to make the correct diagnosis, and, finally, to provide appropriate treatment in a timely fashion.

To address these challenges, we set out 15 years ago to write a simple, practical clinical guide to benefit practitioners and their trainees. We made the guide symptom based; i.e., listen to the patient's concern (e.g., "I see double"; "the vision in my left eye is slowly worsening"), turn to the appropriate chapter (e.g., Chapter 6, "Double vision"; Chapter 3, "Blurred vision or field loss"), and let the book guide you every step of the way to the correct diagnosis and treatment without presuming that you have any previous neuro-ophthalmic training.

In the 5 years since the second edition of this book was published, there have been many advances in our ability to diagnose and treat neuro-ophthalmic conditions. Accordingly, this third edition of *The Neuro-ophthalmology Survival Guide* provides an updated but still carefully structured approach. Specifically, it tells you what questions to ask, what to look for during the examination, what diagnostic tools might be useful to make the correct diagnosis, and, depending on the diagnosis, what the management options are, all using clear and simple bullet points and flowcharts. Also unique to this book are 60 videos showing various important eye movement and pupil abnormalities and some important examination techniques.

Neuro-ophthalmology is the "needle in the haystack" in the busy clinics of all practitioners who see patients with visual complaints. We hope this book helps you avoid sitting on too many of these needles.

Anthony Pane
Neil R. Miller
Michael Burdon

INDEX OF KEY MANAGEMENT FLOWCHARTS

INDEX OF KEY CLINICAL DIAGNOSTIC CRITERIA

As ophthalmologists, optometrists, or neurologists, we all need to know a few things about neuro-ophthalmology. Why? Here are six reasons:

1. You Can't Avoid Neuro-ophthalmology!

Whether you're a generalist, subspecialist, or trainee, you will see, from time to time, patients with vision "worse than it should be," double vision, ptosis, or orbital pain. You need to know what to do when you encounter these problems. Your great abilities in your chosen ophthalmic subspecialty will mean little to a patient if you fail to diagnose their brain tumor, aneurysm, or giant cell arteritis (GCA)!

2. Neuro-ophthalmology Is Special!

Neuro-ophthalmology is unusual as an ophthalmic subspecialty in that looking in the eyes may be the least useful part of the clinical assessment. There are none of the "spot diagnoses" on slit-lamp examination that we enjoy in other areas: intraocular examination is usually normal or (when there are optic disc changes) nonspecific and nondiagnostic. In fact, diagnosis of neuro-ophthalmologic disorders often is dependent on particular symptoms that can only be elicited on careful ophthalmic and systemic history taking; subtle signs discovered on a structured examination not only of vision but also of the pupils, eyelids, eye movements, and cranial nerves; and often specific investigations including neuroimaging, optical coherence tomography, and electrophysiology. We're not used to approaching most eye patients in this manner, so you need to know what to ask and what to look for as regards each common neuro-ophthalmic complaint.

3. You Want Your Patients to See Well!

Hundreds of potentially treatable diseases can affect the optic nerves, chiasm, and post-chiasmal visual pathway, as well as the extraocular muscles, ocular motor nerves, and their neural connections, and pupillary abnormalities may be the first signs of such diseases. If the correct diagnosis is made and appropriate treatment begun, sight can often be saved or double vision eliminated; if not, unilateral or bilateral blindness or permanent diplopia may be the result.

4. You Want Your Patients to Stay Healthy!

Serious (often life-threatening) diseases present more often with neuro-ophthalmic complaints than with symptoms related to any other ophthalmic subspecialty. Blurred or double vision may be the first symptom of an orbital or brain tumor, an undiagnosed intracranial aneurysm, myasthenia gravis, a chronic infectious disease, or systemic vasculitis. You will often be the first medical specialist to see these patients and, thus, their best chance for early diagnosis. If you know what "warning" symptoms and signs to look for, you are more likely to diagnose the patient promptly, and their chance of long-term survival without major neurologic or systemic disability is likely to be much greater than if the diagnosis is delayed.

5. You Want to Stay Out of Trouble!

The most dangerous mistake that can be made by any ophthalmologist is not identifying a life-threatening but potentially treatable disorder. Many patients with treatable brain lesions or systemic diseases will first present to you with purely ophthalmic complaints, and they will be frustrated, angry, and litigious if you miss the diagnosis.

The second most dangerous mistake is not referring patients with suspected neuro-ophthalmic disease with the appropriate urgency. You might say, "I don't need to know anything about neuro—I just send everything like that to a neuro-ophthalmologist"; this is reasonable to some extent, but you have to be able to clinically triage your patients to know how urgently to refer them. Your next "otherwise well" patient with new-onset double vision could have an expanding aneurysm and die within hours of seeing you if he or she is not immediately admitted and treated; conversely, the patient could have an ischemic nerve palsy due to atherosclerosis and safely wait several months to be seen by a neuro-ophthalmologist after routine written referral. Through a careful history and examination, you have to decide who to worry about and who can wait.

6. You Want to Pass Your Exam (if You Still Have It Ahead of You)

Neuro-ophthalmic cases are old favorites for examiners for both written and clinical exams, including recertification exams, and one of the most common causes for candidate failure. For the written exam, you need to know something about the clinical features, appropriate investigations, and correct treatment of the common neuro-ophthalmic diseases, but more importantly, you need to have a practical management plan for patients with suspected neuro-ophthalmic problems for "clinical scenario" type essays. In the clinical component, a simple but structured approach to examining patients with acquired strabismus, nystagmus, ptosis, and visual sensory pathway disease is essential to your success.

How Can This Book Help?

This is not a book for neuro-ophthalmologists: it is designed to be of everyday practical use to all other ophthalmologists, optometrists, and neurologists. Despite (or perhaps because of) the many recent advances in neuro-ophthalmology, most general ophthalmologists, optometrists, and neurologists remain quite confused regarding the diagnosis and management of conditions commonly seen by neuro-ophthalmologists. Randomized clinical trials and large detailed textbooks are crucial for providing evidence-based information regarding diagnosis and treatment, but when it comes down to you and a new patient with an optic nerve or motility problem facing each other in the clinic, what should you actually DO?

We have designed this book to be a practical, symptom-based, "how-to" guide to neuro-ophthalmology and acquired strabismus for the non-neuro-ophthalmologist. Each chapter targets a specific clinical symptom, such as blurred vision or double vision, and includes:

- an introduction to the clinical assessment of each symptom
- an examination checklist reminding you which key features to check for on history and examination for each symptom
- a management flowchart to follow
- clinical diagnostic criteria checklists to ensure safe clinical diagnosis of common conditions, e.g., typical optic neuritis and ischemic sixth nerve palsy
- diseases that can cause the symptom, including a brief discussion of the symptoms, signs, and management of each
- when to refer, how urgently to refer, and how to investigate further if you choose not to refer.

In addition, Chapter 1, "Staying out of trouble," is a concise list of practice guidelines to help you avoid serious mistakes with your neuro-ophthalmic patients.

If you read this book straight through, great. If not, read Chapter 1 and look at the flowcharts, then keep the book with you in the clinic for your next "Oh no—neuro!" patient.

Please note:

- This book is not meant to be a substitute for referral to a neuro-ophthalmologist when necessary. There is nothing like experience and, as there are many rare conditions that can present with neuro-ophthalmic symptoms, you should refer early or urgently if you are uncomfortable investigating or managing a patient or if their clinical course seems atypical.
- Neuro-ophthalmology is a fascinating but complex field; the most comprehensive neuro-ophthalmic reference text, the sixth edition of *Walsh and Hoyt's Clinical Neuro-ophthalmology*, is 3573 pages long. For this reason, a brief book such as this must rely on extensive summarization, and many rare conditions are not mentioned here at all. Please see "Suggested reading" for more detailed reference texts.
- This book does not cover pediatric neuro-ophthalmology; for information on the management of visual pathway disease and strabismus in infants and children, we recommend one of the pediatric ophthalmology texts listed in the "Suggested reading" section.
- We necessarily err on the side of caution in investigating and managing patients; following the flowcharts may sometimes lead to the ordering of investigations that an experienced neuro-ophthalmologist would not request, based on having seen many hundreds of similar cases. However, in general, the "over-investigation" of a few patients will lead to less harm than underinvestigation, which unfortunately is all too common and often leads to the late diagnosis and treatment of serious disease.

- Neuro-ophthalmic practice varies considerably internationally and even region-ally within a single country. Different neuro-ophthalmologists will hold differ-ent opinions regarding the investigation and treatment of various diseases, often based on their own previous clinical experience. We believe that the approach pre-sented here represents safe, "mainstream" clinical practice with which most neuro-ophthalmologists would agree. However, it cannot be denied that some issues in neuro-ophthalmology remain highly controversial.

Staying Out of Trouble

If you read only one chapter in this book, read this one. It covers the most common and most serious mistakes made by ophthalmologists and ophthalmic trainees when dealing with neuro-ophthalmic patients.

Twenty Neuro "Rules" to Keep You Out of Trouble

The following 20 practice guidelines have a good chance of keeping your patients (and you) safe. Naturally, as with all "rules," there are rare exceptions to all of these, but they are still useful to keep in the back of your mind in the clinic or ophthalmic emergency department.

PATIENT PRESENTATION

1. Beware the "silent" neuro-ophthalmic patient!
   - patients with optic nerve or brain tumors will sometimes be referred to you as "cataract," "glaucoma," "optic neuritis," "ischemic sixth nerve palsy," "senile ptosis," or other benign-sounding diagnoses (Fig. 1.1)

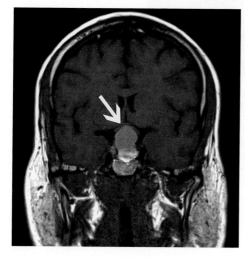

Fig. 1.1 This 37-year-old patient was referred to an ophthalmologist "for treatment of cataracts." On initial examination, visual acuity was right 20/30 and left 20/50, with only very early cataracts being present; neither color vision nor visual fields were assessed, and no pupillary examination was performed. It was only when vision did not improve after bilateral cataract surgery and subsequently worsened that another cause was suspected; this pituitary tumor was diagnosed as the real cause of the patient's blurred vision 1 year after first ophthalmic assessment. Final visual acuity after tumor resection was only 20/100 in each eye; visual outcome could have been improved by earlier diagnosis of the tumor. Note that the tumor is midline and bows the optic chiasm upward *(arrow)*.

EXAMINATION

2. Every new eye patient complaining of blurred vision should have:
   - confrontation field testing (peripheral and central)
   - a "swinging torch test" for a relative afferent pupillary defect (RAPD) before dilation
   - perimetry if either of these is abnormal, the patient describes a field defect, or the degree of visual loss is not consistent with the ocular examination (Fig. 1.2)

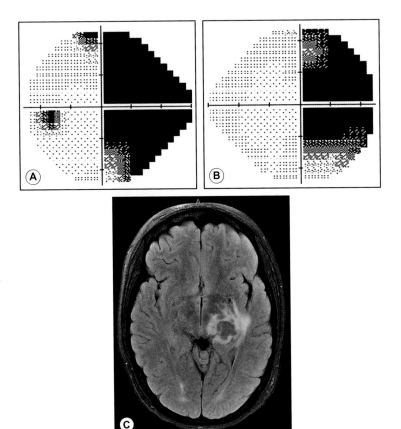

Fig. 1.2 This 16-year-old girl presented to the ophthalmology department complaining of headaches, blurred vision in her right eye, and flashing lights. Visual acuity was 20/20 in each eye and intraocular examination was normal. No visual field testing was performed, and the patient was told her symptoms were due to migraine. Reexamination by another doctor revealed a right homonymous hemianopia (**A**, **B**) that was easily detected with confrontation testing; (**C**) a left thalamic mass lesion was diagnosed on magnetic resonance imaging; further investigation showed this to be a cryptococcal abscess.

BLURRED VISION OR FIELD LOSS

3. You can never diagnose the cause of optic nerve dysfunction just by looking at the disc (Fig. 1.3).

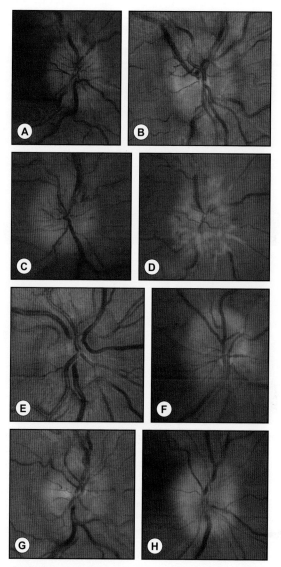

Fig. 1.3 Hundreds of different diseases can present with a similar optic disc appearance. For example, these swollen discs have been caused by (**A**) sarcoid optic neuritis, (**B**) optic nerve infiltration by lymphoma, (**C**) nonarteritic anterior ischemic optic neuropathy, (**D**) papilledema, (**E**) Leber hereditary optic neuropathy, (**F**) cat-scratch disease,(**G**) idiopathic optic neuritis, and (**H**) optic nerve sheath meningioma. In no case was the disc appearance diagnostic; diagnosis was made on careful history, other examination, perimetry, and other investigations as suggested in the management flowchart on p. 63.

4. All patients with nontraumatic ACUTE optic nerve dysfunction who do not meet all the clinical diagnostic criteria for either:

- typical optic neuritis (p. 66), or
- anterior ischemic optic neuropathy (AION) (p. 67)

require urgent referral to a neuro-ophthalmologist (or, if this is not possible, urgent investigation as suggested on p. 68) (Fig. 1.4).

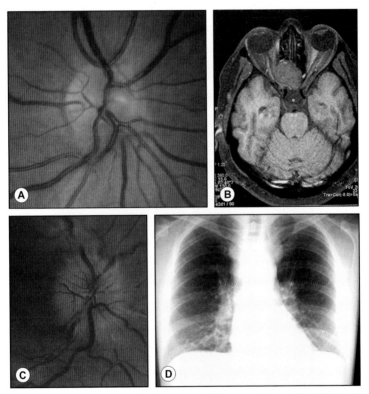

Fig. 1.4   Not all acute optic neuropathies in young adults are optic neuritis! (**A**) This 32-year-old woman presented with progressive visual loss in the right eye over 3 weeks (right 20/60), pain behind the right eye, a right relative afferent pupillary defect (RAPD), and normal optic discs. Her ophthalmologist diagnosed "retrobulbar optic neuritis" and reassured the patient that her vision would return spontaneously. Three months later, vision had worsened (20/200) and optic atrophy had developed. (**B**) Magnetic resonance imaging showed this large nasal tumor compressing the right optic nerve. Vision did not improve after removal of the tumor. Visual outcome would probably have been better with earlier diagnosis. For how to safely diagnose typical optic neuritis, see p. 66.

Not all acute optic neuropathies with a swollen disc are anterior ischemic optic neuropathy! This 55-year-old man with hypertension complained of progressive loss of vision in his right eye over 7 days. His ophthalmologist found (**C**) right visual acuity to be 20/40, a right RAPD, and right optic disc swelling. A right inferior altitudinal scotoma was detected on perimetry. The ophthalmologist diagnosed "anterior ischemic optic neuropathy" and advised the patient that there was no treatment. Ten weeks later, right visual acuity (VA) had deteriorated to 20/400 and the right disc had become pale; further investigation revealed an increased serum angiotensin-converting enzyme (ACE) and (**D**) hilar lymphadenopathy on chest x-ray. Biopsy of a lower eyelid conjunctival granuloma confirmed the diagnosis of sarcoidosis. Because diagnosis was delayed, right VA only returned to 20/80 with steroid treatment. For how to safely diagnose anterior ischemic optic neuropathy, see p. 67.

5. All patients with CHRONIC optic nerve dysfunction who do not meet all the clinical diagnostic criteria for glaucomatous optic neuropathy (p. 68) require referral to a neuro-ophthalmologist (or, if this is not possible, investigation as suggested on p. 68) (Fig. 1.5).

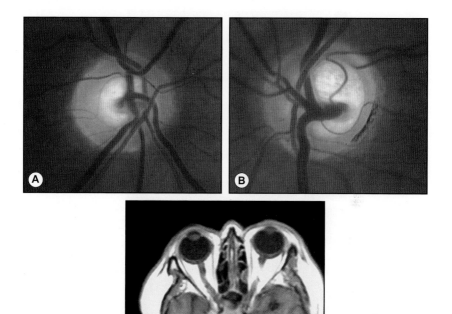

Fig. 1.5 Not all chronic optic neuropathy with a "cupped" disc is glaucoma! This 48-year-old patient asked her optometrist for a change of glasses because of blurred vision. The optometrist found (**A**, **B**) visual acuity right 20/30, left 20/60, intraocular pressures of right 25, left 29, and bilateral disc "cupping" and referred the patient to an ophthalmologist for treatment of possible glaucoma. Perimetry was attempted but fields were said to be "unreliable"; the ophthalmologist commenced glaucoma eye drops. One year later, visual acuity had decreased further to right 20/60, left 20/200, and optic disc pallor was noted; (**C**) Magnetic resonance imaging revealed a large suprasellar meningioma. Visual outcome would probably have been better with earlier diagnosis. For how to safely diagnose glaucoma, see p. 68.

6. Amblyopia is a specific diagnosis, with specific diagnostic features; never use a history of "lazy eye" as the explanation for worsening vision. Features of optic nerve disease should be absent and a demonstrable cause for the amblyopia should be present (Fig. 1.6).

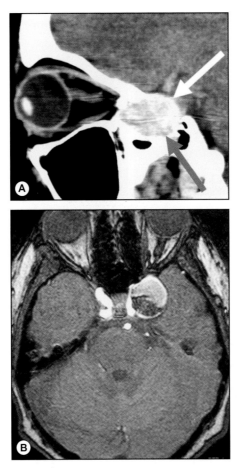

Fig. 1.6 A 38-year-old woman presented to her ophthalmologist complaining of blurred vision in her left eye and the left eye "turning in." She said that the left eye had always been "a bit lazy" so the ophthalmologist recorded "left amblyopia" as the cause of the blurred vision without checking for an relative afferent pupillary defect. The ophthalmologist diagnosed "decompensated congenital esotropia" and attributed the poor vision in the left eye (20/80) to "strabismic amblyopia." Eventually another ophthalmologist investigated the patient and found (**A**, **B**) a large internal carotid artery aneurysm causing compressive optic neuropathy and sixth nerve palsy. Unfortunately, by this time, the left eye was blind.

7. Whenever you look in an eye, think: is the level of vision explained by visible intraocular disease? If not, there could be disease behind the eye. Unexplained poor vision, optic atrophy, disc cupping, or field loss always requires investigation (Fig. 1.7).

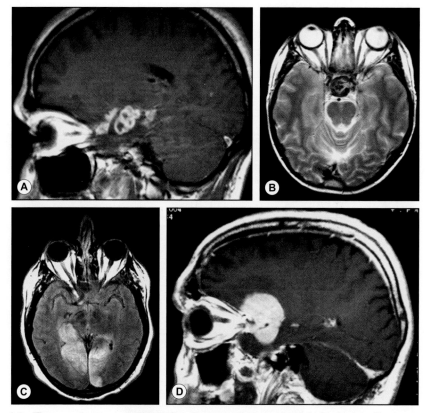

Fig. 1.7 These patients were all initially referred to their local ophthalmologists "for treatment of cataracts": **(A)** tuberculous meningitis and optic neuritis, **(B)** craniopharyngioma, **(C)** bilateral occipital lobe stroke causing "cortical blindness," and **(D)** sphenoid wing meningioma. Suspect that the patient is not "just another cataract" if he or she has one or more of the following: visual acuity loss greater than that expected from the density of the cataracts, color vision loss, relative afferent pupillary defect, or visual field loss (described by the patient or identified on confrontation testing). Optic disc pallor is helpful only when present (the discs may look entirely normal in early optic neuropathy); by the time pallor develops, irreversible damage has often occurred.

8. Compressive optic neuropathy from an orbital or brain tumor (including pituitary tumors) can present with:
- ANY optic disc appearance (normal, swollen, pale, or "cupped")—one or both eyes
- ANY sort of field loss (including arcuate scotoma or altitudinal field defect)—one or both eyes (Fig. 1.8).

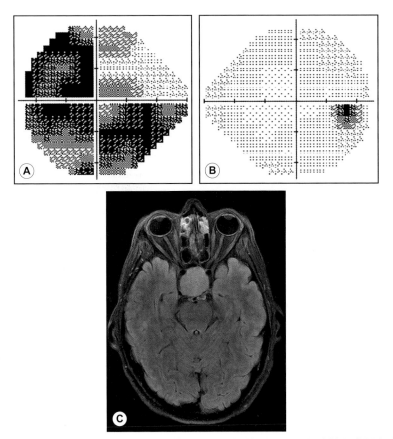

Fig. 1.8 This patient with a pituitary tumor (**C**) presented with visual acuity (VA) 20/200 in the left eye associated with a diffuse scotoma (**A**). The right eye VA was 20/20 with a normal visual field (**B**). It is actually fairly uncommon for pituitary region tumors to present with a "textbook" bitemporal hemianopia; they more commonly cause a unilateral or bilateral optic neuropathy or a combination of optic neuropathy and chiasmal dysfunction.

9. Just because both eyes look completely normal and there is no RAPD, do not assume the patient has nonorganic ("functional") visual loss; diagnose this only if you have thoroughly examined the patient, performed perimetry and have been able to "trick" the patient into demonstrating completely normal vision (see p. 128) (Fig. 1.9).

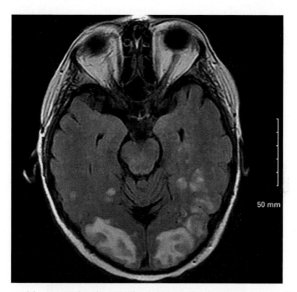

Fig. 1.9 This 60-year-old woman developed bilateral blurred vision associated with a mild headache while on high-dose steroids after a bone marrow transplantation. Because she had normal pupillary reactions and normal optic discs and retinas on funduscopic examination, the patient was thought to have "functional visual loss." The patient was referred to a neuro-ophthalmologist, who obtained a magnetic resonance imaging that revealed a posterior leukoencephalopathy affecting the optic radiations and striate cortex bilaterally.

BILATERAL DISC SWELLING

10. Bilateral disc swelling could be papilledema (disc swelling due to raised intra-cranial pressure). The first investigation should be urgent (same-day) magnetic resonance imaging (MRI) plus magnetic resonance venography (MRV) or computed tomographic (CT) scanning with CT venography (CTV) to exclude a brain tumor or dural venous sinus thrombosis (see p. 112) (Fig. 1.10).

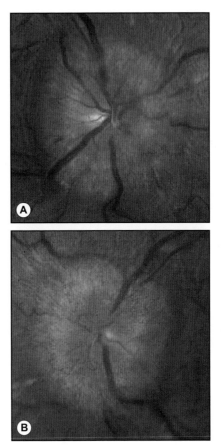

Fig. 1.10 This 38-year-old man presented to an ophthalmic emergency department complaining of blurred vision and headaches. Examination revealed visual acuity 20/20 right and left and bilateral moderate disc swelling (**A, B**). Because vision was good and there were "no other neurologic signs," the patient was allowed to go home and was scheduled for neuroimaging as an outpatient. Two days later, while driving, the patient experienced a generalized seizure, resulting in severe injuries to himself and another driver. Magnetic resonance imaging revealed a brain tumor, which was found at surgery to be an astrocytoma. For how to safely manage disc swelling with normal vision, see p. 137.

11. The diagnosis of primary pseudotumor cerebri (PTC), also called idiopathic intracranial hypertension (IIH), is based on specific diagnostic criteria (p. 141). MRI plus MRV and lumbar puncture must be performed in all cases of suspected IIH; not all women with disc swelling have IIH (Fig. 1.11).

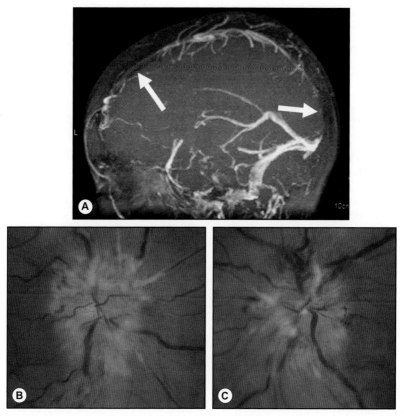

Fig. 1.11 Not all women with disc swelling have "idiopathic intracranial hypertension!" This 28-year-old, markedly obese woman presented to her ophthalmologist complaining of headaches and transient blurring of vision when she bent over or coughed. The ophthalmologist found visual acuities of 20/20 in both eyes and bilateral moderate optic disc swelling, diagnosed "benign intracranial hypertension," and requested a computed tomography brain scan that was normal. The patient was treated with acetazolamide tablets and told to lose weight. One week later, the patient collapsed at home and was admitted to the neurologic intensive care unit; magnetic resonance imaging plus magnetic resonance venography revealed a superior sagittal sinus thrombosis (**A**) and papilledema was noted to be very severe (**B, C**). Despite intensive treatment, the patient suffered bilateral optic disc infarction secondary to the severe papilledema and final visual acuity was 20/200 in both eyes with bilateral postpapilledema optic atrophy. She was also left with permanent right-sided weakness due to secondary cerebral venous infarction. Earlier diagnosis might have resulted in a better visual and neurologic outcome. For how to safely manage disc swelling with normal vision, see p. 139.

DOUBLE VISION

12. Beware the "spot diagnosis" in acquired strabismus. Many diseases that cause motility disturbance can present with the same clinical picture (Fig. 1.12).

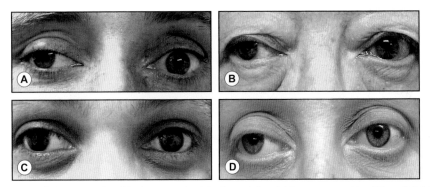

Fig. 1.12 Right exotropia with decreased adduction of the right eye caused by (**A**) partial third nerve palsy due to aneurysm, (**B**) myasthenia, (**C**) right lateral rectus myositis, and (**D**) internuclear ophthalmoplegia. Eye appearance and pursuit "eye movement" testing was not diagnostic in any case; diagnosis was made by a careful history, a detailed examination including saccade testing, and other investigations. See p. 197 for a management flowchart for diplopia.

13. All cases of unexplained double vision (in which you are unable to make a definite diagnosis) require neuro-ophthalmic referral, urgently if of acute onset. There could be a serious underlying cause such as aneurysm, tumor, or myasthenia (Fig. 1.13).

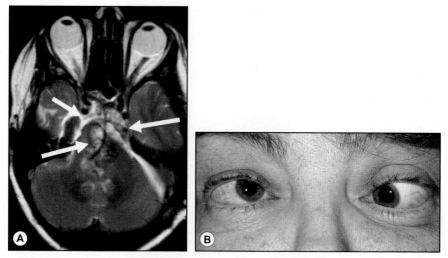

Fig. 1.13 This 42-year-old woman initially presented to her local ophthalmologist complaining of gradual-onset horizontal double vision. At first examination, she had a small esotropia in primary position; however, eye movements were noted to be "full" (no restriction was seen in any direction). The ophthalmologist diagnosed "decompensated esophoria" and prescribed prism to be ground into the patient's spectacles. Although this relieved the diplopia, the amount of prism required gradually increased over the next 18 months until the spectacles were too heavy for the patient to wear comfortably; at this stage, it was noted that abduction was visibly limited in both eyes. Magnetic resonance imaging revealed a large clival tumor that on biopsy was found to be a chordoma (**A**). The tumor had caused gradually progressive bilateral sixth nerve palsies that initially presented as a small comitant esotropia with no visible limitation of abduction. Further tumor spread eventually led to a vertical deviation being superimposed on the esotropia (**B**), due to partial third nerve palsy.

14. All patients with partial or complete third nerve palsy require urgent MRI and magnetic resonance angiography (MRA) or CT and CTA to exclude an aneurysm, except patients who meet all the clinical diagnostic criteria for ischemic third nerve palsy (p. 199) (Fig. 1.14).

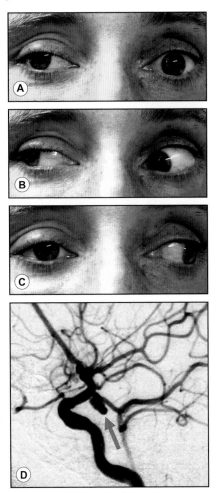

Fig. 1.14 This 35-year-old woman with diabetes presented with acute-onset horizontal diplopia. Her ophthalmologist noted a right exotropia, limitation of adduction of the right eye with normal elevation and depression, and a mild right ptosis (**A–C**). The pupils were equal in size and both were briskly reactive to light. The ophthalmologist diagnosed a partial right third nerve palsy. He thought that this was "ischemic" in origin because the right pupil was "spared" and the patient had diabetes. "To rule out any other cause," a computed tomography (CT) scan of the brain was obtained that was normal; the patient was reassured the diplopia would resolve spontaneously and a return appointment was made for 3 months' time. The following day, the patient collapsed at home; an urgent magnetic resonance imaging and magnetic resonance angiography showed a right posterior communicating artery aneurysm that had ruptured, causing subarachnoid hemorrhage; this was confirmed on angiography (**D**). The patient underwent urgent neurosurgical intervention and survived but was left with a dense left hemiplegia. Earlier diagnosis of the aneurysm before it ruptured could have prevented her serious permanent disability. For how to safely diagnose ischemic third nerve palsy, see p. 199.

15. Patients with fourth nerve palsy require an MRI to exclude a brain tumor or vascular malformation, except patients who meet all the clinical diagnostic criteria for either:
- congenital fourth nerve palsy (p. 201), or
- ischemic fourth nerve palsy (p. 200) (Fig. 1.15)

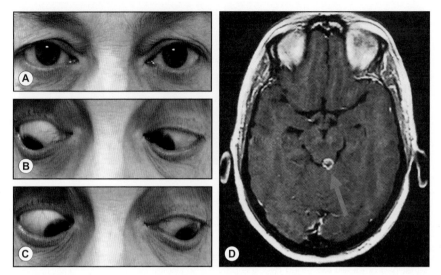

Fig. 1.15 This 56-year-old woman with hypertension presented with a 2-week history of vertical and torsional diplopia. She was initially diagnosed with a "right ischemic fourth nerve palsy" and reassured that the diplopia would resolve spontaneously. However, closer examination revealed 12 degrees of excyclotorsion on double Maddox rod testing, a right hypertropia in left gaze that changed to a left hypertropia in right gaze, and mild bilateral superior oblique underaction (decreased depression of each eye in adduction) (**A–C**). A diagnosis of bilateral fourth nerve palsy was made. Magnetic resonance imaging with contrast revealed a small enhancing lesion in the collicular area (**D**), biopsy of which diagnosed a glioma. For how to safely diagnose ischemic or congenital fourth nerve palsy, see p. 201.

16. All patients with sixth nerve palsy require an MRI to exclude a brain tumor, except patients who meet all the clinical diagnostic criteria for ischemic sixth nerve palsy (p. 202) (Fig. 1.16).

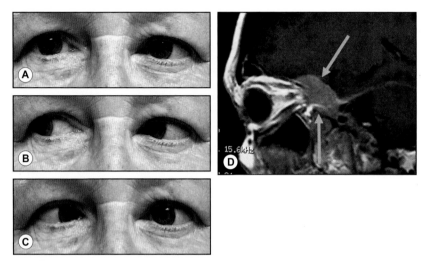

Fig. 1.16 This 62-year-old woman with diabetes and hypertension presented with horizontal diplopia that had gradually worsened over the previous 2 weeks. Her ophthalmologist found a left esotropia with reduced abduction of the left eye and diagnosed an "ischemic" left sixth nerve palsy. However, over the next 6 months, the diplopia did not resolve and in fact worsened; the patient was eventually examined by a neuro-ophthalmologist who found reduced left corneal and supraorbital sensation in addition to a marked esotropia with left abduction weakness consistent with a left sixth nerve palsy (**A–C**). Magnetic resonance imaging revealed a large left sphenoid wing meningioma that had invaded the cavernous sinus (**D**). The patient was angry that she had been initially observed instead of investigated. For how to safely diagnose ischemic sixth nerve palsy, see p. 202.

GIANT CELL ARTERITIS

17. Don't miss giant cell arteritis (GCA) (Fig. 1.17): think of it in every patient over 50 with:
    - transient visual loss (including "amaurosis fugax")
    - sudden, persistent visual loss
        - with optic disc swelling (e.g., AION)
        - with evidence of a central retinal artery occlusion
        - with a normal fundus but other evidence of an optic neuropathy (retrobulbar ischemic optic neuropathy)
    - transient double vision (even if your examination is normal)
    - persisting double vision (including third, fourth, or sixth nerve palsies)

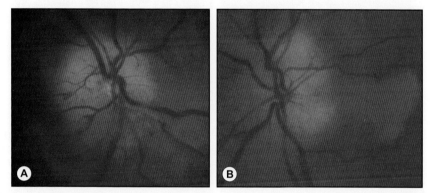

Fig. 1.17 A 68-year-old woman was referred to her local ophthalmologist with vague visual complaints of 2 weeks' duration. She complained of "seeing double" for minutes at a time and of loss of vision in her right eye lasting minutes and then resolving. The ophthalmologist found ocular motility and intraocular examination to be entirely normal and reassured the patient that there was "nothing wrong with the eyes." Three days later, the patient suddenly went blind in the right eye, followed an hour later by loss of vision in the left eye, due to anterior ischemic optic neuropathy (**A, B**). Specific questioning revealed a 3-month history of a new type of headache, fatigue, myalgias, and scalp pain when she tried to brush her hair. Despite urgent treatment with intravenous and then oral steroids, the final visual acuity was right no perception of light, left light perception. Temporal artery biopsy confirmed giant cell arteritis.

NEUROIMAGING

18. MRI is far superior to in detecting most of the causes of neuro-ophthalmic disease and is the investigation of choice. A normal brain CT does NOT exclude serious disease (Fig. 1.18).

   - you need to know what sort of MRI to order, and in some cases you need to push to have it done urgently
   - MRI should always be requested "with contrast" as many orbital and brain lesions are difficult to detect unless contrast injection is given.

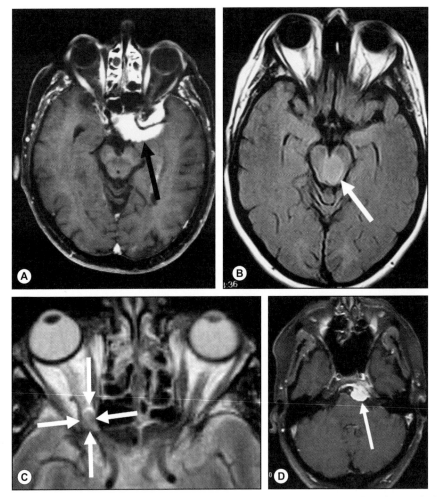

Fig. 1.18 These tumors were all missed on brain computed tomography scan but detected with contrast-enhanced magnetic resonance imaging. (**A**) Sphenoid wing meningioma. (**B**) Pontine glioma. (**C**) Orbital apex meningioma. (**D**) Clival meningioma.

OPHTHALMIC EMERGENCIES

19. The prime ophthalmic emergencies, in order of importance and urgency, are:

Life-threatening:
- double vision due to possible partial or complete third nerve palsy in which an aneurysm cannot be clinically excluded
- bilateral optic disc swelling due to brain tumor or dural venous sinus thrombosis
- acute unilateral or bilateral ophthalmoplegia from acute myasthenia, pituitary apoplexy (Fig. 1.19), cavernous sinus thrombosis, carotid-cavernous fistula, or orbital cellulitis
- ptosis or diplopia with dyspnea, dysphagia, or severe systemic weakness due to severe myasthenia
- ptosis and ipsilateral small but reactive pupil from Horner syndrome related to an acute internal carotid artery dissection

Bilateral sight-threatening:
- acute loss of vision from GCA, pituitary apoplexy, or neuromyelitis optica

Unilateral sight-threatening:
- acute glaucoma, endophthalmitis, penetrating eye injury, sphenoid sinus mucocele

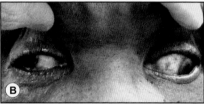

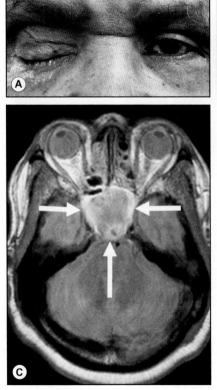

Fig. 1.19 This 42-year-old man presented to the ophthalmic emergency department complaining of the sudden onset of blurred vision, diplopia, right ptosis, and headache of 3 hours' duration (**A**, **B**). The ophthalmology resident was informed but was too busy with other patients to see him immediately. Six hours later, the patient collapsed in the waiting room and was admitted via the general emergency department. Urgent magnetic resonance imaging revealed pituitary apoplexy (sudden infarction of a previously undiagnosed pituitary tumor) (**C**). Urgent medical therapy and neurosurgical treatment saved the patient's life. In retrospect, this patient's case was much more urgent than the retinal detachments and penetrating eye injury with which the resident had been occupied.

THREE COMMON MISTAKES

20. Three common mistakes made by ophthalmologists that lead to permanent blindness, disability, or death of patients with neuro-ophthalmic disease are:

- ■ not suspecting the possibility of serious orbital or brain disease as the cause of a patient's "eye" complaints
- ■ not performing a thorough history and examination
- ■ not referring to a neuro-ophthalmologist early and urgently when necessary

These three mistakes cause much more harm than not knowing all the details of rare neuro-ophthalmic diseases (Fig. 1.20).

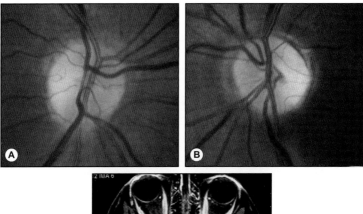

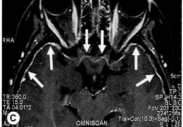

Fig. 1.20   This 33-year-old woman was referred to her local ophthalmologist complaining of blurred vision in both eyes for the past 2 months. Examination revealed visual acuity of 20/30 in each eye, reduced color vision in both eyes, and temporal pallor of both optic discs (**A, B**). The ophthalmologist requested a magnetic resonance imaging (MRI) (but did not specifically ask for contrast enhancement) and ordered the following blood tests: vitamin B12, folate, erythrocyte sedimentation rate, c-reactive protein, and complete blood count. The MRI was said to be normal, as were the blood tests, except for the B12 level that was slightly low; the patient was told she had "nutritional deficiency optic neuropathy" and was given multivitamins and B12 injections. Despite this treatment, her vision worsened to 20/200 in both eyes over the next 12 months. At this stage, the patient was advised that she might have "optic neuritis" and was given a 3-day course of intravenous methylprednisolone without effect. A blood test was then performed for Leber hereditary optic neuropathy, which was negative. Eighteen months after first seeing the ophthalmologist, the patient's visual acuity had decreased to "light perception" in each eye and she was finally referred to a neuro-ophthalmologist. (**C**) A contrast-enhanced MRI revealed diffuse meningeal enhancement *(arrows)* suggestive of a chronic granulomatous meningitis; and serum angiotensin-converting enzyme (ACE), computed tomography of the mediastinum, and lumbar puncture resulted in a diagnosis of chronic sarcoid meningitis and optic neuritis. Because of the severe optic atrophy, vision did not improve despite immunosuppressive treatment. If, at the start, the patient had been promptly referred to a neuro-ophthalmologist or investigated thoroughly, rather than investigated inadequately and "piecemeal" over a long period, it is likely that she would have retained good vision in both eyes.

CHAPTER 2

Neuro-ophthalmic History and Examination

Introduction

The majority of neuro-ophthalmic disorders are not "spot diagnoses"; that is, they are not apparent with a brief slit-lamp or fundoscopic examination. However, many can be diagnosed clinically or with a minimum of investigations, provided that a full history has been taken and an accurate examination performed.

The aims of the history and examination are to:

- clearly define the presenting complaint
- quantify the degree of impairment
- localize the site of the disease process
- establish the diagnosis or differential diagnosis
- identify possible precipitating factors or risk factors
- guide further investigations

Having a structured plan for your history and examination of patients with suspected neuro-ophthalmic problems means you are much less likely to miss important clues to their underlying disease.

History

The structure of the history is similar to that for any medical condition.

PATIENT DETAILS

- age

PRESENTING COMPLAINT

- This must be asked in terms the patient can understand (e.g., it may be appropriate to ask a patient with transient visual loss if they have ever had migraines but also ask if they have ever had a "sick headache").

- A detailed description of the problem, including:
  - nature of the problem (e.g., double vision, visual loss, blurred vision, headache)—why are you here today?
  - Time course
    - time of onset: it is important to distinguish between time of onset and when the problem was first noticed (e.g., a patient who only incidentally notices visual loss in one eye when covering the other eye cannot clearly define time of onset)
    - speed of onset and development over time
    - variability throughout the day or from day to day
    - "warning signs" prior to the onset of permanent loss of function (e.g., transient visual loss preceding permanent visual loss)
    - status: is it still present or was it transient?
    - associated symptoms/signs (e.g., numbness, weakness, headache)
  - previous episodes
    - frequency
    - duration
    - triggering/predisposing factors
  - investigations/treatment so far

OTHER OPHTHALMIC SYMPTOMS

- pain (site, timecourse, worse on moving eyes?)
- visual loss
- double vision

OPHTHALMIC HISTORY

- glasses or contact lenses
- eye drops, surgery, or laser
- eye patching or strabismus surgery as a child ("did you ever have a lazy eye?")
- previous history of eye disease (e.g., age-related macular degeneration, cataract)
- details of last eye test: this may help to date the onset of visual loss

MEDICAL HISTORY

- cancer
- autoimmune disease
- diabetes, hypertension, high cholesterol
- trauma, particularly to the head or neck
- surgery

MEDICATIONS

- often give clues to systemic diseases forgotten by the patient

- many medicines may cause or exacerbate neuro-ophthalmic disorders including:
  - optic neuropathy: ethambutol, isoniazid, amiodarone, drugs for erectile dysfunction
  - raised intracranial pressure (ICP): corticosteroids, oral contraceptive pill, tetracyclines, vitamin A derivatives used for acne
  - retinopathy: vigabatrin, tamoxifen, hydroxychloroquine
  - double vision: penicillamine, aminoglycosides, others (drug-induced myasthenia)
  - nystagmus: phenytoin, lithium

FAMILY HISTORY

- particularly of ophthalmic or neurologic disease
- if a positive history, it is useful to draw out a family tree

SOCIAL AND OCCUPATIONAL HISTORY

- marital status
- occupation and potential occupational hazards (e.g., exposure to toxic substances, foreign bodies)
- recent travel
- visual requirements (e.g., driving)
- current or previous smoking or alcohol use
- current or previous use of illicit drugs
- diet/nutrition (if poor nutrition suspected, ask specifically what the patient ate yesterday, day before, etc.)

SYMPTOMS OF GIANT CELL ARTERITIS

- All patients over 50 with a history of transient or permanent visual loss or double vision should be asked about:
  - new or unusually severe headaches
  - scalp and/or temple tenderness
  - ache or pain in the jaw muscles on chewing food
  - ear pain or ache
  - tongue ache on talking or chewing
  - fevers, fatigue, decreased appetite, weight loss, chronic cough
  - muscle aches and pains.

SYSTEMS REVIEW QUESTIONS

- Symptoms (past or present) revealed by systems review questioning may either suggest an underlying systemic disease or help localize the site of a neuro-ophthalmic problem. Detailed questioning may not be necessary in all cases but for many, it provides important clues to the etiology of the disorder

General

- recent infections (infectious or postinfectious diseases)
- fevers, night sweats, fatigue, weight loss, poor appetite (cancer, chronic infection, giant cell arteritis [GCA])
- recent head or neck trauma, chiropractic neck manipulation (traumatic visual loss or nerve palsy; internal carotid artery or vertebrobasilar dissection)

Neurologic

- headache (GCA, tumor, aneurysm, raised ICP)
- persistent hemifacial or hemicranial pain, numbness, or "pins and needles" (tumor, aneurysm)
- "fits, faints, funny turns" (tumor, stroke, transient ischemic attacks)
- numbness or weakness (tumor, stroke, multiple sclerosis [MS])
- difficulties with speech, balance, micturition, bowel control (MS)
- fatigable weakness (myasthenia)
- transient episodes of numbness, weakness, or vertigo in the past (MS, transient ischemic attacks)

Ear, Nose, Throat

- deafness (vestibular schwannoma)
- tinnitus (vestibular schwannoma; if pulsatile, suspect carotid-cavernous fistula [CCF] or raised ICP)
- sinus congestion or nosebleeds (nasopharyngeal carcinoma, Wegener granulomatosis)
- problems swallowing (myasthenia, oculopharyngeal dystrophy)
- mouth ulcers (Behçet)

Respiratory

- cough, short of breath, wheeze, "adult-onset asthma" (sarcoidosis, tuberculosis, cancer)

Cardiovascular

- history of "heart murmur" (embolic risk)
- chest pain (vasculitis, thrombosis)

Gastrointestinal

- abdominal pains, change in bowel habits, passing blood (cancer, inflammatory bowel disease, possible nutritional deficiency due to malabsorption, periarteritis nodosa)

Genitourinary

- burning or stinging on passing urine, genital ulcers or discharge, past history of a sexually transmitted disease (syphilis, HIV, Behçet)
- blood in urine (vasculitis, cancer)

- prostate symptoms (cancer)
- galactorrhea/amenorrhea (pituitary tumor)

Musculoskeletal

- muscle aches? (GCA, vasculitis)
- joint pain or swelling? (chronic infections, autoimmune diseases, e.g., systemic lupus erythematosus [SLE])

Skin

- skin rash (syphilis, sarcoid, Lyme, vasculitis)
- new-onset easy bruising (leukemia)

Infectious Risk Factors

- friends or family with infectious disease (e.g., tuberculosis)
- recent travel to any regions where unusual infections possible?
- pets (cat scratch disease)
- tick bites (Lyme disease)
- intravenous drug use or blood transfusion (infectious diseases including HIV)

Examination

For most neuro-ophthalmological conditions, the history indicates the likely diagnosis or at least points the examiner in the right direction, and the examination is merely confirmatory. At the very least, the history indicates if a patient has a visual sensory disturbance (afferent pathway), double vision or abnormal eye movements (efferent pathway), a difference in the size of the pupils, drooping of the eyelid, or headaches/facial pain. Therefore, it is often appropriate for the examination to focus on one of these areas. By doing so, however, there is a danger that other potentially diagnostic or localizing signs may be missed; for example, failing to notice decreased corneal sensation, anisocoria, or even optic disc swelling in a patient with a sixth cranial nerve palsy. Similarly, it is frequently assumed that patients with transient symptoms will have a normal examination, but a careful search may, for example, reveal peripheral retinal emboli in a patient with monocular transient visual loss (i.e., amaurosis fugax).

To avoid missing important signs, we recommend that a minimum neuro-ophthalmic examination (see Summary box) be performed on all patients, supplemented where appropriate by a more detailed examination of the area suggested by the history. **Instead of expecting that a particular part of the examination will yield normal findings, always assume that the examination results are going to be abnormal until you have proved that they are normal**.

Patients with symptoms of previously undiagnosed systemic disease or a generalized neurologic disorder also require a full systemic and neurologic examination. You may wish to consider enlisting the assistance of a neurologist or internist.

MINIMUM NEURO-OPHTHALMIC EXAMINATION

- visual acuity (VA) at distance and near (best-corrected or with pinhole)
- color vision (Hardy-Rand-Rittler or Ishihara plates best)
- confrontation visual fields (finger counting, finger wiggling, red test object)
- perimetry, i.e., formal visual field testing before dilating drops if there are symptoms or signs of afferent pathway disease
- eye movements
  - fixation holding (is there nystagmus?)
  - primary position deviation (observation, cover test)
  - ductions/versions (if limited in both eyes, test doll's-head maneuver)
  - pursuit
  - saccades
  - convergence (to an accommodative target)
- pupils
  - size
  - response to light (if poor, also test near response)
  - swinging light test (for relative afferent pupillary defect [RAPD])
- lid position: ptosis, retraction
- orbits: proptosis (pulsatile?), enophthalmos, injection, chemosis, bruit
- corneal and facial sensation to light touch
- orbicularis oculi and facial muscle strength
- if patient over 50 and history consistent: palpate the temporal arteries for pulsatility and tenderness
- slit-lamp examination (before and after dilation)
- intraocular pressure (IOP)
- ophthalmoscopy after dilation, including careful optic disc, macular and peripheral retinal examination
- vital signs including blood pressure (in appropriate setting)

VISUAL ACUITY

- distance visual acuity (VA) with the optimal refractive correction (or at least a pinhole) is an obvious first examination step
- however, remember that normal VA does not exclude serious visual pathway disease (patients can have dense bitemporal or hemianopic visual field defects with absolutely normal VA)
- test reading VA at 30 cm with the appropriate refractive correction as well (if the patient has to bring the reading card closer to see the print, indicate at what distance the chart was held)
- using a reading card with text rather than a card that just has individual letters or numbers provides an indication not only of the patient's near acuity but also a sense of the patient's cognition!
- if patient has poor near vision, can use a plus lens or a pinhole (as with distance vision) to see if it improves

COLOR VISION (VIDEO 2.1)

- color vision is often decreased earlier, or more severely, than VA in optic neuropathies of many causes
- therefore, decreased color acuity is an important neuro-ophthalmic "warning sign" even if VA is normal

- however, congenital "color blindness" is common
    - patients with congenital dyschromatopsia can be recognized because their color loss is bilateral, symmetric, and asymptomatic; they have normal VA (or decreased VA explained by visible intraocular disease) and normal visual fields
    - by contrast, patients with acquired dyschromatopsia usually have a visual field defect and/or decreased VA, often have asymmetric color loss and sometimes the color loss is symptomatic (colors look "washed out" or faded)
- the following are simple tests of color acuity

Subjective Color Desaturation (Fig. 2.1)

- in cases of a unilateral or asymmetric optic neuropathy, a colored target (such as the red top of an eyedrop bottle) will seem less colorful to the affected (or worse) eye than the unaffected eye (e.g., red appears brown or there is no color at all!)

Color Plate Tests (e.g., Ishihara or Hardy-Rand-Rittler Pseudoisochromatic Color Plates)

- many color plate tests were designed to detect congenital color defects (that occur in approximately 8% of men and 1% of women)
- they have a number of limitations when applied to acquired visual pathway disease
    - patients with reduced acuity may not be able to see the plates (the Ishihara plates are unreliable if the acuity of the eye being tested is 20/120 or worse)
    - patients with a field defect may only see half of each plate (this may alert you to the presence of a field defect)
    - patients with cognitive impairment may not be able to recognize a number formed out of dots (as seen in the Ishihara plates) even if they can identify the color of each dot on the plate individually

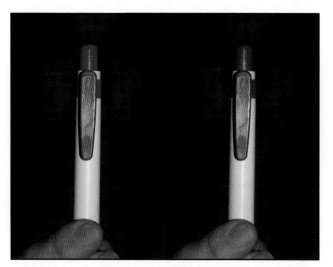

Fig. 2.1 Subjective color desaturation. *Left:* red target as seen by a normal eye. *Right:* desaturated red target as seen by an eye with an optic neuropathy.

- nevertheless, color plate tests can provide a useful measure of color vision in acquired visual pathway disease
- it is important to choose one of the tests and to become familiar with its use and its limitations
  - compare the number of plates seen with each eye
  - if the patient is able to see all the plates with either eye, turn to a plate with no visible number and ask the patient to compare the saturation of color with each eye
    - ask the patient to look at the plate with their better eye and to assess the brightness of the colors (like adjusting the color on a television)
    - ask the patient to change to their other eye and compare the brightness of colors: "if you give the first eye 10 out of 10 for color brightness, would you give the second eye more, the same, or less?"
  - if patient cannot see any figures on color plates, can use objects or colors on a smartphone to check gross color perception

VISUAL FIELDS TO CONFRONTATION (FIG. 2.2 AND VIDEO 2.2)

- confrontation testing is a useful qualitative test capable of detecting hemianopic, quadrantic, altitudinal, and some central defects; however, a normal test does not rule out a more subtle defect
- confrontation testing cannot be used to monitor field loss
- it is important to develop a consistent technique

Descriptive

- the patient looks at your nose with one eye at a time
- ask "are all parts of my face equally clear or is a part blurred or missing?"
- this is a quick and surprisingly sensitive technique and can often detect subtle defects like central or paracentral scotomas which can be missed on standard confrontation testing

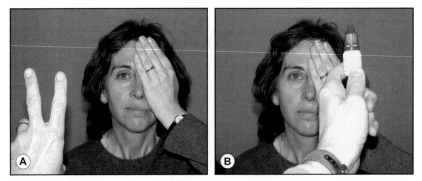

Fig. 2.2 Visual fields to confrontation. (**A**) Finger counting in four quadrants. (**B**) Assessment of red saturation in central field and four quadrants.

Finger Counting in Quadrants

- the patient covers their left eye, you close your right, they stare into your open eye
- holding both hands in the upper midperiphery area, hold out one or two fingers of each hand and ask "how many fingers in total?"
- then move both hands to the inferior midperiphery area and repeat
- repeat for the other eye

Red Target for Central Field

- the patient covers their left eye, you close your right, they stare into your open eye
- you place a red target (hat pin or similar) in the middle of their field and ask "what color is this?"
- if the patient says red then you repeat the test with their other eye and ask them if the target is a brighter red in one eye compared with the other eye
- if the patient reports that the color of the target is not red or less saturated in one eye, move the target away from the center of their affected eye and ask "is the red becoming brighter or duller?"

Red Target for Hemianopic Defect

- particularly useful if a chiasmal defect is suspected
  - ask the patient to compare the color saturation of a red target held in each quadrant
  - if the patient reports desaturation in one quadrant, move the target toward the vertical and horizontal meridians and say "tell me when the red becomes brighter"

Perimetry

- all patients with suspected visual pathway disease should have static or kinetic perimetry in order to:
  - localize the site of the lesion in the visual pathway
  - obtain a quantitative baseline against which future changes can be compared

FIXATION, ALIGNMENT, AND EYE MOVEMENTS (VIDEO 2.3)

A full ocular motility assessment may involve some or all of the following:

Fixation

- observation (p. 30)
- assessment of nystagmus (p. 30)
- assessment of inappropriate saccadic movements (p. 31)

Eye Alignment in Primary Position

- cover test (pp. 31–32)
- alternate cover test (pp. 32–33)
- prism cover test (p. 33)

Eye Movements

- range of movement (ductions and versions) (p. 34)
- pursuit (p. 36)
- saccades (pp. 36–37)
- convergence (pp. 37–38)
- vestibulo-ocular reflex (VOR) (pp. 38–39)
- optokinetic nystagmus (OKN) (p. 39)

Special Tests

- prism fusional amplitude (p. 40)
- head tilt test (p. 41)
- double Maddox rod test (p. 42)
- forced duction testing (pp. 42–43)

Fixation

- acquired abnormalities of fixation (nystagmus or saccadic intrusions) frequently present with oscillopsia
- patients with congenital/early-onset fixation disorders do not usually complain of oscillopsia; they are more likely to be referred because they have been incidentally noticed to have abnormal eye movements

Observation

- the patient should be asked to look at a fixation target, initially in the primary position, then in eccentric gaze and finally on return to the primary position
- the eyes should be observed for continuous or intermittent oscillations; if the patient complains of oscillopsia but no oscillations are seen with the naked eye, he or she should be re-examined at the slit-lamp or with a direct ophthalmoscope

Assessment of Nystagmus

(See also Chapters 8 and 9.)

- waveform
  - pendular (sinusoidal)
  - jerk (slow movement away from fixation and a fast corrective movement in the opposite direction)
  - mixed
- plane
  - horizontal
  - vertical
  - torsional
  - mixed
- direction
  - the direction of the fast phase is used to describe jerk nystagmus (e.g., left-beating nystagmus has fast phase to the patient's left)
  - patients with horizontal jerk nystagmus should be observed for several minutes to see if the direction changes—the defining feature of periodic alternating nystagmus

- conjugacy
  - conjugate: the fast and slow (if jerk) or slow (if pendular) phases of both eyes are in the same direction
  - disconjugate: the fast and slow phases are in different directions (e.g., the right eye has slow phases to the right and fast phases to the left, whereas the left eye has slow phases to the left and fast phases to the right as in convergence-retraction nystagmus)
- influence of eye position
  - is the nystagmus present in the primary position or only on eccentric gaze?
  - does the plane vary with direction of gaze?
  - does the intensity (amplitude times frequency) vary with direction of gaze or with convergence?
  - is there a position where the intensity is least (null zone) or where the direction of jerk nystagmus reverses (neutral zone)?
- influence of fogging or occlusion
  - is the intensity increased by fogging (use Frenzel goggles or a thin-rimmed +11D or greater spherical lens)?
  - does the nystagmus only occur or change direction when one eye is occluded?
- influence of nystagmus on eye movements: does the nystagmus break up pursuit eye movements?

Assessment of Inappropriate Saccadic Movements
- plane
  - horizontal
  - vertical
  - oblique
- amplitude
  - small (less than 5 degrees)
  - large (more than 5 degrees)
- frequency
  - high vs low
- duration
  - intermittent (bursts)
  - continuous (oscillations)

Eye Alignment in Primary Position
- abnormalities of ocular alignment usually present with persistent or intermittent double vision, unless the patient has poor vision or a childhood strabismus
- the cover test is the basic test of ocular alignment; it should be performed on all patients with neuro-ophthalmic symptoms
- the choice of further tests depends on the patient's symptoms and the results of the cover test

Cover Test (Fig. 2.3)
Purpose
- to detect manifest deviation (tropia) in the horizontal and vertical planes

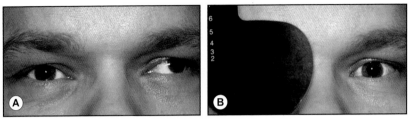

Fig. 2.3 Cover test. (**A**) Patient with left exotropia and hypertropia; note decentered light reflex in left eye. (**B**) On covering the right eye, the left eye moves inward and downward to take up fixation.

Technique
- if the patient wears glasses they should be appropriate for the distance being tested
- the patient should look straight ahead at a distant target such as a letter on an acuity chart with both eyes open
- briefly cover then uncover the right eye while watching the left eye
- if the left eye moves when the right eye is covered, the patient has a manifest deviation of their left eye
  - if the left eye moved outward: it was turned in (left esotropia)
  - if the left eye moved inward: it was turned out (left exotropia)
  - if the left eye moved downward: it was turned up (left hypertropia)
  - if the left eye moved upward: it was turned down (left hypotropia)
- if no movement of the left eye is observed, briefly cover and uncover the left eye while watching the right eye: if the right eye moves when the left eye is covered, the patient has a manifest deviation of their right eye
- if there is no movement of either eye, the patient has no manifest deviation in the primary position
- repeat while the patient looks at a near target (e.g., a reduced Snellen chart)
- if the patient's history suggests that their double vision varies with direction of gaze (or is only present on eccentric gaze), the test should be repeated in those eye positions
Note: this test does not detect torsional misalignment
- if the history suggests that torsional diplopia is present, ask the patient to look at a linear target (e.g., a pencil) held horizontally and to describe what they see
- if the patient reports torsional diplopia (typically also separated vertically), ask them to describe the torsion, for example "are the images closer together on the right or on the left?"

Alternate Cover Test

Purpose
- to detect a latent deviation (phoria) that may only become manifest when the patient becomes fatigued or sick

Technique
- this test should be preceded by the cover test
- if the patient wears glasses, they should be appropriate for the distance being tested

- the patient should look straight ahead at a distant target such as a letter on an acuity chart with both eyes open
- swing the occluder back and forth between the two eyes, covering each eye for a few seconds at a time
- repeat for near
- if there was no movement of the eyes with the cover test, movement of the eyes detected on alternate cover test indicates latent strabismus (phoria)

Note:

- most people have a small phoria, particularly in the horizontal plane
- some patients with a tropia have a larger angle of deviation when tested by the alternative cover test because this test fully dissociates the two eyes

Prism Cover Test

Purpose

- to measure the amount (in prism diopters) of ocular misalignment detected by the cover test or alternate cover test
- to determine the direction of maximum deviation (by testing in all directions of gaze)
- to document changes over time

Technique

- measure for both distance and near (with the appropriate glasses if used) and eccentric positions of gaze, if required
- put a (free or bar) prism oriented in front of the deviated eye, with the base of the prism pointing opposite to the direction to the deviation
  - esotropia/phoria: base out
  - exotropia/phoria: base in
  - hypertropia/phoria: base down
  - hypotropia/phoria: base up
  - oblique deviation: combine vertical and horizontal prisms
- perform an alternate cover test and adjust the strength of prism until the eyes no longer move to take up fixation
- if patient has both horizontal and vertical deviation, you can stack the prisms; i.e., you can put one over the other; however, you should never stack two or more horizontal or vertical prisms; instead, place one horizontal prism over one eye and the other over the fellow eye

Note:

- if poor vision prevents the patient from fixating with one or other eye, the angle of deviation can be estimated from the position of the corneal reflection of a point source of light
  - ask the patient to look at a light in primary position (e.g., a small torch positioned at your nose)
  - if no significant deviation is present, the corneal reflection on each side will be central
  - if strabismus is present, the reflection will be decentered (e.g., toward the temporal limbus in an esotropic eye)

- the angle of strabismus is then estimated by:
  - Krimsky test: put the prism in front of the deviated eye and adjust its strength until the corneal reflection is centered
  - Hirschberg test: estimate the size of the strabismus from the position of the corneal reflection in the deviated eye:
  - reflection at pupil margin: approximately 30 prism diopters
    - reflection at mid-iris: approximately 60 prism diopters
    - reflection at limbus: approximately 90 prism diopters

Eye Movements

- to see clearly, the visual system must be able to rapidly fixate on an object of interest and to maintain fixation despite movements of either the object or the observer. In general, the visual system uses saccades—fast eye movements—to get a target onto the fovea and pursuit—slow eye movements—to keep it on the fovea. These movements are co-ordinated by horizontal and vertical/torsional gaze centers in the brainstem and cerebellum. These centers connect to the nuclei of the third, fourth, and sixth cranial nerves, thereby directing the activity of the six extraocular muscles of each eye
- it is therefore insufficient to simply assess the range of movement of each eye. A routine eye movement examination should also assess pursuit, saccadic, and vergence movements. Occasionally, it may also be necessary to test vestibulo-ocular and optokinetic movements

Testing Range of Movement (Ductions and Versions) (Fig. 2.4)

Monocular eye movements are called ductions; binocular eye movements in the same direction are called versions; binocular eye movements in opposite directions are called vergences (e.g., convergence versus divergence)

Purpose

- to determine if there is limitation of movement in one or both eyes

Technique

- ask the patient to follow a target from the primary position into each of the six cardinal positions (see Fig. 2.4A) with both eyes open
- if there appears to be limitation of movement of one eye, reassess that movement with the other eye covered

Note:

- limitation of movement ("underaction") in any particular direction can be caused by a "weak" agonist muscle or a "tight" antagonist muscle (see Fig. 2.4B)
  - for example, limited abduction can be caused by a weak lateral rectus (e.g., from a sixth nerve palsy) or a tight medial rectus (e.g., from thyroid eye disease)
  - movements limited by muscle weakness usually appear to be better when tested monocularly because the muscle will be driven harder to reach the target (the occluded eye will be overacting), whereas movements limited by a restrictive process will be the same whether tested monocularly or binocularly

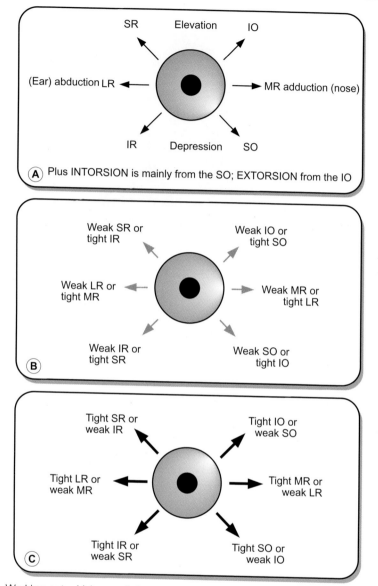

Fig. 2.4 Working out which muscle/s are under- or overacting (right eye, patient facing you). (**A**) The principal muscles acting in each direction of duction. (**B**) Reasons for underaction. (**C**) Reasons for overaction.

- greater than normal movement ("overaction") in any particular direction can be caused by an "overacting" or "tight" agonist muscle or a "weak" antagonist muscle (see Fig. 2.4C)
  - for example, overaction of the right eye looking up and to the left can be caused by an "overacting" or "tight" inferior oblique or a weak superior oblique

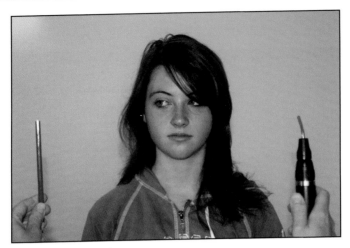

Fig. 2.5   Testing horizontal saccades.

Testing Pursuit

Purpose
- to assess how well the patient can follow a moving target
- normal speed of pursuit is about 30 degrees/second, although many patients can pursue faster than this

Technique
- observe the patient following a target in the horizontal and vertical planes
- assess the quality of these movements

Note:
- normal pursuit movements are smooth, without breaks or saccades
- if a patient has cerebellar problems, their pursuit may break down and become "cogwheel" or "saccadic" (composed of a series of catch-up saccades following the object, rather than a single smooth motion)

Testing Saccades (Fig. 2.5)

Purpose
- to assess how rapidly and accurately the patient can fixate on an eccentric target
- it is important to test saccades routinely because:
  - in some diseases, saccades can be abnormal whereas pursuit is entirely normal or nearly so (e.g., in the early stages of progressive supranuclear palsy [PSP] or dorsal midbrain syndrome)
  - in other cases, saccades may be more severely affected and easier to detect than a subtle pursuit abnormality (e.g., a mild internuclear ophthalmoplegia [INO] may have apparently normal pursuit movements but adducting saccades may be slow)
  - where eye movements are obviously limited, saccades may help you decide the cause of the limitation (e.g., in an esotropia with limitation of abduction)

- if limitation is due to a tight medial rectus (e.g., thyroid eye disease), abducting saccades will be fast up to the point of restriction, then the eye will come to an abrupt stop
- if limitation is due to a weak lateral rectus (caused by muscle disease or sixth nerve palsy), abducting saccades will be slow and the eye will come to a gradual stop
- if limitation is due to neuromuscular disease (e.g., myasthenia gravis), saccades will be faster than normal for the distance the eye travels

Technique
- hold two targets (e.g., a red pen in one hand and a handlight in the other) in front of and on either side of the patient's head such that the patient will make approximately 20–30 degree movements from the primary position
  - say to the patient "without moving your head, look at the handlight"; then, after a few seconds, say "look at the pen"
  - repeat this several times in the horizontal plane and then in the vertical plane
  - assess the quality of these movements for speed of initiation, velocity, and accuracy
- saccadic initiation
  - normally, there is only a very short delay between a command to move the eyes and the onset of the movement
  - some conditions (e.g., Parkinson disease) may cause a considerable delay
- saccadic velocity
  - saccades are normally very fast movements; if a saccade is slow, the cause could be disease in the brain, nerve, or muscle
  - saccadic speed is usually normal in a restrictive myopathy such as thyroid eye disease (up to the point of restriction), slow in an ocular motor nerve palsy, and may be normal or fast in neuromuscular disease such as myasthenia gravis
- saccadic accuracy
  - saccades that "undershoot" the target (too small) are called hypometric; the eyes then have to make one or more extra smaller saccades to reach the target
  - saccades that "overshoot" the target (too large) are called hypermetric; the eyes then have to make one or more extra smaller saccades back to the target
  - saccades are often inaccurate in brainstem or cerebellar disease
  - note that when you first begin to test saccades, the patient may make a few overshoots or undershoots, but in a normal person, the saccades rapidly become accurate, whereas in a person with a pathologic process affecting saccades (e.g., brainstem or cerebellar disease), the saccades remain inaccurate throughout the testing

Testing Convergence

Purpose
- to assess how well the patient can follow a target moving in depth; it is particularly important to test convergence if:
  - the patient complains of double vision at near only

- the patient has an acquired exotropia with limited adduction on smooth pursuit testing
    - this could be a partial third nerve palsy, myasthenia, or INO
    - if attempted convergence produces a much better adduction movement than smooth pursuit adduction, INO is the likely diagnosis (although this is not present in all cases of INO)
- the patient has nystagmus (to see if the nystagmus lessens on convergence)

Technique
- ask the patient (wearing the spectacles they normally use for reading) to look at an accommodative target (i.e., not your finger or a pencil but something they can focus on, such as a letter or number) about 30 cm away, held perpendicular to their nose
- move this target slowly toward the bridge of their nose, urging the patient to "keep it single for as long as you can"
- observe how far the eyes adduct toward each other
- measure the distance from the eyes at which the patient says the target becomes double (repeat this several times): this distance is the "near point of convergence" (NPC); this is different from the near point of accommodation (NPA), which is the distance at which the patient reports that the target printing becomes blurred
    - the NPC is normally around 10 cm and does not vary greatly with age
    - the normal NPA is approximately 8 cm at the age of 10, increasing to 50 cm by the age of 50

Testing Vestibulo-ocular Reflex

Purpose
- to assess how well the patient can maintain fixation during brief head or body movements (rotations, tilts, or translations); it is particularly important to test vestibulo-ocular reflex (VOR) if:
    - there is bilateral partial or total ophthalmoplegia (including horizontal or vertical gaze palsies)
        - in supranuclear ophthalmoplegias, the eye excursion elicited by VOR testing is better than that found on pursuit or saccadic testing
        - in nuclear, ocular motor nerve, neuromuscular junction, or extraocular muscle disease, the limitation of movement is the same on VOR as it is with pursuit and saccades
    - a patient complains of oscillopsia, either spontaneously or only on movement or walking, but no nystagmus is present (subtle or early cerebellar or brainstem disease can cause loss of VOR without overt nystagmus)

Technique
- to compare the range of movement on VOR with the range of movement on pursuit in patients with limitation of motility ("doll's-eye" or "doll's-head" test):
    - first ask the patient if they have any neck problems (if so, don't do the test, or, instead, rotate the patient in a swivel chair, with the neck held still)

- to test horizontal VOR, ask the patient to keep looking at your nose; then gently but rapidly rotate their head from side to side
- to test vertical VOR, ask the patient to keep looking at your nose, and tilt their head forward and backward
- observe how well the patient maintains fixation
  - the normal response is for the patient's eyes to remain fixed on your nose, despite quite rapid head movements; note how far the eyes move (and if this is a larger range of movement than that seen with pursuit and saccades)
  - an abnormal result is for the patient's eye movements to lag behind their head or (if severe) for no eye movement to be elicited at all
- to test if VOR is normal in patients with oscillopsia but apparently normal motility
  - measure the distance VA with distance glasses and both eyes open
  - with both eyes open, ask the patient to read down the chart again, while they rapidly shake their head from side to side (testing horizontal VOR) or rapidly nod their head up and down (for vertical VOR)
  - a patient with normal VOR can read down to within two lines of their "head still" VA with this test; patients with abnormal VOR have their VA severely degraded by head movement
- remember that if the patient is awake and alert, the patient MUST cooperate with the testing by fixating on the target. If the patient cannot or will not fixate, the VOR will appear abnormal even though the vestibulo-ocular system is normal!

Testing Optokinetic Nystagmus

Purpose

- to assess how well the patient can maintain fixation during sustained head or body movement (rotation or translation)
- optokinetic nystagmus (OKN) is the normal response of the ocular movement system to sustained self-rotation or to a scene moving in constant linear translation; it is a form of jerk nystagmus with the fast phase directed toward the oncoming scene and the slow phase maintaining fixation
- it is particularly useful to test OKN if the patient is suspected of having nonorganic "blindness" (OKN is difficult to suppress consciously)
- OKN also may help localize the site of a lesion causing a homonymous hemianopia; parietal lesions may have reduced ipsilateral OKN response (i.e., when targets are moved or rotated toward the side of the lesion)

Technique

- OKN should ideally be a "full visual field" test, but it only rarely is performed this way as most clinics do not have a large rotating drum or curtain for the patient to sit in
- the two main ways of testing in most clinics are:
  - rotating OKN drum: have the patient look at the stripes or figures on the drum (held fairly close to their face); beginning with slow rotations, observe whether or not OKN is elicited; test with the drum rotating to the right, left, up, and down
  - "OKN strip": this is a long strip of fabric with a repetitive stripe or figure pattern that is moved in front of the patient's eyes; this is probably less accurate and tests smooth pursuit rather than OKN

Special Tests

Prism Fusional Amplitude (Fig. 2.6)

Purpose

- to measure amount of motor fusion in the horizontal and vertical planes
- approximate normal values
  - horizontal
    - distance: convergence >15 prism diopters; divergence >6 prism diopters
    - near: convergence >30 prism diopters; divergence >15 prism diopters
  - vertical: upward (sursumvergence) 2–3 prism diopters; downward (deorsumvergence) 2–3 prism diopters
- an important test for:
  - patients with intermittent horizontal diplopia: they may have a phoria taking them to the edge of their fusion range
  - patients with a vertical deviation: a high vertical fusion range (combined upward and downward measurements) indicates that the deviation is long standing
    - a high vertical fusion range suggests that the cause of a fourth nerve palsy is "congenital" rather than acquired
    - patients with long-standing vertical deviation due to other causes may also have a large vertical fusional amplitude

Technique

- ask the patient to look at a small letter on the distance acuity chart in primary position (use a letter two lines above the VA of their worse eye)
- place an appropriately oriented low-strength prism (either part of a prism bar or a rotary prism) in front of one eye
  - base out for convergence
  - base in for divergence
  - base down for sursumvergence
  - base up for deorsumvergence
- ask the patient if they can see one or two letters
- gradually increase the strength of the prism, encouraging the patient to try to "keep it one," until he or she is no longer able to fuse the two images
- record the power of prism causing the patient to see double—the breakpoint
- allow the patient to rest between prism orientations (e.g., base in and base out)
- repeat horizontal measurements using a near target

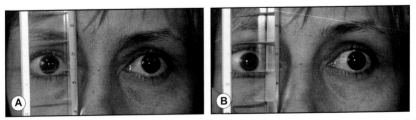

Fig. 2.6   Prism fusional amplitude. **(A)** Within horizontal fusion range; note symmetric pupil light reflexes. **(B)** Beyond horizontal fusion range; note right pupil light reflex displaced temporally.

Head Tilt Test

Purpose

- to determine the influence of head tilt (ear to shoulder) on ocular alignment
- the normal compensatory ocular response to head tilt is intorsion of the ipsilateral eye and extorsion of the contralateral eye (e.g., head tilt to the right causes intorsion of the right eye and extorsion of the left eye)
- intorsion is produced by the combined action of the superior rectus and superior oblique muscles; their opposing vertical actions cancel each other out
- extorsion is produced by the combined actions of the inferior rectus and inferior oblique muscles; again, their opposing vertical actions cancel each other out
- if there is weakness of one of the vertically acting muscles, head tilt will cause a change in the vertical alignment of the eyes because the affected muscle will not be able to cancel the vertical action of its fellow intorter/extorter

Technique

- usually performed as part of the Parks or Bielschowsky three-step test; the size of the vertical deviation is assessed by performing alternate cover tests in the following eye and head positions
  - step one: determine which is the higher eye in the primary position
  - step two: determine if the vertical deviation increases on right or left gaze
  - step three: determine if the vertical deviation (in the primary position) increases on head tilt to the left or right

Note:

- this test is most frequently performed if a fourth nerve palsy is suspected; a right fourth nerve palsy (for example) will cause a right hyperphoria/tropia that increases on left gaze, and on head tilt to the right
- a skew deviation, the most common differential diagnosis of a fourth cranial nerve palsy, may cause a positive head tilt test (hypertropia increasing on head tilt to the ipsilateral side)
  - however, a skew deviation causes intorsion of the hypertropic eye, whereas a fourth nerve palsy causes extorsion of the hypertropic eye
  - the two conditions often can be differentiated by examining the fundus and determining if intorsion or extorsion is present by assessing the relative positions of the disc and fovea or by measuring torsion with the double Maddox rod test
  - another way of differentiating between a fourth nerve palsy and a skew deviation is to perform the Wong Upright-Supine Test
    - first, measure the vertical misalignment with the patient sitting upright
    - next, have the patient lie down supine and measure the vertical misalignment with a target held at 1/3 meter
    - a 50% or greater decrease in vertical misalignment when the patient changes from the upright to the supine position indicates a skew deviation (76% sensitive; 100% specific)

Double Maddox Rod Test (Fig. 2.7)

Purpose
- to measure the amount (in degrees) and direction of ocular torsion

Technique
- the patient wears a spectacle trial frame with degree markings
- place a 5-prism diopter prism trial lens base down on one side
- place Maddox rod lenses on each side (red on the right and white on the left) with their grooves running vertically
- dim the lights and ask the patient to look at a point white light source (e.g., a torch) in primary position
- if no torsion is present, the patient will see white and red horizontal parallel lines, one above the other
- if subjective torsion is present, it can be measured by rotating the appropriate Maddox rod lens; when both lines are horizontal and parallel, read the number of degrees of extorsion or intorsion present off the trial frame

Forced Duction Testing

Purpose
- to differentiate between paretic and restrictive eye movements

Technique
- advise the patient that the test may be uncomfortable and that there is a chance of causing transient eye irritation or a subconjunctival hemorrhage
- instill several drops of local anesthetic into both eyes
- with two pairs of sterile toothed forceps, firmly grasp the eye to be tested near the limbus on each side
- ask the patient to look in the direction of limitation
- try to move the eye with the forceps in the direction of limitation

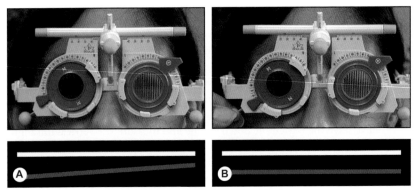

Fig. 2.7 Double Maddox rod test with diagrams showing the view seen by a patient with a right fourth nerve palsy when looking at a point white light source. (**A**) Starting position, Maddox rods orientated vertically. (**B**) Adjusting orientation of right Maddox rod.

- the test is positive (indicating restrictive disease of the antagonist muscle) if either:
  - you can't manually move the eye as far as it should go, or
  - you can move the eye fully but it requires significant force
- the test is negative (indicating that the strabismus is due to a weak agonist muscle) if you can easily move the eye with the forceps to its normal full extent
- if you are unsure, repeat the test on the other ("normal") eye to see if you can feel any difference
- the test is usually also combined with the "active force generation" test:
  - holding the eye with the forceps in primary position, ask the patient to look in the direction of limited movement
  - if restrictive disease is present, there will be a strong tug on the forceps as the normal-strength agonist muscle activates
  - if paretic disease is present, there will only be a weak tug from the muscle

Note:

- in patients with significant limitation of movement, forced duction testing can be performed simply by having the patient attempt to look in the direction of limitation and using a cotton-tipped applicator to try to push the eye in the direction of limitation rather than using forceps as described above
- regardless of the technique used, forced duction testing is subjective and requires practice to obtain consistent results
- a common mistake is to push the globe into the orbit while performing the test; this tends to slacken any restrictive muscles, giving a false-negative result

PUPILS (VIDEO 2.4)

Note the size and shape of the pupils in room light, then dim the lights and note their constriction to light and whether or not there is an RAPD on the swinging light test.

Remember that optic nerve disease, which often causes an RAPD, never causes a difference in pupil size (anisocoria). Likewise, disease of the pupil constrictor pathway (third nerve or ciliary ganglion) or pupil dilator pathway (sympathetic chain) causes anisocoria but never by itself an RAPD.

Measure Pupil Size in Room Light

- ask the patient to look at a distant target (to prevent miosis due to the near response) and assess the size of the pupil in each eye
- if anisocoria is present, also assess the size of each pupil in dim light

Assess Pupil Constriction to Light

- dim the room lights, ask the patient to look at a distant target (to prevent miosis due to the near response) and observe the magnitude and speed of contraction of each pupil to a bright light shone in one eye and then the other
- for patients with darkly pigmented irises, either ask the patient to look straight but shine the light from below or have the patient look up and then shine the light straight ahead. Either technique will allow you to see the pupillary response to light more clearly than if the patient looks straight ahead and the light is directed straight ahead (Fig. 2.8)

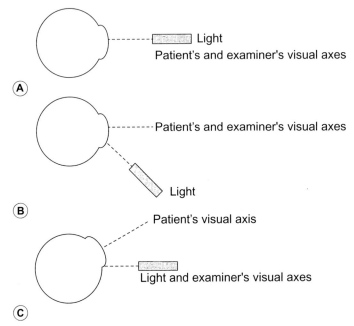

Fig. 2.8 Schematic diagram showing the appropriate techniques for assessing pupil reactivity in patients with darkly pigmented irises. **(A)** The normal technique, with the patient looking straight ahead and the examiner's visual axes in the same plane. **(B)** In a patient with darkly pigmented irises, the patient can look straight ahead, and the examiner's visual axes can be in the same plane, but the light can illuminate the pupils from below. **(C)** The optimum technique for patients with darkly pigmented irises is for the patient to look up while the examiner's visual axes and light source remain in the horizontal plane. Both techniques B and C allow optimum viewing of pupillary reactions.

- if a pupil constricts poorly to light, check if its constriction is greater when viewing a near target (light-near dissociation); if this is present, also check for the speed of constriction to near, and the speed of redilation when the patient looks back to a distant target

The Swinging Light Test (Fig. 2.9)

- the presence of an RAPD may be the only objective sign of a lesion in the afferent visual pathway
- the swinging light test is therefore an essential part of the afferent pathway examination
- the test may be performed on patients who are unconscious

Technique

- dim or turn off the room lights
- use a bright, uniform light source
- have the patient stare at a distant target to prevent pupil miosis from the near response

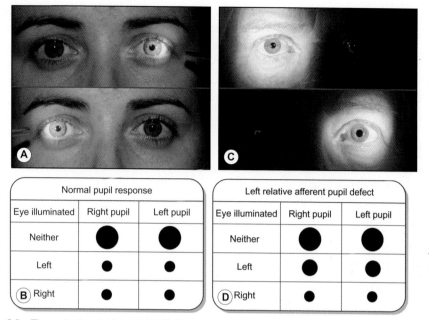

Fig. 2.9 The swinging light test. (**A, B**) Normal pupil response. (**C, D**) Left relative afferent pupil defect.

- swing the light source from eye to eye, remaining on each eye for about a second
- make sure you shine the light for an equal time on each eye or you can create an artifactitious RAPD by bleaching one eye's retina more than the other's
- look for the initial movement of each pupil when illuminated: this is normally a small constriction
- an RAPD is present if one pupil consistently dilates rather than constricts
- in cases of "equivocal" RAPD, also perform a subjective brightness comparison between the two eyes (ask the patient to compare the brightness of a light when viewed with one eye at a time)

Interpretation

- the presence of an obvious RAPD in an eye without extensive retinal disease almost always indicates optic nerve disease, but the absence of an RAPD can either mean that both optic nerves are healthy or that both optic nerves are equally damaged
- less commonly, an RAPD is a sign of contralateral optic tract disease
- a clinically detectable RAPD is never caused by media opacities (even a dense cataract or vitreous hemorrhage will not cause an RAPD)
- although amblyopia can cause a very slight RAPD, a clinically detectable RAPD in an eye with poor vision should always be assumed to be due to an optic neuropathy unless proved otherwise
- the presence of an RAPD can still be detected even if one pupil is immobile (e.g., due to third nerve palsy or iris damage) by observing the mobile pupil

- if the mobile pupil constricts when the light is shone directly on it but dilates when the light is shone on the other eye, there is an RAPD in the other eye
- if the mobile pupil dilates when the light is shone on it but constricts with the light on the other side, there is an RAPD on the side of the mobile pupil

EYELIDS

Is there ptosis or lid retraction on one or both sides? If there is, assess the following:

Assess Eyelid Position

- measure vertical palpebral fissure distance with eyes in primary position (normally 10–11 mm in adults)
- assess lid position with respect to the cornea (normally the upper lid covers 1 mm of the cornea)
- look for variability of ptosis with direction of gaze (Duane syndrome, congenital ptosis, aberrant regeneration of third cranial nerve)
- look for jaw winking (congenital ptosis)

Examine Upper Lids

- lid contour
- position of skin crease (normally 6–7 mm above the lid margin)
- skin and tarsal surface for tumors or thickening due to inflammation

Measure Range of Upper Lid Movement

- ask the patient to look down
- align a ruler with the upper lid margin
- press firmly on the eyebrow to prevent frontalis action
- ask the patient to look up and measure range of movement (normally 14–15 mm)

Look for Fatigability

- ask the patient to maintain upgaze for 2 minutes
- measure the palpebral aperture pre and post upgaze; more than 2 mm worsening of ptosis post upgaze is suspicious for myasthenia

ORBITS

Is there proptosis, enophthalmos or ocular injection on one or both sides? If so, perform the following:

- exophthalmometry
- retropulsion (is there resistance)?
- if proptosis is present: is it pulsatile or is there an audible bruit when the closed eyelids are auscultated with the bell of a stethoscope? (CCF)

CRANIAL NERVES (VIDEO 2.5)

Routine testing of all the cranial nerves is not necessary. However, testing the fifth and seventh cranial nerves, and asking about symptoms of eighth cranial nerve dysfunction,

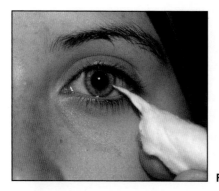

Fig. 2.10   Testing corneal sensation.

is very important in all patients with neuro-ophthalmic problems because these nerves are often compressed, stretched, or infiltrated by tumors or inflammatory conditions that can also cause blurred vision or diplopia.

If abnormalities are found in any of the following, the diagnosis is not typical optic neuritis, anterior ischemic optic neuropathy (AION) or "ischemic" third, fourth, or sixth nerve palsy so investigations for another cause are mandatory.

Corneal and Facial Sensation Testing (Fifth Nerve) (Fig. 2.10)

Testing
- corneal sensation: warn the patient what you are about to do, then gently touch the central region of each cornea (it has the most nerve fibers) in turn with a wisp of tissue; observe the blink reflex and ask "did that feel the same on each side?"
- facial sensation: touch each side in turn of the patient's forehead, cheek, and chin; ask "did that feel the same on each side?"

Significance of Reduced Sensation
- diplopia: possible tumor in the cerebello-pontine angle (CPA) (causing a sixth nerve palsy) or cavernous sinus (causing a third, fourth, and/or sixth nerve palsy)
- blurred vision: possible pituitary region or orbital apex tumor (causing an optic chiasmopathy or neuropathy)
- seventh nerve palsy: probable CPA tumor (e.g., vestibular schwannoma)

Orbicularis and Facial Strength Testing (Seventh Nerve) (Fig. 2.11)

Testing
- orbicularis strength: ask the patient to close both eyes as tight as they can (observe that full closure is possible); then say "keep your eyes closed, don't let me open them" and try to pry open the closed lids with your fingers on each side
- other facial strength: observe for facial asymmetry; tell the patient "show me your teeth" and "puff out your cheeks"; ask the patient to raise the eyebrows

Significance of Orbicularis or Facial Weakness
- ptosis: possible myasthenia gravis or myopathy
- diplopia: possible myasthenia gravis or myopathy; possible CPA tumor (causing sixth and seventh nerve palsies)

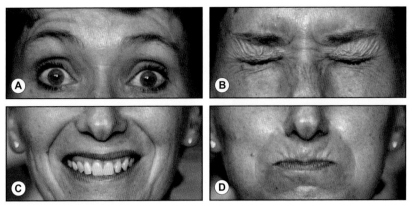

Fig. 2.11   Testing the facial nerve. (**A**) "Lift your eyebrows." (**B**) "Close your eyes tight." (**C**) "Show me your teeth." (**D**) "Purse your lips and blow out your cheeks."

Auditory and Vestibular Symptoms (Eighth Nerve)

Testing
- ask the patient if they have had "any deafness, ringing in the ears, or episodes where the world spins around you?"

Significance of Eighth Nerve Dysfunction in a Patient with Diplopia or Seventh Nerve Palsy
- diplopia: possible CPA tumor (causing sixth and eighth nerve palsies)
- seventh nerve palsy: probable CPA tumor (causing seventh and eighth nerve palsies)

TEMPORAL ARTERIES (FIG. 2.12)

Palpation of the temporal arteries for tenderness and pulsatility is important in patients with suspected GCA, although it is a somewhat unreliable sign and both false positives and false negatives can occur. However, its inclusion in the examination of any patient over age 50 with transient diplopia, persistent diplopia, transient blurred vision, or persistent blurred vision reminds you to think: "Could this patient have GCA?" and to investigate further to exclude this if necessary.

SLIT-LAMP EXAMINATION (FIG. 2.13)

It is important to resist the temptation to get the patient in front of the slit-lamp until all the previously described examination steps have been performed. If you perform slit-lamp examination too early, you will temporarily "blind" the patient with the light (making color acuity and motility assessment inaccurate), and you may forget to perform other important steps in the examination.

When slit-lamp examination is performed, a thorough examination of the whole globe should be performed (not just a quick look at the optic discs undilated). Dilating drops should always be used to give the best possible view of the optic discs and retina unless the patient has an acute-onset neurologic problems (in which case, the pupils should be left undilated to allow their observation as part of neurologic monitoring).

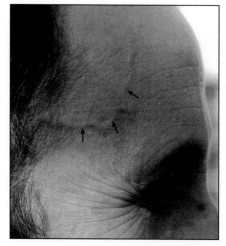

Fig. 2.12 The right superficial temporal artery *(arrows)*.

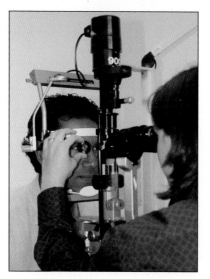

Fig. 2.13 Slit-lamp examination.

Eyelids

Are there follicles or granulomas on the conjunctival surface of the upper or lower lids? (These may rarely represent sarcoidosis.)

Gonioscopy

This should be performed in all cases of transient monocular visual loss or unexplained ocular pain to exclude intermittent angle-closure glaucoma.

Iris and Pupil

- note pupil shape and position
- look for damage/atrophy of iris, particularly of the iris sphincter

- compare iris color for possible heterochromia
- look for uneven (segmental) contraction of the iris to light or near
- always assess pupil reactivity at the slit-lamp if, on testing of general pupillary reactivity to light/near, one or both pupils appear to be nonreactive

Cornea, Anterior Chamber, and Vitreous

Is there intraocular inflammation?

Macula

Could macular disease be the cause of, or contributing to, blurred vision?

Peripheral Retina

Are there retinal changes of posterior uveitis (e.g., perivascular sheathing in sarcoidosis), ocular ischemic syndrome (e.g., midperipheral blot hemorrhages), or previously undiagnosed diabetes?

Optic Discs

Size and Shape
- relative size can be measured, if necessary, by the vertical height of the slit beam while viewing through a 78D or similar lens
- lumpiness suggests drusen; buried drusen may be more easily observed by transilluminating the disc with a slightly decentered slit beam and a 78D or similar lens

Cup:Disc Ratio
- this should be compared with the size of the disc to determine if nerve fiber loss has occurred

Color
- pallor may be due to infarction or to any long-standing optic neuropathy (note that a normal optic disc may appear pale in patients who have had cataract surgery and are either aphakic or have an intraocular lens; it is also often difficult to assess pallor in infants and children who have a pale fundus)
- hyperemia may be due to ischemia, impaired venous outflow (e.g., vein occlusion, nonarteritic AION, papilledema), or even Leber hereditary optic neuropathy.

Margins
- indistinct margins (optic disc swelling or infiltration)
- irregular but distinct margins (optic disc drusen)

Vessels
- dilated and/or tortuous veins (vein occlusion or papilledema)
- anomalous branching (optic disc drusen)
- indistinct vessels due to swelling of the adjacent axons (optic disc swelling or infiltration)
- venous retinochoroidal collaterals: indicate chronically raised venous pressure (advanced optic nerve sheath meningioma, glioma, papilledema, or previous retinal vein occlusion)

- the presence of spontaneous venous pulsations (SVPs) suggests that ICP is normal; the converse is not necessarily true because SVPs are not always seen in otherwise normal discs, and loss of SVPs may occur from venous outflow obstruction

Peripapillary Changes
- hemorrhages, exudates and/or cotton-wool spots are all pathologic
- retinal and chorioretinal folds (e.g., Paton folds) are usually pathologic

OTHER EXAMINATION

It is essential to remember that the eye is connected to the body! Often, systemic disease (vasculitis, severe hypertension, infection, tumors) can first present with ophthalmic symptoms, so it is important that a doctor examines any neuro-ophthalmic patient "head to toe." Usually, as ophthalmologists, we don't feel comfortable performing a full systemic exam, so ask an internist to see the patient for you. Finding lymphadenopathy, hepatomegaly, a breast lump, a high temperature, or very high blood pressure could be the vital clue to the cause of the patient's visual complaints.

PERIMETRY

Performing formal visual field testing is an essential part of the assessment of any patient with possible visual pathway disease, even if confrontation visual field testing is normal. Clues to the site of disease may be found and a baseline field can be established to monitor the efficacy of treatment.

The results of perimetry must be considered together with all other aspects of the history and examination to help localize the site of visual pathway disease (Table 2.1).

Notes for Table 2.1

1. Localizing the lesion further in partial homonymous hemianopia
   - if there is a complete homonymous hemianopia, no further localization is possible
   - if there is only partial homonymous field loss, this can help you further localize the lesion in two ways (however, neither is completely reliable):
     - the more congruous the field defect (i.e., the more similar the field defect is in both eyes), the more posterior the lesion is likely to be; e.g., anterior optic radiation field defects are often moderately different in size and shape between the two eyes, whereas occipital cortex lesions cause an identical or nearly identical defect in both eyes
     - if the partial defect is predominantly superior or inferior:
       - partial superior homonymous defects are probably from damage to the inferior parts of the posterior visual pathway: the inferior optic radiation (often damaged in temporal lobe lesions), or the inferior part of the occipital visual cortex
       - likewise, partial inferior defects occur from damage to the superior parts of the pathway: the superior optic radiation in the parietal lobe, or the superior part of the visual cortex

TABLE 2.1 ■ **Localizing Value of Visual Field Defects**

Any of These Visual Field Defects	Plus These Other Signs	Localizes the Lesion to	Why?	What Lesions Can Cause This?
Bilateral homonymous field loss	Normal or bilateral decreased acuity, normal pupils, no RAPD, normal discs	Bilateral optic radiation or visual cortex	Acuity may be normal due to macular sparing; or may be reduced bilaterally because the cortical macular representations (or their supplying fibers) have been destroyed—there is also a variable amount of homonymous field loss on each side, depending on how extensive the lesions are	Usually ischemic stroke
Homonymous hemianopia or quadrantanopia	Normal acuity normal pupils, **no RAPD**, *normal discs*	Optic radiation or visual cortex	The optic radiation and cortex on one side of the brain contain the visual information from the contralateral binocular visual hemifield; you only need "half a macula" working for normal acuity; hence, these patients still have normal VA *(localizing the lesion further: see note 1)*	Stroke or tumor
Homonymous hemianopia	Normal acuity normal pupils, **ipsilateral (to the field defect) RAPD**, *pale discs* if long-standing severe lesion *(see note 2)*	Contralateral optic tract	Each tract contains retinal ganglion cell axons from the ipsilateral temporal hemiretina and the contralateral nasal hemiretina *(explanation of why an RAPD is present: see note 3)*	Stroke or tumor
Bitemporal hemianopia	Normal or reduced acuity, ±RAPD; *pale discs if long-standing severe lesion (see note 2)*	Chiasm	Nasal hemiretinal fibers cross (decussate) in the chiasm; these fibers (which supply the temporal field on each side) are most vulnerable to compression of the chiasm by tumors	Usually pituitary region tumors or aneurysms *(see note 4)*

TABLE 2.1 ■ Localizing Value of Visual Field Defects—cont'd

Any of These Visual Field Defects	Plus These Other Signs	Localizes the Lesion to	Why?	What Lesions Can Cause This?
Unilateral nasal or temporal hemianopia ◐○ ◐○ ◑○ ◐○	Normal vision, RAPD in the affected eye; ±pale disc in the affected eye	Immediately prechiasmal part of one optic nerve	Just before the optic nerve joins the chiasm, the nasal and temporal hemiretinal fibers line up "ready to cross" in the chiasm—a lesion of one optic nerve at this point can therefore damage just the nasal or temporal fibers and cause a unilateral hemifield defect	Usually pituitary region tumors
Any field defect in one eye; superotemporal field defect respecting the vertical midline in the opposite eye ("junctional scotoma") ◉◔ ●◔ ◐◔	RAPD ± reduced acuity ± pale disc	Immediately prechiasmal part of one optic nerve	Axons from the right inferonasal retina ("seeing" superotemporal field) crossing in the chiasm may loop anteriorly into the most posterior portion of the left optic chiasm ("Wilbrand knee") before continuing posteriorly into the left optic tract—damage to this region thus causes both a left eye field defect of any kind, plus a small right eye superotemporal defect (an alternative explanation is that the superotemporal defect is just due to early chiasmal damage)	Usually pituitary region tumors or aneurysms

Continued

TABLE 2.1 ■ Localizing Value of Visual Field Defects—cont'd

Any of These Visual Field Defects	Plus These Other Signs	Localizes the Lesion to	Why?	What Lesions Can Cause This?
Any other visual field defect, one or both eyes—including these scotomas: ⬤ ⬤ ◖ ◗ ⬤ ⬤ ⬤ ⬤ Central scotoma, cecocentral scotoma, superior altitudinal defect, superior arcuate defect, diffuse patchy defects, peripheral field loss, diffuse loss of sensitivity, diffuse severe field loss	Normal or reduced acuity; RAPD if unilateral, or bilateral but asymmetric; sluggish pupil response to light without RAPD if bilateral, symmetric and severe Disc/s normal, swollen, pale, or "cupped"	One or both optic nerves at any point from optic nerve to chiasm	There is imprecise topographic organization of retinal ganglion cell axons for most of the extent of the optic nerve, and any one disease can cause a wide variety of field defects—for this reason *the pattern of the field defect is NOT DIAGNOSTIC* for either the cause or the location of the lesion in optic nerve disease: the same disease in the same location may produce many different patterns of field loss in different patients many different types of disease may produce an identical pattern of field loss *NOTE: COMPRESSIVE optic neuropathy from orbital or brain tumors can produce ANY of these field defects*	Ischemia, inflammation, tumors, infections, many others

RAPD, relative afferent pupillary defect; *VA*, visual acuity.

2. Patterns of disc atrophy in chiasm and tract lesions
   - "bow-tie" or band atrophy of the disc may be seen in the eye/s with temporal field loss
     - if there is damage to the retinal ganglion cell axons from the eye's nasal hemiretina, which "sees" the temporal visual hemifield (as occurs in both eyes in chiasmal lesions, and the contralateral eye in optic tract lesions), the disc may develop a horizontal band of pallor (rather than diffuse pallor)
     - this occurs because nasal hemiretinal fibers enter the disc closer to the horizontal meridian (compared with temporal hemiretinal fibers, which enter more superiorly and inferiorly)
     - this usually takes several weeks or even a few months to develop
   - hence, in chiasmal compression causing bitemporal hemianopia, both discs may show "bow-tie atrophy"; in a left optic tract lesion, the right disc (the eye which has lost the temporal hemifield) may show bow tie atrophy (the left disc is likely to have diffuse pallor)
   - however, the absence of band pallor certainly does not exclude a chiasmal or tract lesion; many patients with such lesions have diffuse disc pallor, temporal pallor, or (if compression is acute, mild, and/or recent) the discs may look absolutely normal, with no visible pallor at all.
3. Reason for RAPD in optic tract lesions
   - there are slightly more nerve fibers from the nasal hemiretina of each eye than from the temporal hemiretina (the nasal hemiretina contains slightly more ganglion cells)
   - a left optic tract lesion will destroy the fibers from the left temporal hemiretina and right nasal hemiretina; this results in a greater loss of pupil response from the right eye (which has lost its nasal hemiretina fibers) than from the left eye, so a small right RAPD will be present
4. Other field defects caused by pituitary region tumors
   - pituitary region tumors frequently present with field defects other than bitemporal hemianopia; they can cause any type of field defect in one or both eyes (due to unilateral or bilateral optic neuropathy, chiasmopathy, optic tract lesion or a mixture of any of these)

Neuroimaging (Table 2.2)

The two principal modes of orbit and brain imaging are magnetic resonance imaging (MRI) and computed tomographic (CT) scanning.

In general, MRI is the preferred method of imaging for patients with suspected neuro-ophthalmic disease. This is because of its much greater sensitivity for detecting brain lesions, especially demyelinating lesions and small tumors. Brain lesions that are detectable on CT are usually imaged in far greater detail on MRI (Fig. 2.14).

MRI is also a safer technique than CT due to the lack of ionizing radiation in MRI, as well as a lower incidence and severity of intravenous contrast allergy. However, CT is superior for imaging the bony orbit (e.g., in suspected orbital fracture or thyroid eye disease).

It has been shown that MRI contrast material can deposit in the basal ganglia and dentate nucleus of the cerebellum; however, the clinical significance of this deposition has yet to be determined. In the meantime, one should never avoid neuroimaging in

TABLE 2.2 ■ **Magnetic Resonance Imaging Versus Computed Tomography**

	Magnetic Resonance Imaging	**Computed Tomography**
Imaging of optic nerve and brain lesions	Excellent	Poor
Imaging of aneurysms	Good (if magnetic resonance angiography requested)	Good (if computed tomography angiography requested)
Imaging of bone (e.g., orbit)	Poor	Good
Radiation dose	Zero	High
Intravenous contrast allergies	Rare (gadolinium contrast)	Not infrequent (iodinated contrast)
Scan time	Long (30–40 minutes)	Short (5–10 minutes)
Cost	High	Relatively low
Contraindications	Implanted metal devices, (e.g., cardiac pacemaker, metal heart valve, recent cardiac stent, inner ear implant, some scleral buckle clips) Renal failure, gadolinium allergy, severe claustrophobia	Iodinated contrast allergy child (radiation dose)

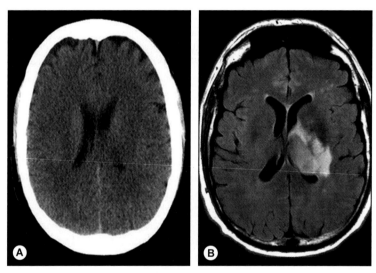

Fig. 2.14   A 38-year-old man presented with a partial right homonymous hemianopia and a "normal" computed tomography (CT) brain scan (**A**). Magnetic resonance imaging (MRI) scan (**B**) revealed a large invasive tumor, diagnosed on biopsy as a malignant glioblastoma. Most brain lesions are seen much more clearly on MRI than CT.

patients in whom it is clinically indicated because of the fear of some unknown problem that might develop in the future.

The particular type of scan to order is specified in the relevant sections of this book— for example, a patient with papilledema should have an MRI plus magnetic resonance venogram (MRV) or a CT and computed tomographic venography (CTV) of the orbits and brain, whereas a patient with an unexplained Horner syndrome requires an MRI plus a magnetic resonance angiogram (MRA) or CT angiogram (CTA). Gadolinium contrast should be requested for all MRI scans, unless there is a medical contraindication (e.g., significant renal disease).

CHAPTER 3

Blurred Vision or Field Loss

Not Explained by Visible Ocular Disease—Optic Disc/s Normal, Swollen, Pale or "Cupped"

Introduction

Blurred vision and/or visual field loss not explained by visible ocular disease can be caused by disease of the:

- eye
- optic nerve
- optic chiasm
- retrochiasmal brain visual pathway
- or (rarely) nonorganic functional visual loss (the patient is simulating visual loss in the absence of real disease)

A careful history and detailed examination will often give important clues as to the location of the disease (Fig. 3.1).

EYE DISEASE

Eye disease is by far the most common cause of blurred vision and is usually obvious on slit-lamp examination. However, some ocular disorders, such as keratoconus and some macular dystrophies, may be difficult to diagnose in their early stages and may be overlooked on a cursory ocular examination (see "occult" ocular diseases, p. 127).

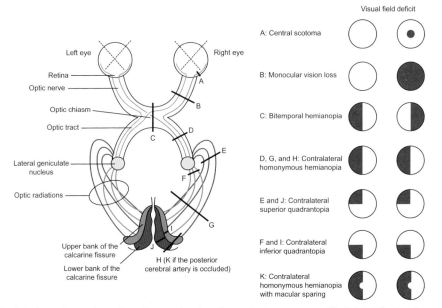

Fig. 3.1 Locations along the afferent visual pathway that cause specific field defect patterns. Courtesy Moises Dominguez, MD, in Mcdbullets Step 1 (podcast). Visual Pathway—Neurology, 22 August 2022. Available at https://step1.medbullets.com/neurology/113086/visual-pathway. Accessed 20 June 2023.

Optic Nerve Disease

Disease of the optic nerve can be recognized by the presence of one or more of the following:

- abnormal visual acuity (VA), color vision and/or visual field, not explained by (or worse than that expected from) visible intraocular disease
- presence of a relative afferent pupillary defect (RAPD) (unless optic nerve disease is bilateral and symmetric)
- pallor, swelling or "cupping" of one or both optic discs (in some but not all cases)

Please note: If the optic disc is swollen, the optic neuropathy is considered "anterior"; if the disc is normal in appearance, the optic neuropathy is considered to be "posterior" or "retrobulbar." If the disc is pale, no distinction can be made between "anterior" and "posterior" as it may be that the disc previously was swollen and subsequently has become pale, or it may be that the disc previously was normal and subsequently has become pale.

Glaucoma is by far the most common optic neuropathy. The next most common optic neuropathies are the acute neuropathies of typical optic neuritis and anterior ischemic optic neuropathy (AION). There are many other causes of optic neuropathy and it is important that they are identified because many are treatable if diagnosed early (before optic atrophy occurs), e.g., compressive, infectious, or sarcoid optic neuropathy.

As ophthalmologists, we all need to know the following four things about optic nerve disease:

1. How to make a safe clinical diagnosis of typical optic neuritis (p. 66).
2. How to make a safe clinical diagnosis of AION (p. 67).
3. How to make a safe clinical diagnosis of glaucomatous optic neuropathy (p. 68).
4. What to do for all other patients with nontraumatic optic nerve disease who cannot be diagnosed clinically as having typical optic neuritis, AION, or glaucoma. We recommend that these patients be referred to a neuro-ophthalmologist for further assessment (urgently if the problem is acute). If prompt referral is difficult due to geographic or patient factors, or if you wish to work the patient up yourself, the necessary initial basic investigations are outlined on pp. 88–89.

Optic Chiasmal Disease

Optic chiasmal disease can be recognized by the presence of bitemporal visual field defects on perimetry (if unilateral temporal field loss is present, suspect immediately prechiasmal optic nerve disease). Because the most common cause of optic chiasmal dysfunction is compression by a pituitary region tumor, all patients with suspected chiasmal disease require urgent, contrast-enhanced magnetic resonance imaging (MRI) or at least a contrast-enhanced computerized tomographic (CT) scan.

Retrochiasmal Disease

Retrochiasmal disease is characterized by the presence of a homonymous visual field defect on perimetry. Because strokes and brain tumors are common causes of retrochiasmal disease, all patients with homonymous field loss require neuroimaging, either a contrast-enhanced CT scan or contrast-enhanced MRI.

Nonorganic Visual Loss

A diagnosis of nonorganic visual loss is frequently considered when inconsistencies are found in a patient's history and examination. Great care must be taken to establish this diagnosis, bearing in mind that some of these patients have "real" organic disease or organic disease plus an overlay of additional simulated visual loss.

Examination Checklist

BLURRED VISION OR FIELD LOSS

Have you asked about, and looked for, all the following key features?

History

☐ blurred vision or field loss
    ☐ one or both eyes? (how did the patient know; did they check each eye separately?)
    ☐ where in the visual field (all over, central, to the side)?
    ☐ when did it start?
    ☐ speed of onset?
    ☐ change over time?

- □ is it getting better, staying the same or still worsening?
- □ any preceding transient visual loss?
- □ other ophthalmic symptoms
  - □ eye or orbital pain? (if so, does it worsen on eye movement?)
  - □ facial numbness?
  - □ double vision? (possible orbital apex or pituitary tumor)
- □ previous medical and surgical history
  - □ cancer? (possible metastasis)
  - □ potentially toxic medications?
  - □ vascular risk factors?
- □ social history
  - □ smoker, alcohol, special diet, difficulty sleeping, snoring, drugs for erectile dysfunction?
- □ family history: unexplained visual loss or brain disease?
- □ if patient over 50: symptoms of giant cell arteritis (GCA)?
- □ system review questions
  - □ neurologic symptoms?
  - □ any clues to the cause anywhere in the body?

Examination

- □ VA
- □ color vision testing
- □ visual field defect to confrontation?
- □ limitation of eye movements? (possible orbital apex or pituitary tumor)
- □ pupils
  - □ RAPD? (unilateral or bilateral asymmetric optic neuropathy, or optic tract lesion)
  - □ is there anisocoria? (possible partial third or Horner's from intracranial tumor)
- □ eyelids
  - □ ptosis? (possible partial third or Horner's from intracranial tumor)
  - □ lid retraction? (possible thyroid eye disease with compressive optic neuropathy)
- □ orbits: proptosis, enophthalmos, injection, chemosis?
- □ decreased corneal or facial sensation to light touch? (possible orbital apex or cavernous sinus tumor)
- □ if patient over 50: palpate temporal arteries for tenderness
- □ measure blood pressure:
  - □ in all cases, especially if disc swelling is present
- □ full neurologic examination if:
  - □ the patient has an unexplained optic neuropathy, unexplained neurologic symptoms or there is suspicion of chiasmal or retrochiasmal disease

Plus: must perform some type of perimetry
- □ IN ALL CASES

Management Flowchart

BLURRED VISION OR FIELD LOSS NOT EXPLAINED BY VISIBLE OCULAR DISEASE

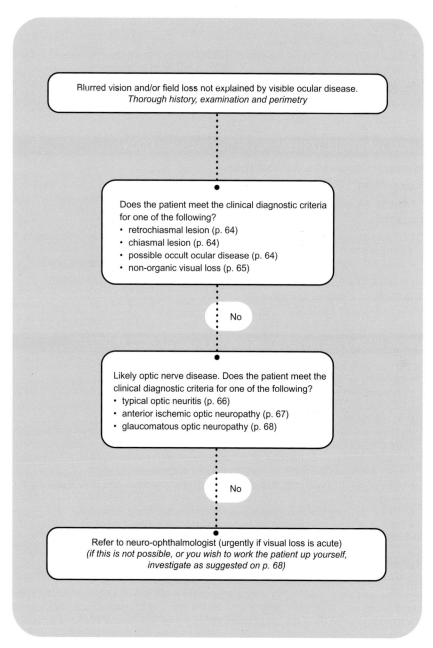

Blurred vision and/or field loss not explained by visible ocular disease.
Thorough history, examination and perimetry

Does the patient meet the clinical diagnostic criteria
for one of the following?
- retrochiasmal lesion (p. 64)
- chiasmal lesion (p. 64)
- possible occult ocular disease (p. 64)
- non-organic visual loss (p. 65)

No

Likely optic nerve disease. Does the patient meet the
clinical diagnostic criteria for one of the following?
- typical optic neuritis (p. 66)
- anterior ischemic optic neuropathy (p. 67)
- glaucomatous optic neuropathy (p. 68)

No

Refer to neuro-ophthalmologist (urgently if visual loss is acute)
*(if this is not possible, or you wish to work the patient up yourself,
investigate as suggested on p. 68)*

CLINICAL DIAGNOSTIC CRITERIA FOR CHIASMAL LESION

The patient must have ALL of the following:

EXAMINATION
- normal or reduced VA

PERIMETRY
- bitemporal visual field defect
- visual field defects stop at the vertical midline (unless there is a superimposed unilateral or bilateral optic neuropathy as well, which is common in pituitary region tumors)

IF THE PATIENT MEETS ALL THESE CRITERIA, SEE P. 120 FOR MANAGEMENT.

CLINICAL DIAGNOSTIC CRITERIA FOR RETROCHIASMAL LESION

The patient must have ALL of the following:

EXAMINATION
- normal VA, unless there is coexistent ocular disease causing blurred vision

PERIMETRY
- homonymous visual field loss: the same (or similar) area of field loss occurring in the same position in each eye
- visual field defects stop at the vertical midline (unless bilateral disease is present)

IF THE PATIENT MEETS ALL THESE CRITERIA, SEE P. 125 FOR MANAGEMENT.

CLINICAL DIAGNOSTIC CRITERIA FOR POSSIBLE OCCULT OCULAR DISEASE

The patient must have ALL of the following:
- no history of neurologic symptoms
- no proptosis or enophthalmos, no ptosis, normal eye movements, normal corneal and facial sensation
- no visible optic disc abnormality
- if there is a field defect on perimetry, it is in keeping with the proposed ocular disease and ONE OR MORE of the following:
- history suggestive of macular or retinal disease, e.g., metamorphopsia, hemeralopia (poor vision in bright light), or nyctalopia (poor vision in dim light)
- signs of keratoconus including abnormal retinoscopic reflex and high astigmatism on keratometry
- signs of macular disease on careful slit-lamp contact lens examination
- signs of occult retinal disease, e.g., vascular sheathing or attenuation

IF THE PATIENT MEETS ALL THESE CRITERIA, SEE P. 127 FOR MANAGEMENT.

CAUTION

Because optic nerve disease carries a higher risk of serious underlying disease (e.g., tumor) than retinal disease, if there is any doubt, the patient must first be investigated with neuro-imaging. If this and other investigations for possible optic nerve disease (e.g., optical coherence tomography [OCT] of the peripapillary retinal nerve fiber layer [PRNFL]) are negative, further retinal investigations such as OCT of the macula, electroretinography (ERG), and fluorescein angiography can then be pursued.

Beware attributing blurred vision or field loss to subtle macular or retinal disease; if the degree of visual loss is out of proportion to the visible disease, there could also be an underlying optic neuropathy.

CLINICAL DIAGNOSTIC CRITERIA FOR NONORGANIC VISUAL LOSS

The patient must have ALL of the following:

EXAMINATION

- inconsistency between different parts of the examination raises the suspicion that vision loss may be partly or completely nonorganic; e.g., there is claimed severe visual loss in one eye with a normal ocular examination, normal optic disc, and no RAPD
- the patient has an up-to-date refraction and this has been checked to be correct
- retinoscopy and keratometry are normal (no signs of keratoconus)
- no RAPD (on careful testing with a bright light in a dark room)
- no proptosis, no ptosis, normal eye movements, normal corneal and facial sensation
- AND you are able to demonstrate in clinical testing that the patient's visual function is actually completely normal (see "clinical tricks," p. 129)

PERIMETRY

- if abnormal, is consistent with nonorganic field loss, e.g., "spiraling" (see p. 132)
- if standard perimetry is normal, central field perimetry (Humphrey 10-2 or similar) should also be performed and also be normal

IF THE PATIENT MEETS ALL THESE CRITERIA, SEE P. 135 FOR MANAGEMENT.

CAUTION

True nonorganic visual loss may be very difficult to diagnose, and it is essential that patients with real but rare diseases are not falsely labeled as nonorganic. If there is any doubt, refer the patient to a neuro-ophthalmologist (urgently if visual loss is acute).

CLINICAL DIAGNOSTIC CRITERIA FOR TYPICAL OPTIC NEURITIS

The patient must have ALL of the following:

HISTORY

- AGE: 15–45 (male or female)
- MEDICAL HISTORY:
  - otherwise well: no history of cancer, vasculitis, or autoimmune disease
- ONE eye only is symptomatic
- TIME COURSE:
  - ACUTE onset of blurred vision
  - worsens rapidly over hours to days
- eye or orbital PAIN (usually, but not always, increased on eye movement)
- no diplopia
- no other systemic neurologic symptoms (apart from those consistent with previous episodes of multiple sclerosis [MS], e.g., an area of numbness that lasts days to weeks then resolves)

EXAMINATION

- no proptosis or enophthalmos, no ptosis, normal eye movements, normal corneal and facial sensation
- affected eye:
  - RAPD
  - normal optic nerve head or mild to moderate swelling
  - no disc pallor, hard exudates, cotton-wool spots, hemorrhages, iritis, vitritis, or other intraocular disease
- other eye: entirely normal intraocular examination

PERIMETRY

- affected eye: any type of field defect
- other eye: an asymptomatic field defect of any type may be present

AND ON FOLLOW-UP

- vision stops worsening within 2 weeks
- vision starts to improve within 4 weeks

If the patient meets all the other diagnostic criteria at the first visit, you can make a provisional diagnosis of typical optic neuritis, but this can only be confirmed as the definite diagnosis if vision behaves as expected on follow-up.

IF THE PATIENT MEETS ALL THESE CRITERIA, SEE P. 71 FOR MANAGEMENT.

CLINICAL DIAGNOSTIC CRITERIA FOR ANTERIOR ISCHEMIC OPTIC NEUROPATHY (AION)

The patient must have ALL of the following:

HISTORY

- AGE: 40 or over (male or female)
- MEDICAL HISTORY:
  - one or more vasculopathic risk factors (e.g., hypertension, hypercholesterolemia, diabetes, smoking, obstructive sleep apnea, amiodarone, erectile dysfunction drugs)
  - no history of cancer, vasculitis, or autoimmune disease
- ONE eye only is symptomatic
- TIME COURSE:
  - VERY SUDDEN VA and/or visual field loss while awake (over seconds or minutes) or visual loss noted first on waking (with normal vision the night before)
  - vision then remains the same, or worsens slowly for up to a week
- no or very mild eye or orbital pain, no diplopia, no other systemic neurologic symptoms

EXAMINATION

- no proptosis or enophthalmos, no ptosis, normal eye movements, normal corneal and facial sensation
- affected eye
  - RAPD
  - mild to severe optic nerve head swelling (hyperemic or pale swelling, sectoral or diffuse); may have disc margin hemorrhages; cotton-wool spots suggests arteritic
  - NO hard exudates, iritis, vitritis or other intraocular disease
- other eye:
  - entirely normal examination (no disc pallor, unless previous documented episode of AION in this eye)
  - "crowded" optic nerve head (with absent or small cup) (unless patient over age 50 and symptoms of GCA present)

PERIMETRY

- affected eye: any type of visual field defect (but often altitudinal or arcuate)
- other eye: entirely normal visual field unless previous attack of AION or other pathology

AND ON FOLLOW-UP

- no progressive worsening of acuity or field beyond a week

If the patient meets all the other diagnostic criteria at the first visit, you can make a provisional diagnosis of AION, but this can only be confirmed as the definite diagnosis if VA and field are found to be stable on follow-up.

NOTE: if the clinical diagnosis of AION is made, it must then be decided (by history, examination, erythrocyte sedimentation rate [ESR], C-reactive protein [CRP] and full blood count) if it could be ARTERITIC (usually due to GCA) or NONARTERITIC: see pp. 85–87.

IF THE PATIENT MEETS ALL THESE CRITERIA, SEE PP. 86–88 FOR MANAGEMENT.

CLINICAL DIAGNOSTIC CRITERIA FOR GLAUCOMATOUS OPTIC NEUROPATHY

The patient must have ALL of the following:

HISTORY

- the patient does not complain of progressive worsening of vision (unless very advanced disc cupping or notching is present)

EXAMINATION

- VA is normal, unless:
  - there is very advanced disc cupping and extensive field loss
  - there is another cause for reduced vision (e.g., cataract) that is consistent with the severity of visual loss
- color testing is normal (except in patients with very advanced disc cupping and reduced VA, or congenital color vision defect)
- intraocular pressure (IOP) may be raised or normal
- increased cup/disc ratio
- focal or diffuse loss of the neuroretinal rim
- the intact areas of neuroretinal rim are not pale

PERIMETRY

- field loss respects the horizontal midline but not the vertical midline
- if the other disc looks normal, it should have an absolutely normal field
- THE DISCS MUST MATCH THE FIELDS (e.g., a superior arcuate scotoma in an eye with an inferior optic disc notch)
- if there is no correlation between discs and fields (e.g., diffuse thinning of neuroretinal rim with a central scotoma on the field), it is not glaucoma

IF THE PATIENT MEETS ALL THESE CRITERIA, TREAT OR REFER AS APPROPRIATE (SEE ALSO P. 97).

SUGGESTED INVESTIGATIONS FOR OPTIC NEUROPATHY THAT CANNOT BE DIAGNOSED CLINICALLY

See p. 111 for details.

These investigations are recommended for patients with optic nerve disease who do not meet the previous clinical diagnostic criteria for typical optic neuritis, AION, or glaucoma and who cannot be referred promptly to a neuro-ophthalmologist, or you choose to investigate yourself. Investigate urgently if acute onset.

1. Basic assessment for all patients: full systemic clinical history and examination, including blood pressure, temperature, and urine analysis.
2. MRI optic nerves and brain with contrast for all patients, unless there is a medical contraindication. MRV (magnetic resonance venography) should also be requested if bilateral disc swelling is present.
3. Blood tests
   - for all patients: full blood count, electrolytes, liver function tests, glucose, ESR, CRP, angiotensin-converting enzyme (ACE), antinuclear antibodies (ANA), syphilis serology
   - plus for atypical optic neuritis: NMO-IgG (neuromyelitis optica) antibodies and MOG (myelin oligodendrocyte glycoprotein) antibodies
   - plus the following blood tests for patients with bilateral symmetric optic neuropathy: red blood cell (RBC) folate, serum vitamin B12
   - plus other tests as required if there is clinical suspicion of a particular disease (e.g., Leber hereditary optic neuropathy [LHON], cat scratch disease, Lyme disease, human immunodeficiency virus [HIV], quantiferon)
4. Chest x-ray for all patients (plus chest CT scan or positron emission tomography [PET] scan if sarcoid or tuberculosis suspected).
5. Lumbar puncture (LP) for selected patients (p. 114).
6. Diagnostic trial of 3 days' intravenous (IV) methylprednisolone for selected patients (p. 114).

Optic Neuropathy

Optic neuropathies may be sudden or insidious in onset, and the visual loss from them may be stable once lost, may be slowly or rapidly progressive, or may spontaneously improve.

Acute Optic Neuropathies

TYPICAL OPTIC NEURITIS

Check that your patient meets ALL the clinical diagnostic criteria on p. 66 before you make this diagnosis!

The term "optic neuritis" just means that the optic nerve is inflamed; it does not indicate the etiology of the inflammation. There are many different types of optic neuritis, including sarcoid optic neuritis, infectious optic neuritis, postinfectious optic neuritis, autoimmune disease-related optic neuritis, and typical optic neuritis. Of these, typical optic neuritis is the only one that can be diagnosed on history and examination alone, and the only one that carries an increased future risk of MS.

Please note:

- not all young adults with an acute optic neuropathy have typical optic neuritis and neither do all patients with optic neuropathy and normal optic discs. Optic neuropathies of many other causes, many of them treatable, are possible in these patients
- typical optic neuritis can only be confirmed in retrospect, after the patient's vision is observed to spontaneously recover as expected over time. At the first consultation, a tentative diagnosis of presumed typical optic neuritis can be made if the patient meets all the clinical diagnostic criteria on p. 66; however, confirmation of the diagnosis can only be made after following the patient over the next few weeks

Demographic

- age 15–45
- men or women (but more common in women)

Symptoms

Ophthalmic

- ACUTE visual loss in one eye that:
    - rapidly worsens for up to 2 weeks
    - then stays stable
    - then starts to improve by 4 weeks after onset of the symptoms
- PAIN in or behind the eye that in most (but not all) patients is worse on eye movement. A minority of cases of optic neuritis (<5%) are painless, so such cases should be considered atypical and investigated

Neurologic

- usually the patient has no other neurologic symptoms at the time of presentation
- some patients have a past history of transient, spontaneously resolving episodes of neurologic dysfunction suggestive of undiagnosed MS, e.g., episodes of numbness or weakness of an arm or leg lasting days or weeks, then resolving, or an episode of unexplained vertigo or loss of balance

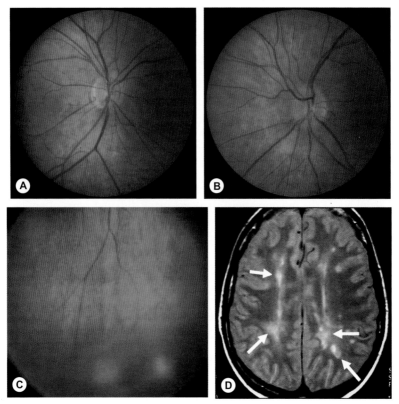

Fig. 3.2 The optic disc in typical optic neuritis can be normal (**A**) or show mild to moderate swelling (**B**). (**C**) Peripheral snowbanking in a patient with multiple sclerosis (MS)–related optic neuritis. (**D**) Magnetic resonance imaging (MRI) showing typical periventricular white matter hyperintensities. In the appropriate setting, these findings are consistent with a diagnosis of MS.

Signs

- variably decreased VA (20/20 to "no perception of light")
- variably decreased color vision (color is usually more severely affected than acuity)
- any type of visual field defect; however, central scotomas and diffuse loss are common
- an RAPD in the symptomatic eye
- optic disc on the affected side (Fig. 3.2):
  - two-thirds of patients have a normal-appearing disc (at least in the Western hemisphere); i.e., a "retrobulbar" or "posterior" optic neuritis (see Fig. 3.2A)
  - one-third have mild to moderate hyperemic disc swelling; i.e., an "anterior" optic neuritis, sometimes referred to as a "papillitis" (see Fig. 3.2B)
  - no hard exudates or cotton-wool spots
- intraocular inflammation:
  - a minority of patients with typical optic neuritis have mild peripheral sheathing of retinal veins ± mild "snowbanking" (similar to that seen in intermediate uveitis [previously called "pars planitis"]) (see Fig. 3.2C)

- however, given that an identical appearance can occur in sarcoidosis, vasculitis, cat-scratch disease, or syphilis, these patients require especially close and careful follow-up, with the appropriate investigations (as suggested on p. 68, plus uveitis opinion) if the vision does not begin to improve within 4 weeks or if the uveitis worsens

Differential Diagnosis

- anti-aquaporin 4 (AQP4) antibody-related optic neuritis (neuromyelitis optica spectrum disease [NMOSD]—see p. 73)
- anti-MOG antibody-related optic neuritis—see page 76
- infectious and postinfectious optic neuritis
- sarcoidosis
- there are many other causes of acute optic neuropathy with normal or swollen disc/s

Investigations

- patients who meet all the clinical diagnostic criteria for typical optic neuritis do not require investigations to confirm the ophthalmic diagnosis
- it is, however, reasonable to obtain an MRI orbits and brain (see Fig. 3.2D) for all patients with first-episode optic neuritis, as the presence and number of brain white matter lesions are powerful prognostic factors regarding the future risk of MS and helps guide discussions as to possible immunomodulatory therapy
- patients with an acute optic neuropathy who do NOT meet the clinical diagnostic criteria for typical optic neuritis or AION should be thoroughly investigated to determine the cause (see p. 68)
  - these tests should include blood testing for anti-AQP4 and anti-MOG antibodies

Visual Prognosis

- the Optic Neuritis Treatment Trial (ONTT) found that 93% of patients (with or without steroid treatment) had recovery of vision to at least 20/40
- even if VA returns to normal or almost low-dose normal, color vision may remain abnormal, and an RAPD persist
- patients usually say that the eye "never sees quite as well again" due to patchy scotomas, color defects, and contrast sensitivity problems
- the chance of recurrent episodes of typical optic neuritis is about 25%; if episodes are severe or many episodes occur, significant and permanent vision loss eventually may result

TREATMENT FOR THE VISUAL LOSS OF TYPICAL OPTIC NEURITIS

No treatment has been shown to improve the final visual outcome. The ONTT found that:

- 1 g IV methylprednisolone daily (i.e., a high dose) for 3 days followed by oral prednisone (1 mg/kg/day—i.e., a low dose) for 11 days often sped up visual recovery, but the eventual visual recovery was the same whether or not steroids were used

- oral prednisone (1 mg/kg/day for 2 weeks—i.e., a low dose) alone (surprisingly) was actually found to be **harmful**, in that it increased the risk of recurrent optic neuritis in the affected eye and new optic neuritis in the fellow eye

Systemic Prognosis—Relationship of Typical Optic Neuritis to Multiple Sclerosis

- one-quarter of MS patients first present with typical optic neuritis
- long-term follow-up suggests that two-thirds of women and one-third of men with typical optic neuritis eventually develop MS
- the risk of developing MS is increased if a patient with typical optic neuritis:
  - has one or more white matter lesions visible on brain MRI
  - has had previous nonspecific neurologic symptoms
  - has recurrent episodes of typical optic neuritis
  - has a family history of MS

Treatment to Delay Development of MS

Corticosteroids

- do not provide any long-term benefit
- in the ONTT, 1 g IV methylprednisolone daily for 3 days followed by oral prednisone (1 mg/kg/day) for 11 days delayed the onset of MS for up to 2 years; however, at 2 years, as many steroid-treated as untreated patients had developed MS

Disease-Modifying Treatments for MS

- A variety of immunomodulatory agents are now available and many more are under development. Examples of these medications include:
  - subcutaneous injections, e.g., beta-interferon (Betaferon, Avonex), glatiramer acetate (Copaxone)
  - oral tablets, e.g., fingolimod (Gilenya), teriflunomide (Aubagio)
  - IV infusions, e.g., natalizumab (Tysabri)
- these treatments may delay the onset of MS in some patients presenting with first-episode typical optic neuritis and white matter lesions on MRI; however, long-term efficacy is unknown, especially with the newer medications
- ophthalmologists should be aware that patients taking fingolimod (Gilenya) tablets may rarely develop uveitis and/or macular edema, usually within the first 6 months of commencing treatment. Therefore, patients about to start fingolimod treatment should have an ophthalmic examination and OCT macula immediately before commencing treatment; 3, 6, and 12 months after commencement; then yearly. Patients should be told to contact their ophthalmologist and neurologist immediately if they develop blurred vision or metamorphopsia at any stage
- patients taking natalizumab (Tysabri) may rarely develop posterior multifocal leukoencephalopathy (PML) with involvement of the posterior visual pathways and homonymous or diffuse visual field loss. Ophthalmologists should therefore perform a careful evaluation, including perimetry, for any MS patients treated with natalizumab who develop new visual symptoms. In general, patients should have a serum PCR for the presence of JC virus before natalizumab is started

Management Recommendations

It would seem reasonable to refer all patients meeting the diagnostic criteria for typical optic neuritis to either a neurologist or neuro-ophthalmologist to discuss:

- the risk of developing MS
- the potential severity of MS when the first sign of which is acute optic neuritis (MS tends to be mild)
- if the patient would like an MRI scan to further assess their risk of MS
- possible steroid treatment (high-dose IV then low-dose oral) for those patients with white matter lesions on brain MRI at presentation, severe visual loss, or an occupational need for rapid return of vision
- possible beta-interferon or other immunomodulatory treatment (where available) for patients with two or more MRI white matter lesions at presentation

Irrespective of other treatment or referral, all patients should be reviewed at 2 and 4 weeks to check that the disease is "still behaving typically." That is:

- vision stops worsening by 2 weeks after the initial onset of symptoms
- vision begins to recover by 4 weeks after the initial onset of symptoms
- no new ophthalmic, neurologic, or systemic symptoms or signs have developed

If atypical features occur at any stage during follow-up, the initial clinical diagnosis of typical optic neuritis should be considered suspect and the patient urgently referred to a neuro-ophthalmologist for further evaluation (or if this is not possible, urgently investigated as suggested on p. 68).

If the disease behaves "as expected" (the patient remains otherwise well and vision rapidly recovers, usually to almost normal), the patient does not require further routine ophthalmic follow-up unless new ophthalmic symptoms occur.

ANTI-AQUAPORIN 4 (AQP4) ANTIBODY-RELATED OPTIC NEURITIS (NEUROMYELITIS OPTIC SPECTRUM DISEASE [NMOSD])

NMOSD is characterized by an immune attack on the optic nerves and spinal cord, as well as some areas of the brain, such as the thalamus and area postrema in the medulla.

It is essential to differentiate NMO-related optic neuritis from the much more common MS-related or idiopathic optic neuritis because:

- NMOSD is, in general, a more severe disease than MS and can lead to severe disability or death if not treated appropriately
- most cases of MS-related optic neuritis will recover without treatment, whereas NMO-related optic neuritis often leads to permanent blindness without urgent treatment; thus, it may be appropriate to treat ALL cases of acute optic neuritis, even those thought to be idiopathic (i.e., with no MRI findings) with high-dose IV corticosteroids, just in case the optic neuritis turns out to be NMO related.
- the treatment for NMO is completely different from that for MS treatment; indeed, if NMO is misdiagnosed as MS, MS therapy may make it worse

A cell-based NMO blood test is available that is >95% sensitive. However, in some cases, clinical features and MRI findings will lead to a diagnosis of NMO, despite a negative blood result.

Demographic

- more common in females than males
- can occur at any age, including childhood, but median age of onset is mid-30s
- affected individuals often have a history of other autoimmune disorders, e.g., Sjögren syndrome

Symptoms

- acute or subacute vision loss in one or both eyes
- bilateral involvement may be simultaneous or sequential
- may or may not have retrobulbar pain
- transverse myelitis from spinal cord demyelination can present with tingling, numbness, and weakness in the limbs, and sometimes bladder control symptoms
- myelitis may occur weeks, months, or years before or after visual loss; or less commonly both may occur simultaneously

Signs

- optic disc/s normal, swollen or (if diagnosis delayed) pale (Fig. 3.3)
- usually markedly decreased visual and color acuity
- RAPD unless neuritis is bilateral and symmetric
- any visual field defect

Differential Diagnosis

- typical or MS-related optic neuritis
- anti-MOG antibody-related optic neuritis
- other autoimmune optic neuritis, e.g., systemic lupus erythematosus (SLE)
- postinfectious optic neuritis

Investigations

- NMO-IgG cell-based blood test:
  - tests for antibodies against the AQP4 astrocyte membrane protein
  - sensitivity of approximately 95%—so if positive, the patient probably does have NMO
  - however, some patients with otherwise typical NMO have a negative antibody test, and non-cell-based tests have a lower sensitivity of about 65%–75% and thus have a high false-negative rate (25–35%)—so if one of these non-cell-based (e.g., enzyme-linked immunosorbent assay [ELISA]) tests is negative, the patient may still have NMO
- MRI (see Fig. 3.3): may show one or more of:
  - optic nerve enhancement, sometimes extending from the orbit through the optic canal to the chiasm
  - "long" (greater than three segments) spinal cord demyelinating lesion/s
  - in most cases the brain itself is normal, without the periventricular white matter lesions of MS
  - however, in some cases, MS-like brain lesions are present, particularly in the thalami, brainstem, and area postrema in the medulla
- LP:
  - if performed, often shows a moderate white cell count (higher than seen in MS)

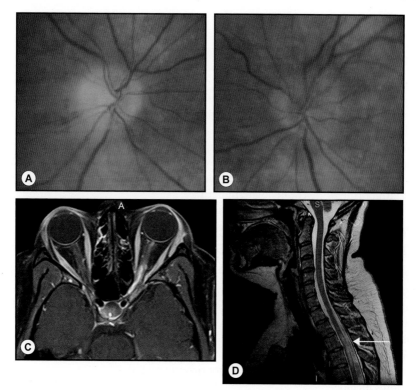

Fig. 3.3 Neuromyelitis optica (NMO)–related optic neuritis. This young woman presented with bilateral sequential atypical optic neuritis, first the right then the left eye. The right disc (**A**) is pale, the left (**B**) is swollen. (**C**) Magnetic resonance imaging shows left optic nerve enhancement, but no other brain lesions. NMO-IgG (aquaporin-4) antibody testing was positive. Some NMO patients also develop myelitis, before or after their optic neuritis, often with "long" spinal cord lesions *(arrow)* (**D**).

Summary—Suspect NMOSD-Related Optic Neuritis If a Patient With Optic Neuritis Has

- "atypical" optic neuritis, i.e., does not meet the clinical diagnostic criteria for typical optic neuritis summarized on p. 66
- severe visual loss in one or both eyes
- bilateral visual loss (simultaneous or rapidly sequential)
- lack of spontaneous recovery of vision
- recurrent optic neuritis
- spinal symptoms as well (either now or in the past)
- a "long" (more than three segments) lesion on spinal MRI
- a history of other autoimmune disorders, e.g., Sjögren syndrome

Prognosis

- untreated, many patients with NMO experience a relapsing-remitting course with progressive severe optic nerve and spinal cord damage, in many cases resulting in blindness, severe disability or death

- with prompt diagnosis and expert treatment, however, visual and neurologic function often can be maintained

Treatment

- acute treatment for NMO-associated optic neuritis usually involves high-dose IV corticosteroids, sometimes also with plasmapheresis or IV gamma globulin, particularly if there is no improvement within 5–7 days despite treatment with high-dose steroid therapy
- long-term immunosuppressive therapy to try to prevent further attacks may include monoclonal antibody therapy, such as rituximab, or other monoclonal antibodies (e.g., eculizumab, satralizumab, tocilizumab) or other agents, such as azathioprine or mycophenolate mofetil

ANTI-MYELIN OLIGODENDROCYTE GLYCOPROTEIN (MOG) ANTIBODY-RELATED OPTIC NEURITIS

Anti-MOG antibody-related optic neuritis is an increasingly recognized syndrome. Several MOG antibody tests are commercially available, with the sensitivity and specificity dependent on the type of test (e.g., ELISA vs. cell-based assay) that is performed.

Clinically, anti-MOG antibody-related optic neuritis seems to be less severe than NMO-related optic neuritis. Nevertheless, some cases cause severe bilateral visual loss that is permanent despite timely and appropriate treatment.

Features include

- usually anterior, sometimes with peripapillary hemorrhages
- often painful; often bilateral
- most common cause of optic neuritis in children (usually have acute disseminated encephalomyelitis [ADEM])
- most common cause of chronic relapsing inflammatory optic neuropathy (CRION; see later)
- recurrences common (especially in Caucasians vs. Asians)
- perineural enhancement on MRI in 50% (i.e., optic perineuritis) (Fig 3.4)
- often requires steroid Rx and/or plasmapheresis acutely
- good visual (6%–7% <20/200) and neurological prognoses?

CHRONIC RELAPSING INFLAMMATORY OPTIC NEUROPATHY (CRION)

Even though the term for this form of optic neuritis includes the word "chronic," this is an acute optic neuritis that may appear to be "typical" but that is both steroid-sensitive and steroid-dependent.

- previously thought to be "idiopathic," but many cases associated with anti-MOG antibodies
- usually requires long-term immunosuppressive therapy such as rituximab

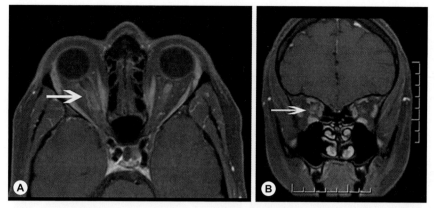

Fig. 3.4 Magnetic resonance imaging in a patient with anti-myelin oligodendrocyte glycoprotein antibody-related optic neuritis. Axial (**A**) and coronal (**B**) images reveal mild enhancement of the right optic nerve and marked enhancement of the right optic nerve sheath.

INFECTIOUS OPTIC NEURITIS

Causes

- direct infection by:
  - bacteria: cat-scratch disease, tuberculosis, syphilis, Lyme disease
  - viruses: measles, mumps, chickenpox, herpes zoster ophthalmicus
  - fungi: mucormycosis extending from the sinuses into the orbit; cryptococcal meningitis
  - rickettsia: tick-borne diseases such as Q fever
  - parasites: toxoplasma, toxocara
- secondary to sphenoid sinusitis, orbital cellulitis, meningitis

Symptoms

- sudden or gradual visual loss in one or both eyes
- painful (with pain increased on eye movement in some cases) or painless
- the patient may be otherwise well or have fevers, lymphadenopathy or meningismus

Signs

- VA may be mildly to severely reduced
- an RAPD is usually present if monocular or bilateral but asymmetric
- the optic disc/s may be normal, swollen or pale at presentation; the same infection may cause different disc appearances in different patients (Fig. 3.5)
- there may be other ophthalmic complications of the disease, including:
  - vitritis
  - retinal vasculitis
  - "stellate neuroretinitis"
    - a clinical term referring to unilateral or bilateral disc swelling associated with a partial or complete hard exudate star around the macula (see Fig. 3.5B)

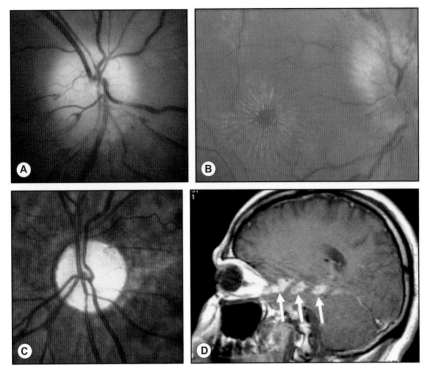

Fig. 3.5 A few examples of infectious optic neuritis. (**A**) Chickenpox optic neuritis. (**B**) Cat-scratch disease optic neuroretinitis with marked optic disc swelling and a complete macular star figure. (**C**) Syphilitic optic neuritis presenting initially with pale flat discs. (**D**) Tuberculous optic neuritis in a patient with tuberculous meningitis and multiple small tuberculous brain abscesses *(arrows)*.

- caused by inflammation of the anterior optic nerve, with secondary leakage leading to the accumulation of hard exudates in the retina
- possible infectious causes include cat-scratch disease, syphilis, toxoplasmosis, tuberculosis (non-infectious causes include sarcoidosis)
- note: this appearance can be associated with and caused by optic nerve head swelling of almost any cause (e.g., papilledema, malignant hypertension). Hence, the presence of "stellate neuroretinitis" is not diagnostic, and patients still require referral or investigation (during investigation, serology for the possible infectious causes listed above should be added)

Investigations

- patients should either be referred urgently to a neuro-ophthalmologist or investigated as suggested on p. 68, with the addition of serology for specific infections suggested by history and examination

Treatment

- specific for the identified organism

POSTINFECTIOUS AND POSTVACCINATION OPTIC NEURITIS

Note: minor infections are common, as are vaccinations. Not all optic neuropathies occurring within a few weeks of these events are causally linked (many are coincidental optic neuropathies of other causes).

Causes

- an autoimmune optic neuritis triggered by infection (typically nonspecific viral or bacterial upper respiratory infections or bacterial gastroenteritis) or vaccination (reported after almost all types of vaccines)

Demographic

- more common in children and young adults but can occur at any age

Symptoms

- acute onset of blurred vision in one or both eyes, days to weeks after an infection or vaccination
- usually painless
- the patient is usually otherwise well; sometimes he or she also has meningitic symptoms

Signs

- acuity may be mildly to severely reduced
- an RAPD is usually present in monocular or bilateral asymmetric cases
- the optic disc(s) may be normal or (more often) swollen (Fig. 3.6)

Investigations

- refer to a neuro-ophthalmologist or investigate as suggested on pp. 111–115.
- work-up is directed at possible/probable cause (e.g., if recent vaccination or self-limited illness, consider antibody testing)

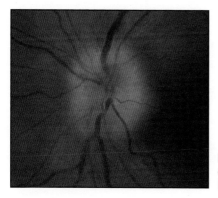

Fig. 3.6 Postinfectious optic neuritis can present with a normal or swollen optic disc in one or both eyes.

Treatment

- treat as suggested on p. 115 with a trial of IV methylprednisolone; many patients with postinfectious or postvaccination optic neuritis will experience a marked improvement in vision with this treatment
- if improvement occurs, continue treatment with oral prednisone; this is tapered and ceased as quickly as possible while maintaining vision
- with or without steroid treatment, many patients recover good vision. However, some patients have steroid-responsive neuropathies and develop optic atrophy without early steroid treatment; it is impossible to identify these patients without a trial of steroids
- patients with steroid-responsive optic neuropathies may also be steroid dependent; such patients may require long-term steroids (months) with very slow taper

SARCOID OPTIC NEURITIS

Demographic

- any age, any race, male or female

Symptoms

- acute, subacute, or slowly progressive blurring of vision in one or both eyes
- painful or painless
- sarcoid optic neuritis may mimic typical optic neuritis (including pain increased on eye movement) except that it does not begin to improve spontaneously within 4 weeks
- symptoms of systemic complications of sarcoid: it may affect almost any part of the body, including the meninges, brain, lungs, joints, skin, and kidneys

Signs

- one or both optic discs may be normal, swollen, or pale at presentation (Fig. 3.7)
- in some cases, there are also one or more of the following:
  - anterior or posterior uveitis
  - iris nodules at pupillary margin or in stroma (Busacca, Koeppe)
  - retinal vascular sheathing
  - vitreous "snowballs" or peripheral retinal "snowbanking" (see Fig. 3.2C)
  - tarsal conjunctival follicles or granulomas (look specifically for these as they can give the diagnosis on biopsy)
- however, none of these is specific for sarcoidosis

Investigations

- refer to a neuro-ophthalmologist or investigate as suggested on p. 68. One or more of the following additional tests may also be necessary if there is clinical suspicion of sarcoid:
- blood tests:
  - serum ACE is elevated in most (but not all) cases of sarcoidosis; however, there are other causes for an elevated ACE level
  - serum calcium may be elevated

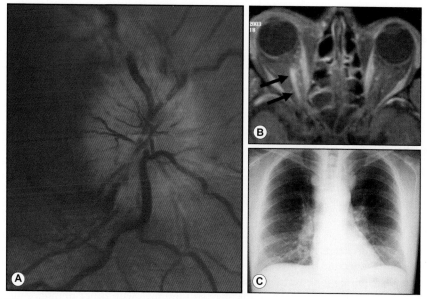

Fig. 3.7 Sarcoid optic neuritis can present with a normal, swollen (**A**) or pale optic disc in one or both eyes. Optic nerve enhancement (**B**) *(arrows)* may be seen on postcontrast magnetic resonance imaging (however, this is a nonspecific change that can be seen in optic neuritis of any cause). Chest x-ray is abnormal in many (but not all) cases of sarcoid optic neuritis (**C**).

- chest x-ray (see Fig. 3.7C); chest CT scan if sarcoid is suspected (chest x-ray alone will miss some cases of sarcoid)
- other tests may be required for diagnosis, including gallium scan, PET scan, bronchial lavage or tissue biopsy (conjunctival follicle, mediastinal lymph node or lung)

Treatment

- consult a neuro-ophthalmologist if sarcoid optic neuritis is suspected
- acute sarcoid optic neuritis often responds dramatically to steroids, e.g., "perception of light" vision returning to 20/30 within a few days of starting treatment
- patients may require immunosuppressive treatment for several years; if they continue to lose vision despite steroid treatment or if prolonged high-dose steroid is required to maintain vision, additional immunosuppression or even radiation therapy may be required

Prognosis

- with early diagnosis and appropriate immunosuppression, many patients with sarcoid optic neuritis have a good prognosis

OPTIC NEURITIS ASSOCIATED WITH AUTOIMMUNE DISEASE

Causes

- systemic autoimmune diseases that may be complicated by optic nerve inflammation include:
  - SLE and other vasculitides
  - inflammatory bowel disease
  - Reiter syndrome

Symptoms and Signs

- painful or painless, monocular, or binocular visual loss
- may mimic typical optic neuritis apart from lack of spontaneous recovery
- optic disc/s may be normal or swollen

Management

- refer or investigate urgently
- many show rapid improvement with steroid treatment and may be steroid dependent, requiring long-term steroid therapy
- if no improvement with steroids, may still improve with other immunosuppressive drugs

ANTERIOR ISCHEMIC OPTIC NEUROPATHY (AION)

Check that your patient meets ALL the clinical diagnostic criteria on p. 67 before you make this diagnosis!

Please note:

- not all middle-aged or elderly adults with a swollen disc have AION. Optic neuropathies from many other causes, many of them treatable, are possible in these patients
- AION can only be diagnosed in retrospect, after the patient's vision is observed to behave as expected over time (sudden initial visual loss, then plateau, sometimes followed by a very slow slight recovery over months). At the first consultation, a tentative diagnosis of AION can be made if the patient meets all the clinical diagnostic criteria on p. 67, but confirmation of the diagnosis can only be made after following the patient over the next few weeks

Causes

Infarction or ischemia in the territory of the short posterior ciliary arteries because of:

- GCA (or rarely vasculitis of other causes): "arteritic" AION
- atherosclerosis: "nonarteritic" AION

Risk Factors

Arteritic AION

- increasing age is the principal risk factor for GCA; most patients with arteritic AION are 60 years of age or older

Nonarteritic AION

- age: most patients are over 55
- the "disc at risk"
  - a small, crowded optic nerve head (with a small or absent central cup) predisposes patients to nonarteritic AION
  - nonarteritic AION is unusual in patients with normal cup/disc ratios
- optic disc drusen
- atherosclerosis of the short posterior ciliary arteries: hypertension, diabetes, hypercholesterolemia, smoking
- rarely: severe hypotension, coagulopathies, sleep apnea, erectile dysfunction drugs (e.g., sildenafil/Viagra, amiodarone)

Symptoms

- VERY SUDDEN acute visual loss, with vision then remaining stable or slowly declining further over the next week
- usually painless or with minimal pain; if pain is present, it almost never worsens with eye movement
- usually unilateral (if bilateral, suspect GCA)

Signs

- variably decreased VA (20/20 to "no perception of light")
- variably decreased color vision (extent of color loss usually consistent with acuity)
- any type of visual field defect, but altitudinal or arcuate defects most common
- an RAPD in the affected eye
- diffusely or segmentally swollen optic disc on the affected side: hyperemic (pink) or pale swelling (Figs. 3.8 and 3.10)

Differential Diagnosis

There are many other causes of acute painless visual loss with a swollen disc, including infectious or postinfectious optic neuritis, sarcoid optic neuritis, and anterior infiltrative optic neuropathy.

Investigations

- no investigations are required to diagnose AION if the patient meets all the clinical diagnostic criteria on p. 67.
- all patients with AION require an urgent complete physical examination, with special attention to underlying systemic vascular disease
- a careful history for symptoms of GCA (see later)
- blood tests for underlying diabetes, hypercholesterolemia, coagulopathy (e.g., antiphospholipid antibody assay, anticardiolipin antibody assay, serum homocysteine level) if nonarteritic AION suspected
- ESR, CRP, and full blood count if arteritic AION suspected
- sleep studies if history suggests sleep apnea (e.g., snoring, insomnia)

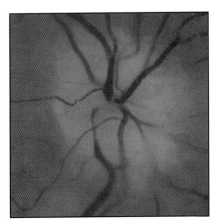

Fig. 3.8 Anterior ischemic optic neuropathy (AION) presents as sudden visual loss with a swollen optic disc.

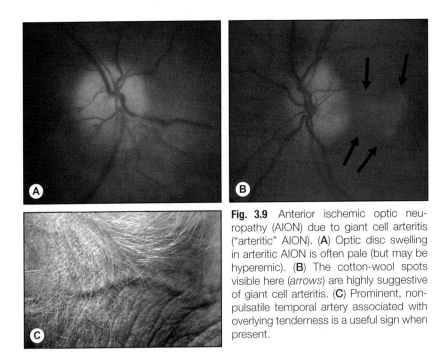

Fig. 3.9 Anterior ischemic optic neuropathy (AION) due to giant cell arteritis ("arteritic" AION). (**A**) Optic disc swelling in arteritic AION is often pale (but may be hyperemic). (**B**) The cotton-wool spots visible here (*arrows*) are highly suggestive of giant cell arteritis. (**C**) Prominent, non-pulsatile temporal artery associated with overlying tenderness is a useful sign when present.

Distinguishing Between Arteritic and Nonarteritic AION

There are no features in the history, examination, or blood test results that can completely exclude GCA. However, the presence of one or more of the following in a patient over 50 who has AION is strongly suggestive of GCA.

Symptoms Suggesting GCA
- ophthalmic
    - transient loss of vision preceding permanent visual loss in the affected eye
    - transient or persistent diplopia
    - bilateral (usually rapidly sequential) visual loss
- systemic
    - onset of a new headache
    - muscle aches, malaise, weight loss, fever, night sweats
    - scalp tenderness (to touch or on hair brushing)
    - jaw or tongue ache on chewing (jaw claudication)
    - neck or ear pain
    - symptoms of systemic complications of GCA: scalp ulceration, Raynaud phenomenon, myocardial ischemia or infarction, transient ischemic attack or stroke, bowel ischemia or infarction

Signs Suggesting GCA
- ophthalmic
    - retinal cotton-wool spots or arteriolar occlusion (Fig. 3.9B)
    - normal (noncrowded) disc in the fellow eye (in most cases of nonarteritic AION, the unaffected disc is small and "crowded" with little or no central cup)
    - signs of ocular or orbital ischemia (uveitis, corneal edema, low IOP, dilated retinal veins, midperipheral retinal blot hemorrhages)
    - motility deficit
- systemic
    - tender and/or nonpulsatile temporal artery on one or both sides
    - scalp tenderness (rarely scalp ulceration)

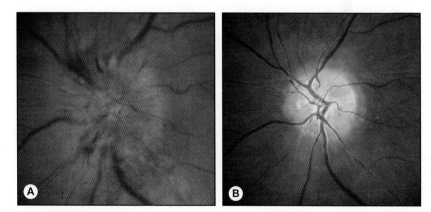

Fig. 3.10 Nonarteritic anterior ischemic optic neuropathy (NAION) presents with sudden loss of vision and a swollen disc (**A**); disc swelling gradually settles and disc pallor results over the subsequent months (**B**).

Blood Test Results Suggesting GCA
- ESR and CRP
  - most patients with GCA have elevation of both ESR and CRP; however, some patients have elevation of only one, so both should be tested but beware of the following:
    - not all patients with GCA have a raised ESR or CRP: a few patients with biopsy-proven GCA have an absolutely normal ESR and CRP
    - not all patients with a raised ESR or CRP have GCA: there are many causes for a raised ESR or CRP, including cancer, acute or chronic infections, renal failure, and other types of vasculitis; some of these other diseases present with headaches and malaise (and sometimes visual loss) that may be mistaken for GCA
- full blood count: increased platelet count (thrombocytosis) and a normochromic, normocytic anemia are common in GCA
- biochemistry: alkaline phosphatase (ALP) is elevated in some cases of GCA

Investigation and Treatment of Suspected Arteritic AION (AION Due to GCA)

Referral

The treatment of suspected GCA may be complex and has significant risks to elderly patients. Refer urgently to a neuro-ophthalmologist at any stage if you are unsure or if the patient is not responding to treatment.

Initial Treatment
- admission to hospital is often advisable, particularly if the patient is unwell or lives alone
- start high-dose steroid treatment as soon as the diagnosis of GCA is suspected: the risk of a few days' steroid treatment is low and you can always cease treatment if the diagnosis is ruled out by temporal artery biopsy
- IV methylprednisolone
  - many neuro-ophthalmologists give this for 3–5 days initially, before starting oral prednisone, if:
    - vision has already been lost in one or both eyes
    - the patient has normal vision but is experiencing transient visual loss
    - there are neurologic, cardiologic, or gastrointestinal symptoms of GCA complications (urgently consult the relevant specialist physicians)
  - dose: 1 g per day for a 70-kg adult (in single or divided doses) for at least 3 days, starting as soon as diagnosis is suspected and blood is drawn for ESR, CRP, etc.
  - monitor blood pressure; daily blood glucose if not diabetic, frequent blood glucose monitoring with sliding-scale insulin if diabetic
- oral prednisone (warn the patient about short- and long-term side effects)
  - 1.5 mg/kg single daily morning dose to start
  - if IV methylprednisolone was given first, start the oral prednisone on the final day of IV treatment

- prophylactic treatment: start the following immediately (continue until steroid ceased):
  - osteoporosis prophylaxis, e.g., calcium plus vitamin D, alendronic acid
  - gastric ulcer prophylaxis, e.g., ranitidine

Temporal Artery Biopsy

- the gold standard test for the diagnosis of temporal arteritis, although in some cases, ultrasound or high-resolution MRI can be helpful in making the diagnosis
- we believe that most patients with suspected GCA should undergo a temporal artery biopsy: if an elderly patient is to be exposed to the risks of steroid treatment for a year or more, a definitive diagnosis must be made, and a biopsy is the best method for doing this
- in general, NEVER wait for biopsy results before starting high-dose steroid treatment
- aim to:
  - perform within a few days of diagnosis
  - obtain a cut artery specimen of at least 2 cm length (specimens less than this length have a decreased yield); avoid crushing the artery
- it is important that the histopathology lab processes and examines the specimen correctly, if false-negative reports are to be avoided: examination of many sections of the artery by an experienced pathologist is ideal
- if the first biopsy is negative, but there is still a high clinical suspicion of temporal arteritis, consider biopsy of the other side (in 1%–11% of cases, the contralateral biopsy will be positive!)
- if adequate bilateral biopsies have been obtained early in steroid treatment and expert histopathologic examination shows no sign of active or healed temporal arteritis, the diagnosis is unlikely, and steroids should be stopped unless there is overwhelming clinical evidence of GCA; have the patient evaluated for other causes of raised ESR and CRP (e.g., atypical meningitis, infections, cancer)

Further Treatment and Follow-up

- natural history
  - temporal arteritis tends to be a self-limiting disease but may persist for many years
  - high-dose IV steroids followed by lower-dose oral steroids usually protect the unaffected optic nerve/s as well as other vessels elsewhere in the body (e.g., heart, brain) while the disease "burns itself out"
  - further vision loss is rare after 1 year, even without treatment, so steroids can usually be safely withdrawn at 12–18 months unless symptoms or raised blood inflammatory parameters persist or recur
- principles of treatment
  - oral prednisone is a life-threatening drug, especially for elderly patients; side effects can be minimized by:
    - educating the patient and their family about the drug and its complications
    - starting osteoporosis and gastric ulcer prophylaxis immediately in all patients

  - regularly monitoring for side effects throughout treatment
  - tapering and ceasing treatment after 12–18 months, if possible
- an initial high dose is essential to protect against early bilateral blindness and to put the disease into remission; the dose is then tapered as rapidly as possible, balancing the risks of treatment against the risk of losing vision
- it is essential that the patient is followed up by a doctor experienced with prednisone treatment for GCA throughout their course: if you do not have this experience, involve a neuro-ophthalmologist or rheumatologist early
- "resistant" or "recurrent" disease: obtain a neuro-ophthalmic opinion; such patients may benefit from addition of tocilizumab; it is unclear if this drug should be used as first-line treatment
- ceasing treatment
  - treatment continues for a minimum of 12 months
  - once prednisone has been withdrawn, the patient needs to be checked for at least a further 12 months to watch for recurrent disease

Visual Prognosis
- recovery of vision in affected eyes is rare
- second eye involvement can occur within hours; hence, if visual loss has already occurred in one eye, urgent action must be taken to save the vision in the other eye
- even patients treated early with high-dose IV steroids after acute visual loss in one eye may lose vision in the second eye, but the risk is much lower with treatment than without

Investigation, Treatment, and Prognosis of Nonarteritic AION

Investigations
- no investigations are required to diagnose non-arteritic AION if:
  - the patient meets all the clinical diagnostic criteria for AION
  - there is no suspicion of GCA on history, examination and blood tests
  - the condition behaves as expected on follow-up (no deterioration of vision beyond a week, no other neurologic symptoms develop); if not, the patient requires investigation as suggested on p. 68)
- however, all patients with non-arteritic AION require investigation for vascular risk factors (by yourself, their family physician or their internist):
  - blood pressure
  - fasting blood cholesterol and lipids
  - blood glucose, full blood count and electrolytes (including calcium)
  - remember to ask about use of possible precipitating medications, e.g., erectile dysfunction drugs and amiodarone
  - evaluate for possible obstructive sleep apnea
  - note: investigations for embolic sources (e.g., carotid ultrasound) are not required for AION unless there are other symptoms suggesting this process
- the "young" patient with non-arteritic AION:
  - if a patient younger than 40 fits all the clinical diagnostic criteria for AION except that of age, he or she should be referred to a neuro-ophthalmologist (or failing this, investigated urgently as suggested on p. 68)

- if no other cause is found (leaving a presumed diagnosis of non-arteritic AION) and the patient is not diabetic, further investigation for vascular disease or coagulopathies should be considered, particularly if the patient has no other known vascular risk factors:
  - the patient could have a familial hyperlipidemia (or just have high cholesterol)
  - hyperhomocysteinemia may be linked to AION at a young age and is treatable
  - vasculitides such as SLE may sometimes cause AION (or an anterior optic neuropathy mimicking AION)
- remember to ask about sleep apnea symptoms (ask patient AND spouse/significant other)
- ask (in private!) about use of drugs for erectile dysfunction (e.g., sildenafil)

Treatment
- no treatment consistently improves the visual outcome once nonarteritic AION has occurred
- treatment to protect the other eye:
  - no treatment is of proven benefit, but many neuro-ophthalmologists will start patients with nonarteritic AION on aspirin in the hope of reducing the chance that the disc in the other eye will also suffer infarction
  - significant ocular hypertension should be treated if present in one or both eyes, with the intention of improving optic nerve head perfusion pressure; however, again there is no proven benefit to this
  - if systemic hypertension is present (or discovered during the work-up for AION), it should be treated:
    - the patient's physician should be advised to avoid a "low" blood pressure or a sudden drop in blood pressure, and to avoid nighttime dosing of antihypertensives because transient systemic hypotension, especially during the night when blood pressure is normally at its lowest, could possibly increase the risk of infarcting the other disc
- treatment to protect the patient against further vascular events
  - nonarteritic AION is a significant "warning sign" that the patient's blood vessels throughout the body are being damaged by vascular risk factors (affected patients have an increased risk of stroke and heart attack)
  - advise patients to stop smoking and to have other identified modifiable risk factors treated by their physician

Follow-Up
- reexamine the patient 2–4 weeks after onset (to check that any slow progression after the initial sudden episode has stopped)
- if acuity or field is still worsening, the diagnosis of AION is suspect and the patient should be investigated
- if ophthalmic findings are stable at 2–4 weeks, reexamine in a further 3–4 months; if still stable, discharge but ask the patient to return immediately if any change occurs

Prognosis
- affected eye
  - it is unusual for the same eye to have a second episode of AION (3%–5%)
  - many patients (about 40%) do have slow recovery of some acuity but improvement in visual field is rare
- fellow eye: patients with nonarteritic AION have about a one in four chance that the other disc will also develop AION; this can happen days to many years in the future

Note: "diabetic papillopathy"
- individuals with diabetes of any age may develop optic disc swelling, with or without visual dysfunction; this is often called "diabetic papillopathy"
  - it may be that some of these cases represent "mild" nonarteritic AION; however, in contrast to most cases of AION, vision often spontaneously recovers to normal as disc swelling resolves over weeks or months
  - patients in whom VA recovers to normal may nevertheless have a persistent visual field defect
  - alternatively, there may be a metabolic cause for the disc swelling in some patients
- it is impossible to exclude the other more serious causes of disc swelling (anterior optic neuropathy of any cause or, in the case of bilateral disc swelling, raised intracranial pressure) without the appropriate investigations
  - remember that persons with diabetes, being functionally immunosuppressed, are at greater risk of atypical infections (e.g., fungal sinusitis), that in some cases can present with unilateral or bilateral disc swelling
- hence, young persons with diabetes with swelling of one or both discs require the same work-up as other patients with unexplained optic nerve dysfunction, even if vision is normal: refer to a neuro-ophthalmologist (urgently if visual loss is acute) or, if this is not possible, investigate as suggested on p. 111

POSTERIOR (RETROBULBAR) ISCHEMIC OPTIC NEUROPATHY

Causes
- postsurgical (after cardiac, major thoracic or abdominal surgery): atherosclerosis plus sudden systemic hypotension and/or blood loss
- spontaneous
  - vasculitis (including GCA)
  - atherosclerosis causing small or large (internal carotid) arterial stenosis or occlusion
  - radiation (see later)

Symptoms
- postsurgical: the patient recovers consciousness to discover painless poor vision in one or both eyes
- spontaneous: acute painless vision loss in one or both eyes

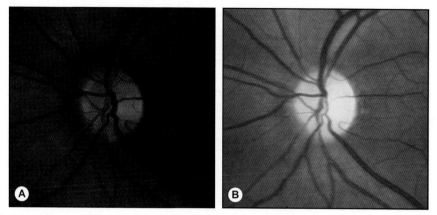

Fig. 3.11 Posterior ischemic optic neuropathy: the optic disc appears normal in the acute phase (**A**), then becomes pale over subsequent months as optic atrophy develops (**B**).

Signs

- optic discs are normal initially, becoming pale after about 6 weeks (Fig. 3.11)
- RAPD on the affected side, unless both eyes affected

Differential Diagnosis

- postsurgical: if both pupils are briskly reactive and there is no RAPD, bilateral posterior cerebral artery distribution infarction is likely (causing "cortical blindness")
- spontaneous: acute posterior optic neuropathy of any cause

Investigations

- postsurgical
  - urgent blood pressure, full blood count, and electrolytes
  - review intraoperative blood pressure measurements and blood loss estimation
- MRI orbits and brain to exclude pituitary apoplexy, occipital infarct or PRES (posterior reversible encephalopathy syndrome)
- spontaneous
  - refer to a neuro-ophthalmologist or investigate as suggested on p. 111
  - a duplex Doppler ultrasound of the carotid arteries is important to exclude potentially treatable internal carotid artery (ICA) stenosis

Treatment

- postsurgical: rapid identification and treatment of causative factors (hypotension and anemia) should be performed but there is no little that this is of benefit
- spontaneous
  - if associated with severe ICA stenosis, surgical treatment of the stenosis usually does not restore vision but may decrease the future risk of stroke
  - if associated with acute nonsurgical anemia, rapid restoration of hematocrit may result in visual improvement

- if associated with acute nonsurgical hypotension, restoration of normal blood pressure may result in visual improvement
- if associated with a systemic vasculitis, urgent immunosuppression (e.g., with IV methylprednisolone) may produce a partial recovery

RADIATION OPTIC NEUROPATHY

Mechanism

- a form of posterior ischemic optic neuropathy caused by delayed radiation damage to vascular endothelial cells within the radiation field

Risk Factors

- high radiation dose per treatment or high total dose
- concurrent chemotherapy
- diabetes mellitus
- irradiation of a tumor that was causing a compressive optic neuropathy (e.g., a pituitary tumor or meningioma)

Symptoms

- acute painless visual loss, most commonly 1–3 years after radiotherapy

Signs

- variable loss of VA and field
  - involvement of the chiasm may produce bitemporal field defects
  - involvement of the optic tract may produce homonymous field defects
- fundoscopy findings vary according to location:
  - anterior optic nerve:
    - the disc may be swollen and show telangiectasia or hemorrhages
    - usually there are also signs of radiation retinopathy (which looks similar to diabetic retinopathy)
  - posterior optic nerve:
    - normal-appearing optic disc until pallor begins to appear in 4–6 weeks or later

Differential Diagnosis

- recurrence of the original tumor causing compressive or infiltrative optic neuropathy
- other causes of acute optic neuropathy

Investigations

- urgent MRI of the optic nerves and chiasm with contrast
- if this shows no tumor recurrence, enhancement of part of the nerve (suggestive of radiation neuropathy) is seen, and the previous radiation dose and field are likely to have caused a neuropathy, no further tests are required

Treatment

- no treatment has been proven to be effective
- steroids, anticoagulation, hyperbaric oxygen therapy, and anti–vascular endothelial growth factor (VEGF) therapy have been tried
- both hyperbaric oxygen therapy and anti-VEGF therapy have been reported to be of benefit in occasional case reports but must be started immediately

Prognosis

- most patients develop severe, permanent visual loss in the affected eye/s

TRAUMATIC OPTIC NEUROPATHY

- traumatic optic neuropathy is "clinically diagnosable" in that there is an obvious cause (eye or head trauma)
- however, beware patients who attribute visual problems to minor eye or head "trauma": the patient often has coincidentally developed a spontaneous optic neuropathy completely unassociated with their "injury"
- if seeing the person as an outpatient, make sure that other more serious injuries (including intracranial injuries) have first been excluded

Mechanism

- indirect (transmitted) blunt trauma, e.g., blow to the forehead
- compression, e.g., by optic nerve sheath or orbital hematoma, or bony fragment
- direct injury, e.g., stab or bullet

Symptoms

- usually unilateral
- blurred vision, ± diplopia if there has been orbital or intracranial injury

Signs

- RAPD in the affected eye
- the optic disc usually looks normal initially
- in rare cases, mild disc swelling is present and may be associated with dilation of retinal veins and some intraretinal hemorrhages (a picture of a central retinal vein occlusion [CRVO])
- ± motility defect
- any type of field defect on perimetry

Investigations

- urgent thin-section CT (Fig. 3.12) or MRI orbit (if the orbit has not already been adequately imaged), looking for potentially surgically treatable lesions: bony fragments compressing the optic nerve at the orbital apex or intraorbital or intraoptic nerve sheath hematomas (particularly in patients with a fundus appearance of a CRVO)

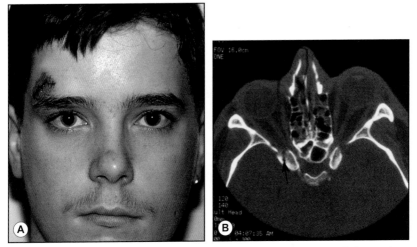

Fig. 3.12 Traumatic right optic neuropathy after motor vehicle accident. (**A**) External appearance of patient; note lack of obvious damage to eye. (**B**) Computed tomography scan shows right optic canal fracture *(arrow)*.

Treatment

- treatment is controversial: ideally involve a neuro-ophthalmologist early
- no treatment is of proven benefit
- many patients improve spontaneously
- management options include:
  - observation
    - IV methylprednisolone—"conventional" dose, i.e., 1 g/day for 2–5 days ("mega-dose" corticosteroid treatment cannot be advocated following the CRASH study findings)
  - surgery:
    - optic nerve sheath fenestration (consider especially if swollen disc and evidence of a hematoma in the optic nerve sheath on CT or MRI)
    - orbital decompression
    - optic canal decompression

LEBER HEREDITARY OPTIC NEUROPATHY

Genetics

- LHON is caused by one of several mutations in mitochondrial DNA, most often at sites 11778, 14484, and 3460
- not all carriers become symptomatic (20% of men, 5%–10% of women)
- the mutation is transmitted only by mothers (affected or carriers) to their children
- although the mutation is present at birth, the disease usually presents in adult life. Risk factors triggering visual loss have yet to be identified. Similarly, there is no explanation as to why men have an increased risk of manifesting the disease

- some families have a strong family history of either LHON or undiagnosed visual loss in young adulthood; however, it is not unusual for a patient to be diagnosed with LHON with no family history of the disease

Demographic

- men and women of all ages but most commonly young adult men

Symptoms

- 50% of patients experience bilateral sequential (within weeks or months) visual loss; 50% experience bilateral simultaneous loss
- visual loss is most commonly acute or subacute (occurring over days or weeks) but in some cases it is gradual and slowly progressive
- visual loss is almost always painless
- most patients have no neurological symptoms; however, rare patients have MS-like symptoms ("Leber-plus disease")

Signs

- severe loss of acuity in most cases
- some patients have an entirely normal-appearing optic disc in the affected eye/s (until disc pallor appears in several weeks' time); others have the "characteristic" disc appearance of mild disc swelling and peripapillary telangiectasia (Fig. 3.13)
- perimetry usually reveals a dense central scotoma in the affected eye/s

Investigations

- a patient who presents with acute visual loss and a known family history of LHON should have a blood test for the LHON genetic mutations
- in the absence of a family history, alternative (potentially treatable) causes of acute optic neuropathy must be excluded: the patient still requires investigation as suggested on p. 68, with the addition of a blood test for LHON if the clinical presentation and perimetry are suspicious for this condition

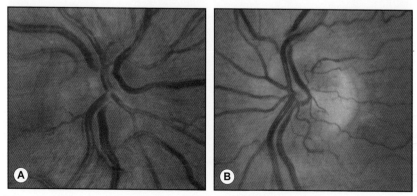

Fig. 3.13 Two different patients (**A, B**) with acute unilateral vision loss from Leber hereditary optic neuropathy, showing the "classic" disc changes of mild hyperemia and peripapillary telangiectasia. In some patients, the discs appear entirely normal until optic atrophy develops.

Treatment

- no treatment has been proven to improve the prognosis of LHON, but some physicians treat with idebenone, a quinol that stimulates adenosine triphosphate (ATP) formation and inhibits lipid peroxidation in the mitochondrial membrane. There is evidence that gene therapy may stabilize or improve visual function, but the evidence is far from conclusive
- suggest that the patient abstain from smoking, and drink alcohol in moderation
- genetic counseling and referral to low-vision specialist
- all patients diagnosed with LHON should be referred to a cardiologist because they may have an asymptomatic cardiac conduction abnormality

Prognosis

Some patients (particularly those with the 14484 and 3460 mutations) experience partial or complete recovery of vision after several months or years.

OPTIC NEUROPATHY FROM SEVERE ACUTE PAPILLEDEMA

- patients with severe papilledema are at risk of rapid bilateral visual loss (within hours or days) from axonal compression or ischemic infarction of the disc (Fig. 3.14)
- hence, all patients with papilledema require careful ophthalmic monitoring (acuity, color vision, pupils, perimetry, disc appearance)
- urgent surgical intervention may be required to save the patient's sight

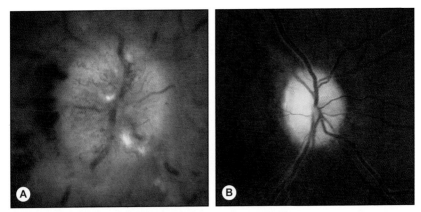

Fig. 3.14 Patients with untreated severe papilledema can become permanently blind from disc infarction within hours or days. Therefore, severe papilledema is an ophthalmic, as well as a neurologic or neurosurgical, emergency. After disc infarction occurs (**A**), swelling decreases due to axon loss and pallor develops (**B**). This reduction in swelling due to the death of the optic nerve should not be mistaken for "improvement" of the papilledema.

OTHER ACUTE OPTIC NEUROPATHIES

- some of the diseases that usually cause slowly progressive compressive or infiltrative optic neuropathies may occasionally present with acute or subacute visual loss, for example:
  - acute optic nerve infiltration from leukemia
  - acute optic nerve compression from pituitary apoplexy

Chronic Optic Neuropathies
GLAUCOMATOUS OPTIC NEUROPATHY

Check that your patient meets ALL the clinical diagnostic criteria on p. 68 before you make this diagnosis!

Glaucomatous optic neuropathy can usually be clinically differentiated from other chronic optic neuropathies by its lack of symptoms and the correlation between optic disc findings and visual field defects.

It is important to note that almost any cause of chronic optic neuropathy (including compressive tumor) can present with a "cupped" optic disc (Fig. 3.15) and an arcuate scotoma; acute optic neuropathy of any cause can also result months later in a "cupped" disc appearance.

Likewise, elevated IOP is not a guarantee that the patient's optic neuropathy is glaucomatous: glaucoma and ocular hypertension are very common and, coincidentally, some patients with these conditions will also develop an optic neuropathy from another cause (e.g., from a pituitary tumor).

Demographic

- glaucoma is mainly a disease of the elderly so beware the young patient diagnosed with "normal-tension glaucoma"

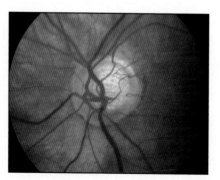

Fig. 3.15 Glaucomatous optic neuropathy with a "cupped" optic nerve head. It should be recognized that optic neuropathy of any cause can result in an arcuate scotoma, and optic neuropathy of many different causes (including chronic compression by tumor) can result in a "cupped" disc.

Symptoms

- in contrast to many patients with other types of slowly progressive optic neuropathy, those with glaucoma usually don't notice blurred vision or field loss until their neuropathy is very advanced
- however, chronic optic neuropathies other than glaucoma (including compressive neuropathy) may also be first detected as incidentally noticed visual field loss

Signs

- VA and color vision are normal, except in patients with very extensive disc cupping and severe field loss; by contrast, patients with nonglaucomatous optic neuropathies, in which the disc is usually only moderately "cupped," often have poor acuity and color vision
- the majority of patients with glaucoma have raised IOP, but raised IOP, like disc cupping, is no guarantee that the optic neuropathy is glaucomatous
- one of the key points in making a clinical diagnosis of glaucomatous optic neuropathy is making sure that "the discs match the fields." In glaucoma, it is usually possible to "match" a visual field defect with a sectoral or focal thinning or notch in the neuroretinal rim, visible clinically or on peripapillary nerve fiber layer OCT. For example, an inferotemporal disc rim "notch" would match a superior arcuate scotoma on the field (Fig. 3.16)
- in glaucoma, the remaining neuroretinal rim should never be pale
  - usually in patients with early or moderate glaucoma, focal shelving or notching of the rim occurs but the rest of the rim remains relatively healthy looking
  - in patients with non-glaucomatous cupping (e.g., due to compressive optic neuropathy), the temporal rim is often diffusely pale without a focal defect, or the whole disc is diffusely pale despite having a well-preserved neuroretinal rim thickness

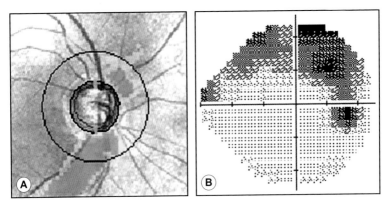

Fig. 3.16 In this case of right glaucomatous optic neuropathy, the optical coherence tomography (**A**) shows an inferior disc notch with inferotemporal nerve fiber layer defect that matches the superior arcuate scotoma on perimetry (**B**).

Differential Diagnosis

- ongoing chronic optic neuropathy of any cause
- previous acute optic neuropathy of any cause

Investigations

- if a clinical diagnosis of glaucomatous optic neuropathy cannot be made by the criteria on p. 68, the patient requires referral to a neuro-ophthalmologist or investigation as suggested on p. 68

Treatment and Follow-up

- treatments available for patients with glaucoma depend on many factors and are constantly changing. Please refer to a textbook or recent article on glaucoma management

COMPRESSIVE OPTIC NEUROPATHY

It is vital to diagnose these patients as early as possible, because:
- early surgical treatment may be curative and also save the patient's life
- if diagnosed before irreversible optic nerve damage occurs, there is a good prognosis for return of vision after surgical treatment

Demographic

- any age, male or female

Causes

Tumors (Fig. 3.17)
- intracranial: unilateral or bilateral optic nerve compression by:
  - sphenoid wing meningioma
  - pituitary region tumor (pituitary adenoma, craniopharyngioma, meningioma)
  - metastases to the orbit or anterior intracranial cavity
- optic nerve: unilateral or bilateral
  - optic nerve sheath meningioma
  - optic nerve glioma
  - optic nerve compression by an orbital tumor of any type

Nonneoplastic
- thyroid eye disease (optic nerve compression can occur with minimal or no proptosis)
- ethmoid or sphenoid sinus mucocele
- aneurysms (internal carotid, anterior cerebral or ophthalmic artery)

Symptoms

- two types of presentation are common:
  - slowly progressive visual loss over months or years
    - including incidentally discovered acuity or field loss on routine optometric screening

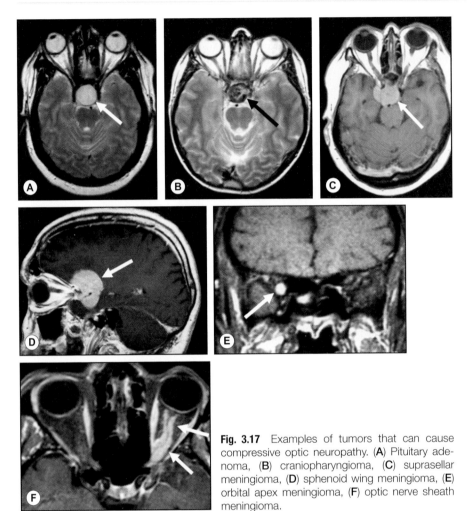

Fig. 3.17 Examples of tumors that can cause compressive optic neuropathy. (**A**) Pituitary adenoma, (**B**) craniopharyngioma, (**C**) suprasellar meningioma, (**D**) sphenoid wing meningioma, (**E**) orbital apex meningioma, (**F**) optic nerve sheath meningioma.

- acute or subacute visual loss may also sometimes occur because of:
    - a sudden expansion of the compressive lesion (e.g., "pituitary apoplexy": acute hemorrhage into a compressive pituitary tumor)
    - vascular compression causing sudden infarction of the optic nerve
- patients may also complain of double vision due to ocular motor nerve compression in the cavernous sinus or orbital apex, or mechanical restriction of the muscles or globe by an orbital tumor or thyroid myopathy

Signs

- VA may be variably decreased; in some cases of early compressive neuropathy, acuity is absolutely normal
- an RAPD will be present if the neuropathy is unilateral or asymmetric (but it may be subtle)

- color vision is usually impaired
- the optic disc/s may look normal, swollen, pale, or "cupped"
- in cases of chronic compressive optic neuropathy, the peripapillary nerve fiber layer may be focally or diffusely thinned on OCT. If severe thinning is present, it is a poor prognostic sign for visual recovery after decompressive surgery
- cavernous sinus or orbital apex invasion may also cause:
  - abnormal ocular motility
  - decreased corneal and/or facial sensation
  - ptosis (from a Horner syndrome or partial third nerve palsy)

Perimetry

- compressive optic nerve lesions can cause ANY pattern of monocular or binocular visual field loss, including:
  - central scotoma
  - cecocentral scotoma
  - arcuate scotoma
  - altitudinal field loss
  - diffuse field loss
  - unilateral temporal or nasal hemifield loss (if the intracranial part of the optic nerve is compressed just before it enters the chiasm)
- in some cases, compression of one intracranial optic nerve just anterior to the chiasm may also cause a "junctional scotoma": any pattern of field loss in the ipsilateral eye, and a superior temporal defect respecting (stopping at) the vertical midline in the contralateral visual field

Investigations

- MRI optic nerves, chiasm, and brain with contrast

Treatment

- options for the treatment of tumors include:
  - observation
  - medical therapy of hormonally active pituitary tumors
  - stereotactic/three-dimensional (3D) conformal fractionated radiotherapy
  - external beam fractionated radiotherapy
  - stereotactic radiosurgery
  - orbital surgery
  - transsphenoidal endoscopic surgery (often used for pituitary tumors)
  - transcranial surgery
- thyroid orbitopathy causing compressive optic neuropathy:
  - high-dose IV or oral steroid treatment is usually started immediately to help preserve the health of the affected nerve
  - steroid treatment may not result in visual improvement or vision may initially improve and then worsen as steroids are tapered, in which case definitive treatment (e.g., orbital decompression, radiation therapy) is required
- sinus mucocele: decompression of the affected sinus
- aneurysms: endovascular treatment (e.g., packing with coils) or neurosurgical clipping may be possible

Follow-up

- patients require regular ophthalmic follow-up, especially in the period immediately before and after treatment; don't forget to organize this

INFILTRATIVE OPTIC NEUROPATHY

Demographic

- any age, male or female

Causes

- infiltration of one or both optic nerves by:
  - leukemia
  - lymphoma
  - most types of solid tumors (e.g., breast, lung, bowel): these may either metastasize directly to the nerve/s or chiasm or have a diffuse metastasis to the meninges ("carcinomatous meningitis"), from which malignant cells invade the anterior visual pathway
  - inflammations, most often sarcoid

Symptoms

- in most cases, the patient is known to have a malignancy, but the optic neuropathy sometimes is the first sign of the cancer
- acute, subacute, or slowly progressive VA or field loss, one or both eyes
- pain may occur if the tumor has also infiltrated sensory nerves; pain may be increased on eye movement in some patients

Signs

- the optic disc/s may be normal, swollen, or pale (Fig. 3.18)
- bilateral disc swelling in carcinomatous meningitis may represent bilateral anterior optic nerve infiltration or papilledema due to raised intracranial pressure
- there may also be other cranial neuropathies (including the ocular motor nerves) due to infiltration
- any field defect, one or both eyes, on visual field testing

Differential Diagnosis

All other causes of anterior or posterior optic neuropathy.

Investigations

- MRI usually shows focal or diffuse enlargement of one or both optic nerves (see Fig. 3.18B)
- LP may show raised protein, decreased glucose and/or malignant cells on cytology

Treatment

- urgent liaison with the oncology team
- chemotherapy and/or radiotherapy

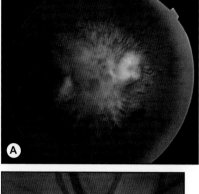
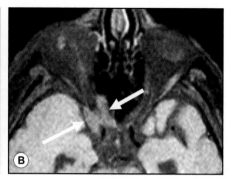
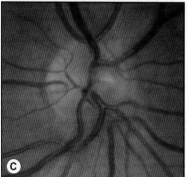

Fig. 3.18 (A) Massive optic disc infiltration by leukemia. (B) Right optic nerve infiltration by bowel cancer metastatic to the orbital apex; the optic disc was initially normal in appearance, (C) but later became pale.

Prognosis

- treatment may restore vision, or slow visual deterioration may occur despite treatment
- however, CNS invasion or metastasis is usually a poor prognostic sign as regards the patient's survival

NUTRITIONAL DEFICIENCY OPTIC NEUROPATHY

Deficiency of vitamin B12, folate, and (rarely) vitamins A and E can cause a reduction in optic nerve function.

Causes

- pernicious anemia causing B12 deficiency
- poor diet, e.g., malnutrition, fad diets
- chronic alcohol use disorder
- extensive small bowel disease or surgery

Symptoms

- usually slowly progressive (but sometimes subacute) bilateral symmetric visual loss

Signs

- VA may be mildly to severely reduced but should be similar in both eyes
- early loss of color vision
- there is usually no RAPD because the disease is almost always bilateral and symmetric
- optic discs usually show temporal or diffuse pallor in established disease, but early on may appear normal or slightly swollen
- perimetry: bilateral central or cecocentral scotomas (but this is not "diagnostic") (Fig. 3.19)

Differential Diagnosis

- all other causes of chronic optic neuropathy, including LHON

Investigations

- refer, or investigate as suggested on p. 68, including blood tests for serum vitamin B12 and red blood cell folate, plus test for vitamin A and E if history of small bowel surgery
- always still perform neuroimaging (don't miss a tumor!)

Treatment

- if B12 is low, ask the patient's physician to:
  - investigate for possible pernicious anemia (unless poor diet is the likely cause)
  - start B12 replacement injections (often monthly for several months, then 3-monthly)
  - prescribe multivitamin tablets (plus folate tablets if this is not included in the multivitamin, even if folate levels are normal)
- if folate is low or poor diet is suspected, commence daily multivitamins (including folate); many neuro-ophthalmologists will also give B12 therapy, even if B12 levels are normal
- in the unusual case of vitamins A or E being low, obtain pharmaceutical advice regarding replacement therapy
- decrease risk factors for a concurrent toxic optic neuropathy (e.g., stop smoking, decrease alcohol intake)

Prognosis

- vision often improves with treatment, unless established optic atrophy is present

TOXIC OPTIC NEUROPATHY

Causes

- medications
  - antituberculosis antibiotics: ethambutol and isoniazid
  - other antibiotics, e.g., chloramphenicol (oral or IV)
  - some cancer chemotherapy and immunosuppressive agents

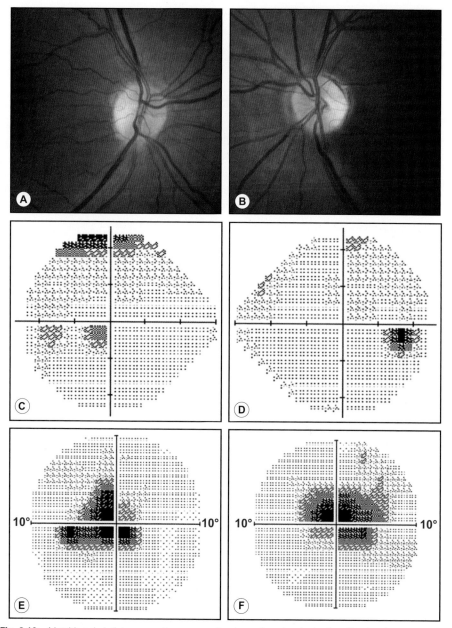

Fig. 3.19 Nutritional deficiency optic neuropathy in a chronic alcoholic with slowly progressive bilateral visual loss and visual acuity 20/120 in each eye. (**A**, **B**) Bilateral symmetric temporal disc pallor. Routine 30-2 perimetry (**C**, **D**) did not show an obvious defect; however, central 10-2 perimetry (**E**, **F**) revealed bilateral dense central scotomas.

- there are also some medications for which a toxic effect is suspected on the basis of case reports, e.g., amiodarone
- substance ingestion or inhalation
  - lead
  - methanol
  - carbon monoxide
  - organic solvents
  - note: alcohol (ethanol) alone is no longer thought to cause a toxic optic neuropathy (but chronic alcohol use disorder may result in nutritional deficiency optic neuropathy)
- there are also many other drugs and substances which are suspected of causing a toxic optic neuropathy; consult a pharmaceutical index if suspicious regarding one or more of your patient's medications or their occupational exposure to toxins

Symptoms

- usually slowly progressive (but sometimes subacute) bilateral symmetric visual loss
- the exception is that methanol drinking and ingestion suicide attempts may cause acute bilateral visual loss

Signs

- VA may be mildly to severely reduced but should be similar in both eyes
- early loss of color vision
- there is usually no RAPD because the disease is almost always bilateral and symmetric
- optic discs may look normal, pale or mildly swollen
- perimetry: bilateral central or cecocentral scotomas (but this is not "diagnostic")

Investigations

- the fact that a patient with gradual visual loss is receiving one of the above drugs does not mean the visual loss is due to the drug
- hence, the patient should be referred to a neuro-ophthalmologist or thoroughly investigated as suggested on p. 68 before their optic neuropathy is called "toxic"
- it is particularly important that patients with tuberculosis or cancer and visual loss be fully assessed for tuberculous or carcinomatous meningitis with secondary invasion of the optic nerves (with MRI and LP) before visual loss is attributed to their drug treatment

Treatment

- suspected medication toxicity: withdraw the suspected medication if possible
- possible nutritional toxicity: decrease alcohol intake, improve diet, treat with multivitamins with folate

Prognosis

- vision may slowly improve with treatment unless advanced optic atrophy is present

AUTOSOMAL-DOMINANT OPTIC NEUROPATHY

Demographic

- equal sex distribution
- the condition probably first becomes visible on examination in mid-childhood; however, most patients present in later childhood or in adult life

Symptoms

- two types of presentation are common:
  - incidentally discovered visual loss on routine optometric examination
  - slowly progressive visual loss over many years

Signs

- this is a bilateral symmetric disease; if the patient has asymmetric visual loss or has an RAPD, suspect another diagnosis
- VA is usually mildly to moderately reduced at presentation, and color vision is abnormal
- the optic discs usually show some pallor at presentation; this may be diffuse or temporal, or, in some patients, there is a wedge-shaped pale excavation of the temporal part of the disc
- perimetry typically reveals bilateral central or paracentral scotomas
- most patients have no other manifestations, but some also have hearing loss, ophthalmoparesis, and/or ptosis

Investigations

- the genes responsible have been identified and a commercial gene test is available for the main mutation (OPA1)
- an essential "test" if you suspect this condition is to examine several first-degree relatives of the patient; if any of them have (symptomatic or asymptomatic) unexplained bilateral symmetric acuity and color loss with temporal disc pallor, this adds weight to the diagnosis
- unless there is a definite family history and relatives show typical features on examination, this is a diagnosis of exclusion, after the patient has been fully investigated for other causes of optic neuropathy (such as compressive tumor or nutritional deficiency)

Treatment

- no treatment is available
- consider referral to low-vision specialist
- genetic counseling is also important

Prognosis

- vision may remain stable for many years or very gradually decline (about one line per decade)
- even in advanced cases, the peripheral field usually remains normal

OTHER INHERITED OPTIC NEUROPATHIES

There are many other rarer types of slowly progressive inherited optic neuropathy (dominant, recessive, and X-linked).

INFECTIOUS OPTIC NEURITIS

Some infections, in particular syphilis and tuberculosis, can cause slowly progressive visual loss in one or both eyes and present with normal, swollen or pale discs. See the section on infectious optic neuritis (p. 77) for further details.

SARCOID OPTIC NEURITIS

- chronic sarcoid optic neuritis is a relatively common cause of slowly progressive optic neuropathy, in male and female adults of all races
- it is important to diagnose, because often there is excellent return of vision with steroid treatment (and no return of vision if the diagnosis is missed)
- see the section on sarcoid optic neuritis (p. 80) for further details

OPTIC NEUROPATHY FROM CHRONIC PAPILLEDEMA

- disc swelling due to raised intracranial pressure (papilledema), if severe or persistent, can cause permanent visual loss (Fig. 3.20)
- typically, patients suffer gradual loss of peripheral field first, with normal VA maintained until late (occasionally acute severe visual loss occurs, possibly because of infarction of the swollen disc)
- all patients with papilledema of any cause require regular ophthalmic examinations, including serial perimetry, until the disc swelling has permanently resolved. This includes patients with brain tumors, head injuries, meningitis, hydrocephalus and dural venous sinus thrombosis, as well as pseudotumor cerebri

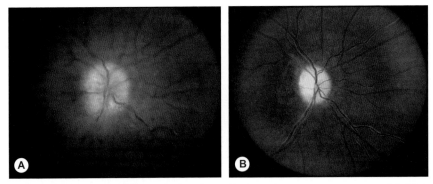

Fig. 3.20   Untreated, or undertreated, chronic papilledema from any cause can result in bilateral blindness. (**A**) Chronic papilledema. (**B**) Postpapilledema optic atrophy.

- in some cases, decline in visual function is the only indication for surgery in these patients
- occasionally, bilateral disc swelling with decreased vision can be due to a combination of papilledema and optic neuropathy of another cause (e.g., tuberculous or cryptococcal meningitis can cause both severe papilledema from high intracranial pressure, plus a direct infective optic neuritis of both optic nerves)

OPTIC NEUROPATHY ASSOCIATED WITH DISC DRUSEN

- optic disc drusen are small concretions that form in the optic nerve heads of 1%–2% of the population; these may be visible ophthalmoscopically or buried (Fig. 3.21)
- drusen can cause problems by:
  - simulating disc swelling (pseudo-disc swelling: see Chapter 4)
  - causing acute, slowly progressive or static field loss (e.g., AION; retinal vascular occlusion)
    - acute events may be ischemic (e.g., AION) in nature (due to small vessel compression in a "tight," "crowded" nerve head)
    - slow loss of the visual **field** may be due to axon compression or chronic ischemia
- cautions:
  - slowly worsening visual field defects from drusen are relatively common but symptomatic progressive loss of VA from them is rare. A patient with progressive loss of VA in the setting of visible or buried drusen should be evaluated for another cause of the visual loss, particularly a compressive lesion!
  - optic disc drusen are common; many patients with optic neuropathy from other causes will incidentally have disc drusen as well

Demographic

- optic disc drusen usually become visible in later childhood and may slowly increase in size throughout life
- there is some tendency for this condition to run in families

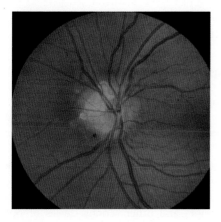

Fig. 3.21   Disc drusen.

Symptoms

- patients commonly present with asymptomatic field defects detected during routine optometric testing (loss of VA is rare with drusen)
- some, particularly children, develop AION due to their "crowded" disc
- others may have a stepwise deterioration or a gradual worsening of the visual field (but NOT acuity!)

Signs

- usually patients with field loss from drusen will have obvious exposed drusen but not infrequently the drusen are buried but detectable on ultrasound

Investigations

- optic nerve dysfunction due to disc drusen is a diagnosis of exclusion. Refer or investigate fully to make sure you're not missing a treatable optic neuropathy of another cause, particularly if there is decreased VA or progressive loss of VA

Treatment

- there is no treatment
- coexistent raised IOP should be treated; in some cases, it is difficult to know whether to attribute field loss to the drusen or to glaucoma, in which case, treatment to reduce IOP is appropriate

Prognosis

- the majority of patients have nonprogressive or very slowly progressive field defects
- it is very rare for patients to suffer loss of central vision

OTHER SLOWLY PROGRESSIVE OPTIC NEUROPATHIES

- some of the diseases that usually cause acute optic neuropathies may occasionally present with slowly progressive or incidentally noticed acuity or field loss, including:
  - MS-related optic neuritis
  - AION
  - LHON
- patients must be fully investigated for other treatable causes; "chronic" MS-related optic neuritis and "chronic" AION are diagnoses of exclusion

PREVIOUS ACUTE OPTIC NEUROPATHY

- previous symptomatic acute optic neuropathy
  - in some cases, a patient will notice acute or subacute vision loss in one or both eyes, but for various reasons will not have an ophthalmic examination until months later
  - it is tempting in these cases to observe the patient's pale disc/s and surmise they "must have" had an AION or typical optic neuritis months ago
  - however, all these cases require either referral to a neuro-ophthalmologist or full investigation, as compressive tumors and other serious causes of optic

neuropathy sometimes cause acute episodes of visual loss superimposed on an otherwise slow decline in vision
- previous unnoticed acute optic neuropathy
  - occasionally, a patient will be incidentally noticed to have a unilateral pale disc, decreased acuity, and/or field defect on routine testing
  - in some cases, this may have been due to a previous acute optic neuropathy that was not noticed by the patient at the time
  - this "presumed" diagnosis can only be made once the patient has been fully investigated for other causes and then shows no further visual loss on extended follow-up

CONGENITALLY ANOMALOUS DISCS

- these can cause problems by:
  - mimicking disc swelling (pseudo-disc swelling—see Chapter 4)
  - causing congenital acuity or field defects that are incidentally discovered in childhood or adult life and need to be distinguished from acquired optic nerve disease
- in some cases, it seems a safe bet to ascribe poor vision or a field defect to an obvious congenital disc defect, such as an incidentally discovered superior field defect to an inferior disc coloboma
- in other patients, without such classic signs (and without the "disc matching the field" as in glaucoma) it is important to refer or investigate the patient to exclude other, potentially treatable, causes for the problem
- progressive VA or visual field loss should never be attributed to a congenital disc anomaly

Suggested Investigations for Optic Neuropathy That Cannot Be Diagnosed Clinically

(See summary box on p. 68.)

The only clinically diagnosable nontraumatic optic neuropathies are typical optic neuritis, AION, and glaucoma. All other patients with optic neuropathy (who do not meet the clinical diagnostic criteria for these three diseases listed on pp. 66–68) require further investigation. We recommend that they be referred to a neuro-ophthalmologist (urgently if the visual loss is acute).

In some cases, there are geographic or patient factors that make prompt referral to a neuro-ophthalmologist difficult, or you may wish to perform the initial investigations yourself. In such circumstances, we recommend the following investigations as an initial basic work-up. However, given that there are many rare causes of optic neuropathy, if these initial investigations do not reveal a cause, we would recommend obtaining specialist neuro-ophthalmic advice.

Investigations for acute optic neuropathies should be urgently pursued for two reasons:
- the patient could have an undiagnosed life-threatening disease (e.g., pituitary apoplexy, neoplastic infiltration of the optic nerve/s or neurosarcoidosis); the patient's

chance of surviving without major neurologic disability is greatest with early and accurate diagnosis

- some diseases have a limited "time window" within which the appropriate treatment can restore vision; if diagnosis is delayed, irretrievable optic atrophy will ensue and visual loss may be permanent

1. REVIEW HISTORY, EXAMINATION AND PERIMETRY

- blood pressure
  - severe hypertension is a rare cause of bilateral disc swelling
  - however, the other investigations should still be pursued even if the patient is significantly hypertensive (the blood pressure could be a coincidental finding, rather than the cause of the ophthalmic presentation)
- temperature: if elevated, can be a clue to systemic infectious disease, e.g., cat-scratch disease
- urine analysis
  - blood or protein can suggest vasculitis
  - glucose can indicate undiagnosed diabetes
- full systemic history and examination (including a systemic neurologic examination)
  - sometimes systemic findings can indicate the likely cause of the optic nerve disease (e.g., lymphadenopathy could indicate systemic infection or hematologic malignancy)
  - remember to ask the "system review" questions (pp. 23–25)
- perform perimetry in all patients as soon as possible after presentation

2. MRI OPTIC NERVES, CHIASM, AND BRAIN WITH CONTRAST (PLUS MRV OR CTV IF DISC SWELLING)

- in the case of acute optic neuropathy, this must be performed urgently
- request specific high-resolution views of the optic nerves and chiasm, as well as brain views
- always ask for contrast (gadolinium) unless there is a medical contraindication: small but important lesions (e.g., small tumors or small areas of inflammation) can be missed if this is not used (Fig. 3.22)
- patients with bilateral disc swelling: request MRV or computed tomographic venography (CTV), as well as MRI, to exclude cerebral venous sinus thrombosis (which may be missed on MRI alone)
- note: "CT orbits and brain" usually does not show enough detail of the optic nerve, chiasm and brain to exclude serious pathology

3. BLOOD TESTS

- for all patients:
  - basic bloods: full blood count, electrolytes, liver function tests, glucose, ESR, CRP
  - autoimmune: ANA

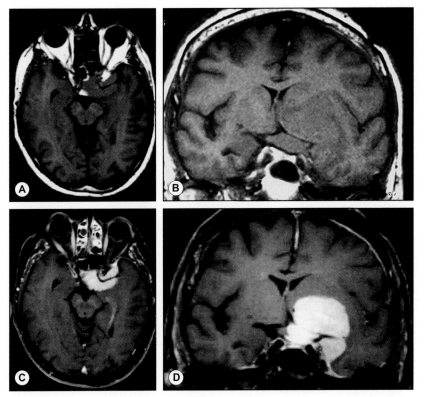

Fig. 3.22 Why "contrast" should be requested for all neuro-ophthalmic magnetic resonance imaging scans: noncontrast (**A**, **B**) and postcontrast (**C**, **D**) scans of a sphenoid wing meningioma. The tumor is much easier to detect after contrast has been given. This is especially important for tumors smaller than this one.

- sarcoid: ACE
- infectious: syphilis serology
- plus for patients with atypical or bilateral optic neuritis: AQP4-IgG antibody testing (for NMO); MOG-IgG antibody testing (for MOG antibody-related optic neuritis)
- plus for patients with bilateral symmetric subacute or chronic optic neuropathy: RBC folate and serum vitamin B12 (nutritional deficiency neuropathy is almost always bilateral and symmetric)
- plus other blood tests as suggested by the specific history, examination, and investigation findings, for example:
  - gene markers for LHON if the patient is a young man with an unexplained unilateral acute dense central scotoma
  - serum quantiferon for tuberculosis, and serology for cat scratch disease, toxoplasma, Lyme disease and HIV if there is the appearance of "stellate neuroretinitis" or evidence of systemic infection on history or examination

4. CHEST X-RAY OR CHEST CT SCAN

- looking for signs of sarcoidosis, tuberculosis, lung cancer, or lymphoma

5. LP (IF NO MASS LESION ON MRI)

- this may be the only way to diagnose:
  - elevated intracranial pressure
  - atypical meningitis (due to leukemia, lymphoma, carcinomatous metastasis, fungal infection, sarcoidosis or tuberculosis) that may first present as an acute or chronic optic neuropathy
- perform LP if no mass lesion or other contraindication on MRI, and one of the following:
  - acute optic neuropathy
  - chronic optic neuropathy with one or more of:
    - unilateral or bilateral disc swelling
    - persisting headaches, meningitic symptoms, unexplained neurologic symptoms or MRI changes suggestive of chronic meningitis
    - progressive visual loss with all other investigations negative
- procedure
  - obtain informed consent
  - in obese patients, should be performed under fluoroscopy (much easier on patient)
  - LP opening pressure in the lateral decubitus position (if this is not possible, perform LP under fluoroscopy in the prone position—cerebrospinal fluid [CSF] pressures are almost equivalent in the two positions) should be measured
  - CSF to be assessed for biochemistry (protein, glucose, oligoclonal bands, myelin basic protein, IgG synthesis), microbiology (microscopy, cell count, culture), and cytology
  - have blood taken at the same time as LP for blood glucose and oligoclonal bands

6. TRIAL OF STEROID TREATMENT

- rationale
  - some patients with acute optic neuropathy for which no cause can be found improve with steroid treatment. Of these, some would have recovered without treatment. However:
    - in many cases, the response to steroids is dramatic and the patient is unlikely to have recovered as fully or as rapidly without treatment
    - it's too late several months after onset, when the patient has developed optic atrophy and not recovered, to think "maybe we should have tried steroids"
  - therefore, give a trial of steroids to all patients with acute optic neuropathy for which no cause can be found who do NOT have:
    - suspected tumor or infection on blood tests, chest x-ray, chest CT, MRI, and/or LP
    - a medical contraindication to steroid use

- indications: give a diagnostic trial of steroid treatment if:
  - no medical contraindication, no sign of infection or tumor on the above investigations, and:
    - acute optic neuropathy, or:
    - chronic optic neuropathy for which no cause can be found and that continues to worsen
- suggested trial
  - obtain informed consent
  - give IV methylprednisolone (1 g in a single daily dose [slow IV infusion] for a patient weighing 70 kg or more) for 3 days
  - continue treatment with oral prednisone (1–2 mg/kg) if:
    - the patient's VA, color vision and/or visual field definitely improves during the 3 days' IV treatment (don't continue long-term steroid treatment if there has been no demonstrable change), or:
    - investigation results are suggestive of a disease (e.g., sarcoidosis) that should be steroid responsive
  - if the patient is steroid responsive, it is ideal to involve a neuro-ophthalmologist early (the patient may benefit from a steroid-sparing immunosuppressive agent to prevent the severe side effects of long-term steroids)
  - the patient must be counseled regarding the side effects of steroids and monitored closely for these
  - prescribe osteoporosis and gastric ulcer prophylaxis for as long as the patient is taking steroids
  - once visual improvement has ceased and vision is stable, try to taper and cease the steroids as rapidly as possible, while still maintaining vision

OTHER INVESTIGATIONS

- note: optic nerve head ultrasound and electrophysiologic testing are usually not helpful
  - they provide nonspecific information that does not further delineate the cause of the optic neuropathy
  - beware any ultrasound or electrodiagnostic report that claims to be able to diagnose the cause or type of an optic neuropathy; it is probably wrong
- examination of relatives
  - this "investigation" can be very useful if there is a family history of visual loss or if other tests are negative in the case of a patient with bilateral chronic optic neuropathy that could possibly be autosomal-dominant optic atrophy

Optic Chiasmal Disease

Optic chiasmal disease (optic chiasmopathy) is characterized by partial or complete bitemporal field loss; pathology affecting the chiasm frequently also involves the adjacent optic nerves or tracts, producing a mixture of field defects.

By far the most common cause of optic chiasmopathy is compression of the chiasm by tumors in the region of the pituitary gland (Fig. 3.23). Rare, noncompressive causes

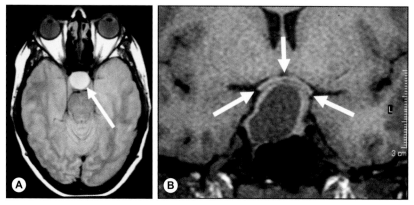

Fig. 3.23 (**A**) Axial view magnetic resonance imaging (MRI)—cystic pituitary adenoma *(arrow)* causing compression of the optic chiasm. (**B**) Coronal view MRI—the optic chiasm *(arrows)* is visible as the thin band of tissue being compressed and stretched upward by the tumor.

of chiasmal disease include infiltration, infection, ischemia, MS, toxins, and nutritional deficiency.

Thus, all patients with suspected optic chiasm disease require an urgent MRI scan to look for a compressive lesion; if no such lesion is found, the patient should then be investigated for other causes of chiasmal dysfunction as you would investigate them for an unexplained optic neuropathy.

COMPRESSIVE CHIASMOPATHY DUE TO PITUITARY REGION MASSES

- pituitary region masses are both sight-threatening and life-threatening
- early diagnosis is associated with a good visual prognosis and minimizes the risk of disability or death
- patients with undiagnosed pituitary region tumors frequently first present to ophthalmologists complaining of blurred vision or field loss; they may be "otherwise well" with no headache and no neurologic symptoms

Causes

- pituitary adenoma
- craniopharyngioma
- suprasellar meningioma
- supraclinoid aneurysm
- metastases to the middle cranial fossa (rare)

Symptoms

Ophthalmic

- VA and/or field loss: patients may present in three ways
    - incidentally discovered field loss on routine screening
    - slowly progressive symptomatic acuity or field loss over months or years

- acute or subacute VA and field loss due to sudden expansion of the compressive lesion or infarction of a compressed chiasm
- diplopia due to:
  - compression of the third, fourth, and/or sixth nerves in the cavernous sinus
  - "hemifield slide":
    - complete bitemporal hemianopia (and, occasionally, bitemporal hemianopic scotoma) causes loss of binocular vision because there are no common points in the visual fields of both eyes
    - the patient can no longer control any underlying phoria and develops a comitant esotropia, exotropia or vertical deviation

Systemic
- the patient may have a nonspecific headache
- symptoms due to pituitary underaction, or overproduction of a single pituitary hormone by a functioning pituitary adenoma, may include:
  - weight loss or gain
  - fatigue, depression
  - in men, impotence
  - in women of child-bearing age, galactorrhea and/or amenorrhea
- pituitary apoplexy
  - a bleed into a compressive pituitary tumor causes a sudden expansion in its size
  - patients usually present to the general emergency department with acute severe headache and/or collapse but may sometimes present to ophthalmologists with headache, visual loss and diplopia

Signs
- VA will be normal unless there is also involvement of the nasal field (often due to involvement of the optic nerve/s as well as the chiasm)
  - sometimes the patient may not see, or struggle with, the letters in the temporal half of each line of the chart
- an RAPD may be caused by:
  - an asymmetric chiasmopathy
  - an associated compressive optic neuropathy
- color vision may be normal or reduced
  - when testing color vision with Ishihara plates, it may be noticed that the patient struggles with, or cannot see, the "temporal" digit of the double-digit plates (e.g., with the right eye viewing, may see a "27" plate as just "2" due to temporal field loss)
- the optic disc/s may appear:
  - normal
  - pale (and sometimes moderately "cupped" as a result of axonal loss) (Fig. 3.24)
  - or (rarely) swollen due to raised intracranial pressure
- abnormal ocular motility in some patients from involvement of ocular motor nerves in cavernous sinus or subarachnoid space
- abnormal corneal and/or facial sensation if a tumor has invaded the cavernous sinus and is affecting one or more trigeminal nerve branches

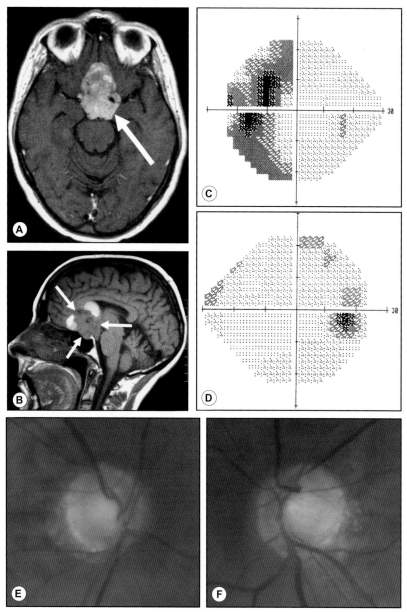

Fig. 3.24 Craniopharyngioma (**A**, **B**) presenting with partial bitemporal field defects (**C**, **D**) and slight temporal pallor of both discs (**E**, **F**).

Perimetry

- pituitary region tumors may compress (see also Table 2.1):
  - one or both optic nerves, causing any type of field defect in one or both eyes (Fig. 3.25)

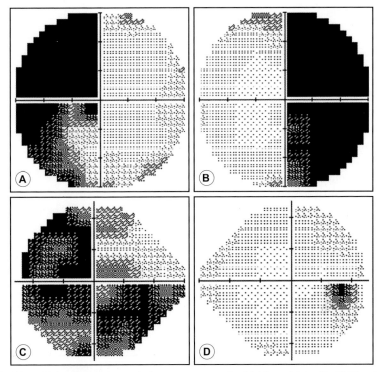

Fig. 3.25 Visual field defects from pituitary tumors can be highly variable. (**A, B**) Classic almost complete bitemporal hemianopia. (**C, D**) Unilateral optic neuropathy with normal other field.

- the chiasm, causing bitemporal field loss
- an optic tract, causing homonymous hemianopic field loss
- most commonly, patients present with a mixed pattern of field loss due to compression of more than one structure
- field loss due to compressive chiasmopathy:
  - complete bitemporal hemianopia is uncommon; most patients present with incomplete and asymmetric bitemporal field loss
  - inferonasal axons are located inferiorly in the chiasm; tumors (typically pituitary adenomas) that compress the chiasm from below hence often initially cause bitemporal superior field loss
  - superonasal axons are located superiorly in the chiasm; tumors (typically craniopharyngiomas and suprasellar aneurysms) that compress the chiasm from above, hence often initially cause bitemporal inferior defects

Differential Diagnosis

- noncompressive causes of chiasmopathy are rare but almost any cause of optic neuropathy may also (rarely) affect the chiasm

Investigations

- *urgent* MRI brain with contrast, with special views of the chiasm (these patients can suffer pituitary apoplexy or collapse from endocrine dysfunction at any time)
- CT brain is not appropriate, as it may miss even moderate-sized pituitary region tumors

Treatment

- patients require urgent referral to both neurosurgery and endocrinology (many of these patients have life-threatening panhypopituitarism)
- treatment options include:
  - medical therapy, for hormone-secreting pituitary adenomas
  - transsphenoidal surgery
  - transcranial surgery
  - conventional, stereotactic or 3D conformal fractionated external beam radiotherapy
  - stereotactic radiosurgery

Prognosis

- vision
  - there is often dramatic and rapid recovery of VA and field after surgery for pituitary adenomas (Fig. 3.26), unless optic atrophy is advanced (patients often report improved vision immediately on waking from the anesthetic)

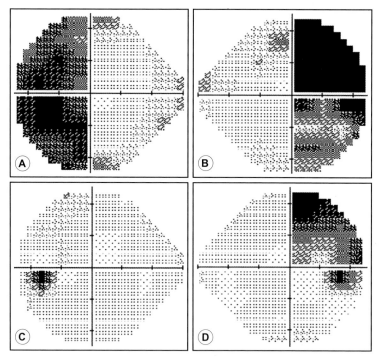

Fig. 3.26 Presurgery (**A**, **B**) and postsurgery (**C**, **D**) visual fields showing partial resolution of bitemporal hemianopia after excision of a large pituitary adenoma.

- other pituitary region tumors are more difficult to treat, and visual recovery is less certain
- morbidity
  - most pituitary macroadenomas cannot be completely excised, but they may be substantially debulked such that they cause no further problem for the patient
  - craniopharyngiomas and pituitary region meningiomas are even more difficult to completely excise, and patients are often troubled with multiple recurrences over many years

Ophthalmic Follow-up

- all patients with pituitary region tumors should have an ophthalmic examination (including perimetry) before as well as after any treatment
- ophthalmic follow-up must be continued for many years; the first (or only) sign of a tumor recurrence may be worsening of the visual fields on perimetry

Retrochiasmal Disease

Retrochiasmal disease (affecting the optic tract, lateral geniculate body, optic radiation or occipital primary visual cortex) causes a partial or complete homonymous hemianopia (Figs. 3.27 and 3.28). The most common etiology is stroke, but brain tumors are also a relatively frequent cause.

There are no clinical features that can reliably distinguish a stroke from a brain tumor in these patients; therefore, all patients with homonymous field loss need neuroimaging.

CAUSES

- stroke: ischemic or hemorrhagic strokes may affect the posterior cerebral artery circulation, causing infarction of part or all of the primary visual cortex on that side (Fig. 3.29)

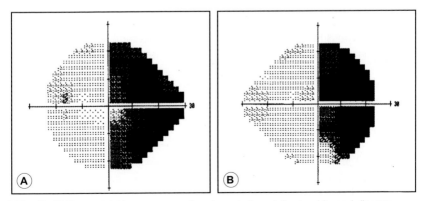

Fig. 3.27   (A, B) Dense right homonymous hemianopia from left retrochiasmal disease.

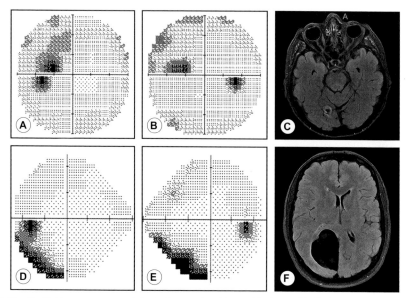

Fig. 3.28 Partial homonymous defects from retrochiasmal lesions. (**A–C**) Superior left homonymous scotoma from right occipital stroke; (**D–F**) inferior left homonmyous scotoma from right occipital cyst.

- tumor: in general, relatively small tumors (most commonly pituitary tumors and craniopharyngiomas) can cause an optic tract lesion; for a dense hemianopia from an optic radiation or cortex lesion, a relatively large tumor must be present
- inflammation: symptomatic optic tract or radiation lesions due to MS are uncommon
- infection: intracranial abscesses (e.g., tuberculosis) are rare
- congenital anomalies including arteriovenous malformations are also rare

SYMPTOMS

- three types of presentation are common:
  - homonymous field loss incidentally discovered on routine screening
  - acute symptomatic field loss: this is most commonly due to stroke but a bleed into a tumor is also possible
  - slowly progressive symptomatic field loss: tumors are a common cause of this presentation

SIGNS

- normal VA and color vision (unless bilateral disease is present (Fig. 3.30), or ocular or optic nerve disease is also present)
- usually no RAPD; if an RAPD is present:
  - either the homonymous field loss is due to an optic tract lesion (on the side opposite the RAPD)

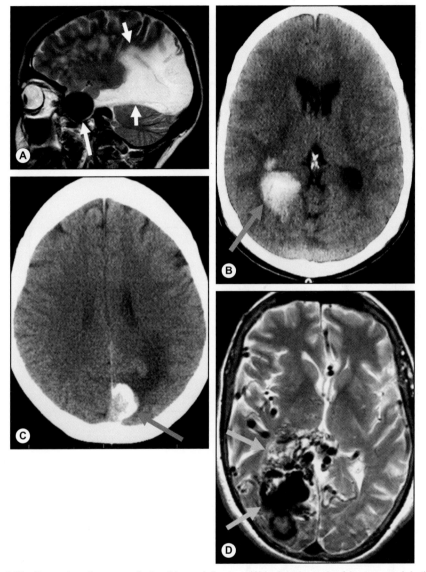

Fig. 3.29 Examples of causes of retrochiasmal disease. (**A**) Ischemic stroke *(short arrows)*, in this case secondary to a middle cerebral artery aneurysm *(long arrow)*. (**B**) Hemorrhagic stroke. (**C**) Tumor (in this case a meningioma). (**D**) Arteriovenous malformation.

- or there is also an optic neuropathy present on the side of the RAPD
- optic discs usually look normal but:
  - tumors or large infarcts may cause papilledema
  - lesions of the optic tract sometimes cause bilateral optic disc pallor
- other localizing neurologic signs (e.g., abnormal gait or hemiplegia)

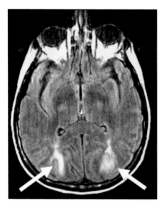

Fig. 3.30 Unilateral retrochiasmal disease causes homonymous hemianopia with normal visual acuity. Less commonly, bilateral retrochiasmal disease can be present causing bilateral homonymous hemianopia; this can cause severe visual acuity and field loss in both eyes ("cerebral blindness" or "cortical blindness"). This patient had severe bilateral visual loss due to bilateral occipital white matter disease caused by chemotherapy. Because the eyes and pupil reactions were normal, the patient was initially misdiagnosed as having nonorganic visual loss.

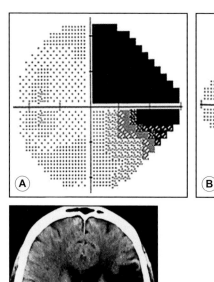

Fig. 3.31 Using the characteristics of a partial homonymous field defect to predict where the lesion could be. Perimetry here shows a right superior incongruous homonymous quadrantanopia (**A**, **B**); this pattern is most commonly caused by a left temporal lobe lesion affecting the inferior part of the anterior optic radiation. Magnetic resonance imaging shows an old left temporal infarct (**C**).

LOCALIZATION

- complete homonymous hemianopia
  - the lesion cannot be further localized; it may be anywhere in the retrochiasmal pathway

- partial homonymous hemianopia (Fig. 3.31 and see Table 2.1)
  - congruity (the amount of similarity between the field defects in each eye):
    - the more posterior the lesion, the more congruous the defects
  - superior or inferior defect:
    - a superior homonymous field defect may be due to a temporal lobe (inferior) optic radiation lesion
    - an inferior homonymous defect may be due to a parietal lobe (superior) optic radiation lesion
  - "macular sparing"
    - the whole visual hemifield is lost except for a small vertical semicircular area around fixation
    - this is difficult to test accurately; many cases of "macular sparing" are caused by the patient's fixation wandering during the field test
    - if truly present, it may be caused by middle cerebral artery "sparing" of the cortical macular representation in a posterior cerebral artery stroke
  - homonymous paracentral scotomas
    - this occurs if only the tip of one occipital lobe (the hemimacular representation) is infarcted or affected by tumor
    - patients with this field loss often present complaining of problems reading (words or parts of words seem to disappear and reappear)
    - routine visual field testing may miss the small paracentral scotomas; they are best detected on Amsler grid testing or with a "central 10-2" field with Humphrey's automated perimeter
    - rarely, wedge-shaped homonymous defects may suggest a lateral geniculate nucleus (LGN) lesion (Fig. 3.32)
    - very rarely, a "checkerboard" pattern of field loss indicated bilateral partial occipital infarction (Fig. 3.33)

INVESTIGATIONS

- MRI brain is the investigation of choice (CT may miss small optic tract or occipital cortex lesions)

TREATMENT

- specific treatment
  - tumors: refer to neurosurgeon
  - stroke: refer to physician for treatment and for investigation of risk factors to try to decrease the chance of further vascular events
- symptomatic treatment
  - a homonymous hemianopia is a significant disability
  - advise the patient that it is illegal to drive if the hemianopic field defect persists and ask them to notify the driving authority
  - referral to a low-vision clinic may help the patient learn practical ways of coping with their field defect (e.g., using a ruler to avoid "losing" the next word or line while reading)

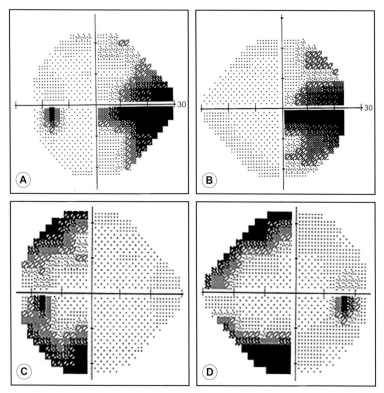

Fig. 3.32　Lateral geniculate nucleus lesions due to stroke are rare, but can produce characteristic wedge-shaped homonymous defects. (**A, B**) Left lateral choroidal artery (from posterior cerebral artery) stroke; (**C, D**) right anterior choroidal artery (from internal carotid artery) stroke.

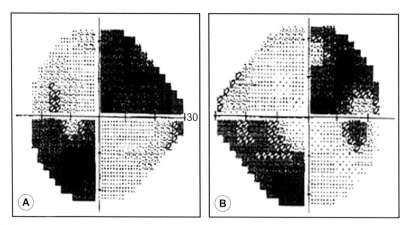

Fig. 3.33　Perimetry (**A, B**) showing rare "checkerboard" visual field defects. There is a left inferior homonymous quadrantanopia from a right superior occipital stroke; and a right superior homonymous quadrantanopia from a left inferior occipital stroke.

Occult Ocular Disease

This is a disease of the globe that is not immediately apparent on routine examination. It is included in the differential diagnosis of "unexplained visual loss" along with optic nerve, chiasmal, and retrochiasmal disease.

However, if there is any doubt, investigate for possible visual pathway disease first, before investigating for an occult retinopathy. It is better to initially "miss" an untreatable cone dystrophy than a treatable (and life-threatening) pituitary tumor.

CAUSES

- cornea: keratoconus (may be missed on routine corneal exam and detected only on retinoscopy or keratometry)
- macula
  - subtle macular edema or epiretinal membrane
  - cone dystrophy or Stargardt disease (the macula may appear normal early on)
  - cancer-associated cone dysfunction
  - other macular degenerations
- peripheral retina ± macula
  - ocular ischemic syndrome
  - retinitis pigmentosa (with or without visible retinal changes)
  - previous retinal vascular occlusions
  - cancer-associated retinopathy
  - "white dot syndromes" e.g., MEWDS (multifocal evanescent white dot syndrome), AZOOR (acute zonal outer occult retinopathy)

SYMPTOMS

- may suggest a particular diagnosis, e.g., progressive hemeralopia (decreased vision in bright conditions) suggests cone degeneration; metamorphopsia suggests macular edema or epiretinal membrane

SIGNS

- look carefully at the cornea, ocular media, macula and peripheral retina
- however, beware attributing poor vision or visual field defects to "subtle" intraocular disease: always think, "Is the ocular disease severe enough to be causing the patient's visual problems?"

INVESTIGATION

- possible macular or retinal disease may be confirmed in some cases by full field or multifocal ERG and/or fluorescein angiography

Nonorganic Visual Loss

Check that your patient meets ALL the clinical diagnostic criteria on p. 65 before you make this diagnosis!

Nonorganic visual loss (also sometimes called "functional" visual loss) means that the patient is simulating poor vision, when in fact their vision is normal. Just because the patient is complaining of blurred vision but there is no RAPD and both eyes look completely normal does NOT mean the patient has nonorganic visual loss; compressive chiasmopathy, bilateral optic neuropathy, bilateral retrochiasmal disease, or bilateral subtle ocular disease frequently presents this way.

Don't hesitate to ask for a neuro-ophthalmic opinion in any case of unexplained visual loss.

APPROACH

- the only way to definitely diagnose nonorganic visual loss is to "trick" the patient into demonstrating normal visual function. "Diagnosis by exclusion" after extensive investigations (MRI, electrophysiology, fluorescein angiography) is not as reliable, because:
    - tests can be "false positive" in patients with nonorganic visual loss: some patients can very accurately and repeatedly "fake" abnormal visual fields, and even electrophysiologic testing (if a patient does not pay attention during a pattern visual evoked potential [VEP], an abnormal VEP will be recorded, raising false concerns of visual pathway disease)
    - tests may be "false-negative" in patients with genuine but early or subtle organic disease
- however, if the patient can't be tricked into demonstrating normal vision, it is always important to perform the relevant investigations to exclude serious organic disease (while appreciating both the "false-positive" and "false-negative" risks of doing so)
- try to separate the patient's personality from their clinical signs
- beware "nonorganic overlay" in addition to genuine organic visual loss
- don't call a patient's symptoms "nonorganic" just because you haven't heard of them before
- be careful regarding what you document in the patient's notes

DISEASES OFTEN MISDIAGNOSED AS NONORGANIC VISUAL LOSS

- pituitary tumors (causing early compressive chiasmopathy or bilateral compressive optic neuropathy with "normal" discs and no RAPD)
- LHON (in the acute phase, before the discs become pale)
- bilateral retrochiasmal disease
- early cone dystrophy or Stargardt disease (the maculae may appear entirely normal despite reduced acuity and color vision)

Causes of Nonorganic Visual Loss

- malingering
  - a psychologically well patient who feigns visual loss for some material benefit (e.g., a medicolegal case or a disability pension)
  - these patients may sometimes become angry and aggressive if they sense that they have been "found out"
- conversion disorder (previously called "hysteria")
  - often a teenager or young adult with significant psychologic or social problems
  - the patient is often very pleasant and may even seem indifferent to their vision problem
  - in some cases, a social precipitant may be discovered on further questioning (school or work stress, parental conflicts); in others, no cause is found
- however, in some cases, an easy distinction cannot be made between these two groups

CLUES THAT A PATIENT'S VISUAL LOSS MAY BE NONORGANIC

A lot of this is experience-based suspicion, based on something "just not adding up" in the patient's examination. For example:
- unilateral severe vision loss with normal acuity and field in the other eye, with normal retinal and disc examination bilaterally, normal retinoscopy and no RAPD seen on careful testing with a bright light in a dark room (the only place the disease can be is in the optic nerve on the affected side, and all significant unilateral optic nerve disease causes an RAPD)
- claimed bilateral complete blindness but the patient is still able to navigate around obstacles when viewed informally (e.g., walking through the waiting room)

"CLINICAL TRICKS" TO TRY TO DEMONSTRATE NORMAL VISION

This sounds unpleasant as we're not supposed to "trick" our patients but it is the safest and best way to confirm the diagnosis of nonorganic visual loss. The key is to have a few "tricks" for each possible scenario, some of which are detailed later, and to use them fluently, without arousing suspicion.

"Bilateral Complete Blindness"
Pupils
- if bilateral blindness is due to severe bilateral retinal, optic nerve or chiasmal disease, both pupils should be sluggishly reactive to light
- if both pupils are briskly reactive to light, the only possible cause for true bilateral blindness is bilateral retrochiasmal disease

Observation
- if the patient can be observed "casually" (e.g., in the waiting room or walking out of the hospital), it may be seen that vision is not as bad as claimed

Tests That Are Independent of Vision (See Video 3.3)

- the patient is asked to sign their name or to follow their own finger with their eyes as it moves side to side
- these are proprioceptive, not visual, tasks that truly blind patients are still able to perform; patients feigning blindness will often make an exaggerated "show" of being unable to do these tasks
- this can demonstrate that the patient has at least some nonorganic overlay but it does not demonstrate normal vision and so does not exclude organic disease

Mirror Test (Video 3.1)

- hold a large mirror in front of the patient and tilt it up and down, right and left. If a patient is completely blind or has only light perception vision from any cause, the eyes will remain stable. In a patient with any useful vision at all, the eyes will move back and forth as the images in the mirror move back and forth

Optokinetic Nystagmus (OKN) (Video 3.2)

- OKN is elicited by a large-field repetitive moving stimulus and is difficult to voluntarily suppress
- the key is to have a large optokinetic target, but these are rarely available; the small drum usually found in clinics may or may not elicit nystagmus and is easier for the patient to "ignore"
- if OKN is seen, the patient is obviously not bilaterally blind, but this does not exclude the possibility of real visual disease with psychologic overlay

"Unilateral Complete Blindness"

Pupils

- if a patient is completely blind from retinal or optic nerve disease in one eye, and has normal VA, color vision and visual field in the other eye, there should be a prominent RAPD in the blind eye

Mirror Test

- with the "good eye" covered, perform the mirror test as described earlier; if a patient is completely blind or has only light perception vision in the eye from any cause, the eye will remain stable. In a patient with any useful vision at all, the eye will move back and forth as the images in the mirror move back and forth

Optokinetic Nystagmus (OKN)

- with both eyes open, rotate the OKN drum or move the OKN target from right to left (or left to right); this should elicit a nystagmus in both eyes
- once you see the nystagmus, bring your hand up to cover the "good eye" (Video 3.3)
- in a patient who is truly blind in one eye, covering the normal eye will result in immediate cessation of the OKN response
- in a patient with nonorganic blindness in one eye, the nystagmus will continue despite covering the "good eye"

"Fogging" or "Crossed Cylinder Technique" With the Trial Frame
- say "I'm going to see if I can improve the vision in your good eye with glasses"
- the vision of the "good" eye is blurred with a high plus (e.g., +5 diopter) lens or crossed +2.5/−2.5 cylinders (that are rotated from being parallel to being crossed as the patient reads down the chart); a plano or +0.25 lens is placed before the "bad" eye so as not to arouse suspicion
- if the patient falls for this trick, he or she will read well down the chart, unwittingly using their "bad" eye

Stereopsis Test
- if the patient demonstrates any stereoacuity on stereovision testing, obviously one eye is not blind; if stereoacuity is normal, both eyes must have normal VA

"Blurred Vision in Both Eyes"

Testing Visual Acuity at Different Distances
- test at 20 feet, 10 feet, and 5 feet; no (or minimal) improvement at the closer distances is inconsistent with organic visual loss (unless large central scotomas are present)

Reading Vision
- some patients with organic visual loss don't realize the connection between reading and distance vision and will happily read fine print at near despite claiming not to be able to see a large letter on the distance chart
- however, check that the reading plates are held the correct distance from the eyes (some patients with genuine severe visual loss can still read well at near if they hold the plates very close to their eyes)

Ishihara or Hardy-Rand-Rittler Plate Color Testing
- say "Were you born with poor color vision? If not, this is a test for color vision problems people were born with and your color vision should be normal."
- if the patient claims "hand movements" vision in both eyes but is still able to see the test plate (which requires an acuity of 20/80 or so), at least some nonorganic overlay is likely
- sometimes patients can be encouraged to "trace" numbers with their finger on the plate, even if they "can't see them well enough to say them"
- "red filter test": patients with 20/80 or better acuity should be able to recognize all the plates if they view them through a red filter (even if they are congenitally red-green color blind)

Perimetry: Demonstrating Entirely Normal Peripheral and Central Visual Fields
- this would be at odds with a patient's claims of severe visual loss
- however, "beware the central scotoma": small dense central scotomas can have a major impact on acuity and be missed on routine perimetry (a dedicated "central" field test, such as Humphrey 10-2 or Amsler grid, should also be performed)

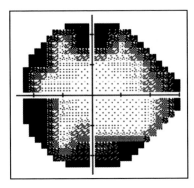

Fig. 3.34 "Cloverleaf" pattern left eye 24-2 perimetry in a patient with nonorganic visual loss. The false negative error rate was very high at 53%.

Perimetry: Responses That Are Not Consistent with Organic Disease

- automated (e.g., Humphrey) perimetry:
  - high false-negative error rate—indicating that at on many occasions the patient saw the stimulus, but chose to not press the button
  - "cloverleaf" pattern visual field defect as shown in Fig. 3.34—this pattern commonly appears due to the testing protocol when patients attempt to feign peripheral vision loss
  - however, patients with nonorganic visual loss can purposely produce ANY visual field defect, including a hemianopia or quadrantanopia in one or both eyes
- manual kinetic (e.g., Goldmann) perimetry:
  - "spiraling": the point responses for a particular size of target "spiral" in toward fixation as the test progresses (rather than remaining at a consistent location on retesting)
  - "crossing isopters": isopter lines for different size targets cross (this does not happen with organic disease if the patient performs the test accurately)
  - "crowded isopters": targets of greatly differing sizes are all seen at a similar position in the visual field (giving a tight "target" appearance in factitious peripheral visual field constriction)
- manual static (e.g., Bjerrum screen) field testing at different distances
  - if a patient with true concentric constriction of visual field plots a field on a Bjerrum screen at the standard distance with a large white target, then retests at twice the standard distance with a target that is half the size, the field should be significantly larger on the second test
  - some patients with nonorganic visual loss will claim to have exactly the same field on both tests (this is sometimes called the "tunnel vision" response)
- any method
  - the persistence of a monocular field defect on testing with both eyes open, when the patient has a normal field in the other eye, is not caused by organic disease
  - for example, if a patient claims to have a right nasal hemianopia and has a normal left monocular field, the nasal hemianopia should disappear on testing with both eyes open

- but remember that:
  - finding inconsistent behavior on field testing does not mean that all the visual loss is nonorganic (and hence is not enough to make a diagnosis)
  - nonorganic visual loss patients may very exactly and repeatedly produce a "fake" visual field defect on any method of visual field testing

"Blurred Vision in One Eye"

Pupils

- usually, if there is unilateral moderate to severe optic nerve or widespread retinal disease, a clinically detectable RAPD will be present
- "Fogging" or "crossed cylinder" technique
- Stereopsis test
- Plus all the techniques for "blurred vision in both eyes" above

Monocular Vertical Prism Dissociation Test

- the key to this test is that the patient perceives that it is their good eye that is being tested
- the patient is asked to look at an acuity chart (ideally a single row of letters) with both eyes open
- a 4-prism diopter prism is placed base down in front of the patient's "good" eye and the patient is asked what they can see
- patients with normal binocular vision will see two equally distinct rows of letters
- patients with genuine visual loss only see one row or, if the vision in their affected eye is reduced rather than completely lost, the lower image will appear less distinct
- patients with monocular functional visual loss, fooled by the fact that the test is being carried out on their "good" eye, almost invariably report seeing two equally distinct rows of letters

"Constricted" Visual Field in One or Both Eyes

The "Saccade" Test

- this is the best and easiest test of true visual field constriction
- the patient is asked if they have any pain or discomfort when moving the eye/s (the answer doesn't matter; the question makes the patient believe that it is the eye movements in which the examiner is interested)
- the patient is asked to look straight ahead and then to follow a slowly moving object (this also gets the patient thinking about eye movement rather than the field)
- the patient is then told to look straight ahead and then to look at a finger or other object suddenly presented in the periphery of the field
- a rapid eye movement to the area of the object indicates that the patient has an intact field in that direction and that the field is not organically constricted
- if the patient states that he or she cannot see the target to the side, the examiner says "I know you can't see it with your side vision, that is why I want you to look directly at it"

Investigations

- these need to be undertaken in every patient you cannot "trick" into demonstrating normal vision. They are done not to prove the patient is nonorganic (no test can do that), but rather to exclude advanced underlying organic disease (but remember that all tests may be normal in early or subtle organic disease)

Optical Coherence Tomography (OCT)

- can be used to assess presence and thickness of both PRNFL thickness (for optic nerve damage) and macular volume and retinal ganglion cell/inner plexiform layer thickness (for optic nerve or retinal damage)
- PRNFL may be thicker than normal with acute optic nerve disease (e.g., acute retrobulbar optic neuritis)
- PRNFL should be thinned with chronic (>4 weeks) optic nerve disease
- if there is long-standing severe retinal, optic nerve, or optic chiasm disease, there will usually be abnormalities visible on OCT imaging
- however, OCT will be normal in bilateral retro-chiasmal disease; and may be normal in early or mild optic nerve or chiasmal disease
- a normal OCT does not exclude organic disease

Visual Evoked Potential (VEP)

- measures the electrical activity of the occipital visual cortex that is triggered when the patient views a reversing black-and-white checkerboard (with variable check size) on a television screen
- the signal recorded is much stronger when the patient is able to resolve ("see") the check size
- if a reliable VEP is performed and is normal down to a small check size, this is reassurance that the patient has at least reasonable vision (but does not exclude mild organic disease)
- however, an abnormal VEP is not definite proof of organic disease: some patients can "fake" an abnormal pattern VEP by not concentrating on the test pattern

Electroretinogram (ERG)

- measures the electrical response of the photoreceptors and Muller's cells of the retina
- full-field ERG measures a massed response and requires at least 25% of the retina to be dysfunctional before it is abnormal; thus, it misses small macular lesions (e.g., macular cone dystrophy)
- multifocal ERG is very sensitive for small central or paracentral scotomas caused by retinal disease

Neuroimaging and Other Tests

- the one cause of poor vision that none of us can afford to miss is visual pathway dysfunction from a brain tumor
- for this reason, if you don't have good evidence that the visual loss is nonorganic, pursue MRI brain imaging with contrast and with special views of the optic nerves and chiasm
- other tests (as suggested on p. 68) may be required if you have only a low suspicion of nonorganic disease, particularly if the patient is worsening

MANAGEMENT OF THE PATIENT WITH SUSPECTED (BUT UNPROVEN) NONORGANIC VISUAL LOSS

- obtain a neuro-ophthalmic opinion in all cases of unexplained visual loss in which nonorganic visual loss is not highly suspected; it is a tragedy when unusual symptoms or the absence of obvious signs lead to real visual pathway disease being misdiagnosed as nonorganic
- if you don't refer these patients, follow them up until such time as you can demonstrate either organic or nonorganic disease

MANAGEMENT OF THE PATIENT *WITH* PROVEN NONORGANIC VISUAL LOSS

Difficult as it sometimes is, diagnosing a patient with nonorganic visual loss is often not nearly as hard as working out what to do next, in particular:

- what do you tell them?
- how do you explain to them "what's wrong" with their eyes when they ask?
- what do you do if they become angry or insult you for "not being able to work out what's wrong with me"?
- what do you do regarding the malingerer's falsified disability pension and sick leave?
- should you refer patients with conversion disorder to a psychiatrist?

These are difficult questions and ones that neuro-ophthalmologists struggle with on a daily basis. In general:

- it is important to personalize your strategy to the particular patient
- offer reassurance that the patient's visual system seems to be quite healthy (i.e., "I am delighted to tell you that I find no evidence of irreversible damage to your eye/s and there is a good chance that your vision will eventually improve")

CHAPTER 4

Swollen Disc/s, Normal Vision

(Note: for swollen disc/s with blurred vision or field loss, see Chapter 3)

Introduction

Swelling of one or both optic discs can be caused by disease of the:
- eye/s
- optic nerve/s
- orbit/s
- brain
- neck
- chest
- blood

There are no clinically diagnosable causes of optic disc swelling with normal vision; all cases require investigation. Investigation of optic disc swelling is urgent because of the high likelihood of serious intracranial disease (that in some cases can kill the patient within hours of them seeing you, if not recognized and treated). Therefore, bilateral disc swelling is a true medical emergency.

As eye care professionals we all need to know:

1. What to do for patients with optic disc swelling with normal vision. We recommend urgent (same-day) referral to a neuro-ophthalmologist or neurologist for further assessment. If prompt referral is difficult due to geographic or patient factors, or if you wish to work the patient up yourself, the necessary initial basic investigations are outlined on p. 140.

2. How to make a safe diagnosis of idiopathic intracranial hypertension (IIH), also called primary pseudotumor cerebri syndrome (PTCS). IIH is overdiagnosed, and women with life-threatening intracranial disease, such as a brain tumor or dural venous sinus thrombosis, are often initially misdiagnosed by an ophthalmologist as having IIH. In fact, IIH is a diagnosis of exclusion! It should only ever be made after the patient has been fully investigated (including magnetic resonance imaging [MRI] and MR venography [MRV] or computerized tomographic [CT] scan and CT venography [CTV] and lumbar puncture [LP] in all cases) and been found to fit all the diagnostic criteria listed on p. 141.

Examination Checklist

SWOLLEN DISC/S, NORMAL VISION

Have you asked about, and looked for, all the following key features?

History

- [ ] ophthalmic symptoms?
  - [ ] how was the disc swelling discovered—on a routine check or was the patient having visual symptoms or headaches?
  - [ ] blurred vision?
  - [ ] transient visual loss?
  - [ ] double vision?
- [ ] headaches?
  - [ ] if so, are they a new type of headache the patient has never had before?
  - [ ] are there features suggestive of raised intracranial pressure (ICP) (e.g., headache worst in morning, nausea or vomiting, pulsatile tinnitus)?
- [ ] other neurologic symptoms, e.g., numbness, weakness, personality change?
- [ ] previous medical and surgical history?
  - [ ] cancer? (possible metastasis)
  - [ ] deep vein thrombosis, pregnancy, miscarriage, recent dehydration? (possible coagulopathy causing dural venous sinus thrombosis)
  - [ ] taking any medications that can cause secondary PTCS? (see p. 167)
  - [ ] history of diseases that can cause secondary PTCS? (see p. 167)
  - [ ] diabetes?
- [ ] social history: smoker, alcohol, special diet?
- [ ] family history: unexplained visual loss or brain disease?
- [ ] if patient over 50: symptoms of giant cell arteritis (GCA)?
- [ ] system review questions: any clues to the cause anywhere in the body?

Examination

- [ ] visual acuity
- [ ] color vision testing
- [ ] visual field testing to confrontation
- [ ] limitation of eye movements? (possible orbital apex or pituitary tumor)
- [ ] pupils
  - [ ] relative afferent pupillary defect (RAPD)? (unilateral or bilateral asymmetric optic neuropathy or optic tract lesion)
  - [ ] is there anisocoria? (possible partial third nerve palsy or Horner syndrome from intracranial tumor)
- [ ] eyelids: ptosis? (possible partial third nerve palsy or Horner syndrome from intracranial tumor)
- [ ] orbits: proptosis, injection, chemosis? (if so, is there a palpable thrill or audible bruit? Suggests carotid-cavernous fistula)
- [ ] decreased corneal or facial sensation to light touch? (possible middle cranial fossa tumor)

☐ if patient over 50: palpate temporal arteries
☐ disc appearance: are there features of pseudo or true disc swelling?
☐ measure blood pressure in all cases: malignant hypertension is a rare cause of disc swelling
☐ full neurologic examination: in all cases of bilateral true disc swelling

Plus: Perform Perimetry

- IN ALL CASES

Management Flowchart

SWOLLEN DISC/S, NORMAL VISION

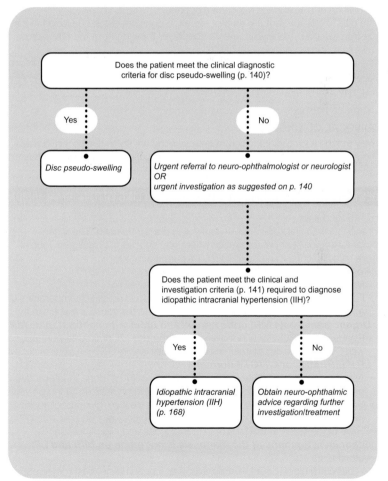

CLINICAL DIAGNOSTIC CRITERIA FOR DISC PSEUDO-SWELLING

The patient must have ALL of the following:

HISTORY

- no blurred vision (except that consistent with visible intraocular disease, e.g., cataract)
- no transient visual loss
- no pulsatile tinnitus ("whooshing" noise in one or both ears in time with the pulse)

EXAMINATION

- normal visual acuity unless there is coexistent ocular disease causing blurred vision
- normal color acuity unless there is a history of a congenital color deficit
- the central disc cup is small or absent or the disc is "tilted"
- the nerve fiber layer over the disc is not opacified or swollen and does not obscure the disc vessels
- the disc is not hyperemic (in true swelling, the disc is usually "pinker" than normal due to dilation of disc surface capillaries) or pale
- the disc is elevated but the area of elevation does not extend beyond the disc margin (in true swelling, the swollen nerve fiber layer extends from the disc across the disc margin to the peripapillary retina)
- the circumpapillary light reflex (the circular "ring of reflection" around the disc margin) is bright and regular (it is lost in true disc swelling due to nerve fiber layer swelling)

PERIMETRY

- normal in both eyes

IF EQUIVOCAL OR UNSURE

- may require fluorescein angiogram (true swelling will show fluorescein leakage), ultrasonography or OCT (may show buried drusen) or urgent referral for neuro-ophthalmic opinion

SUGGESTED INVESTIGATIONS FOR OPTIC DISC SWELLING WITH NORMAL VISION

See p. 146 for details.
    For patients with unilateral or bilateral swollen discs who cannot be urgently referred to a neuro-ophthalmologist or neurologist or whom you choose to investigate yourself.
    These investigations must be URGENTLY pursued.

1. *Review history, examination, and perimetry*
   - Make sure it is true disc swelling, not pseudo-swelling.
   - Full systemic history and examination including blood pressure, temperature, urine test, and systemic neurologic exam; are there clues to the cause anywhere in the body?
2. *Urgent (same-day) MRI optic nerves and brain with contrast, plus MRV brain*
   - If same-day MRI/MRV is not available, same-day CT brain with contrast combined with CTV can rule out a large tumor or vascular lesion. CT scan alone is not adequate.
3. *LP if MRI/MRV or CT/CTV normal*
   - Ask for opening pressure to be recorded (should be done in lateral decubitus or prone position; cannot be certain of true opening pressure in sitting position).
   - Send cerebrospinal fluid (CSF) for biochemistry (protein, glucose, oligoclonal bands), microbiology (microscopy, cell count, culture), cytology.
   - Have blood taken at the time of LP, for glucose and oligoclonal bands.
4. *Other investigations (if the diagnosis is not made on MRI and LP)*
   - blood tests
     - basic: full blood count, electrolytes, liver function tests, erythrocyte sedimentation rate (ESR), c-reactive protein (CRP)
     - inflammatory: angiotensin converting enzyme (ACE), antinuclear antibody (ANA), aquaporin-4 antibody assay (cell-based)
     - infectious: syphilis serology
     - others if history or exam suggests
   - chest x-ray or CT scan

CLINICAL AND INVESTIGATION CRITERIA REQUIRED TO DIAGNOSE IDIOPATHIC INTRACRANIAL HYPERTENSION (IIH)—ALSO KNOWN AS PRIMARY PSEUDOTUMOR CEREBRI SYNDROME (PTCS)

The patient must have ALL of the following:

HISTORY

- No neurologic symptoms other than headache (in most patients) or horizontal diplopia (in some patients).
- On specific questioning, no history of systemic disease, therapeutic drugs, vitamins, foods, or toxins that can cause secondary PTCS (see list p. 167), other than obesity and venous sinus stenosis.

EXAMINATION

- visual acuity normal unless macular hemorrhages/exudates/subretinal fluid, tumor compressing optic nerves/chiasm and obstructing third ventricle, or chronic/severe optic nerve damage
- bilateral (or, very rarely, unilateral) optic disc swelling
- no other abnormalities on examination other than (in some cases) unilateral or bilateral sixth nerve palsy
- normal blood pressure, temperature, and urine analysis

PERIMETRY

- Any visual field defect, one or both eyes; earliest defect is often an enlarged blind spot or midperipheral scotoma.

INVESTIGATION RESULTS

- Normal MRI and MRV or CTV brain (other than dilated optic nerve sheaths or slightly narrowed ventricles in some cases) (CT brain alone is not adequate).
- LP shows raised opening pressure and absolutely normal CSF constituents (normal microbiology, biochemistry, and cytology) (IIH should never be diagnosed without an LP).
- Normal full blood count, glucose, electrolytes, liver function tests, ESR, CRP, ACE, ANA.
- Normal chest x-ray or CT scan in appropriate setting.

IF THE PATIENT MEETS ALL THESE CRITERIA, SEE P. 168 FOR MANAGEMENT.

Disc Pseudo-swelling

(See summary of clinical diagnostic criteria on p. 140.)

DEFINITION

- One or both optic discs appear elevated or have unclear margins, but there is no optic nerve axon swelling (the cause of true disc swelling).

CAUSES

- small disc (Fig. 4.1)
- tilted disc (Fig. 4.2)
- elevated disc with superficial but unappreciated drusen (Fig. 4.3)
- elevated disc with deep (buried) drusen (Fig. 4.4)
- elevated disc without drusen (Fig. 4.5)

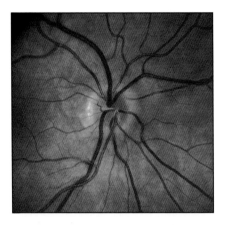

Fig. 4.1 Congenital optic disc hypoplasia with disc elevation that mimics true disc swelling.

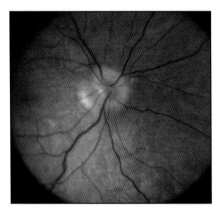

Fig. 4.2 Congenital tilted optic disc in patient with myopic astigmatism causing nasal (but not temporal) disc elevation mimicking true disc swelling.

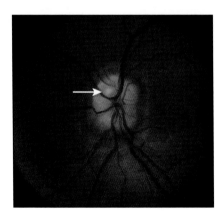

Fig. 4.3 Pseudo-disc swelling from superficial but unappreciated superficial drusen *(arrow)*.

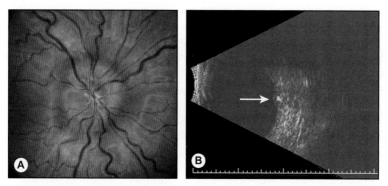

Fig. 4.4 Pseudo-disc swelling from buried drusen. (**A**) Appearance of elevated optic disc. (**B**) Ultrasound showing drusen *(arrow)*.

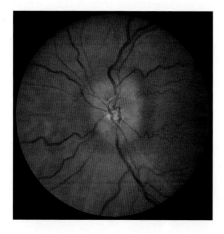

Fig. 4.5 Pseudo-swelling of optic disc without drusen. The patient had no evidence of drusen on ultrasonography and had normal intracranial pressure by lumbar puncture. The appearance of the optic disc did not change over time.

CHARACTERISTICS

- no obscuration of large or small vessels as they pass across disc
- disc vessels not dilated
- anomalous branching of retinal vessels
- nerve fiber layer reflexes normal
- no flame-shaped hemorrhages but a subretinal hemorrhage may be present
- cup absent
- this compares with true disc swelling, that shows:
    - blurred nerve fiber layer
    - flame-shaped hemorrhages
    - disc vessels obscured
    - cup retained
    - dilated retinal veins

SPONTANEOUS VENOUS PULSATIONS (SVPs)

- The central retinal vein or one of its branches on the disc can be seen to pulsate in about 80% of normal subjects (however, is absent in 20% of normal subjects).
- If SVPs are observed in a patient with possible disc swelling, ICP is probably within the normal range at the time of observation, however:
  - ICP can vary markedly during each day or from day to day, so just one observation of SVPs is not reassurance that ICP is not elevated at other times.
  - Therefore, the presence of SVPs should not be relied upon in isolation.
- Caution: "induced" venous pulsation:
  - In cases where SVP is not visible, it is possible to induce visible venous pulsations by pressing on the globe through the eyelid while observing the disc.
  - It is sometimes said that if venous pulsations are easily induced with minimal pressure, this is evidence that ICP is "probably normal" or "almost normal"; however, this is not a reliable sign to differentiate true swelling from pseudo-swelling.

DIFFERENTIATION FROM TRUE DISC SWELLING

- Consider the setting: pseudo-swelling is often seen:
  - on a routine exam
  - in an asymptomatic patient

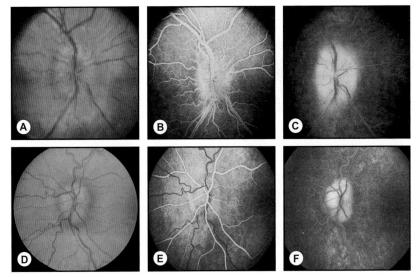

Fig. 4.6 Fluorescein angiography in true optic disc swelling versus pseudo-swelling. (**A**) Appearance of an optic disc thought to be swollen. (**B**) Arteriovenous phase of angiogram shows diffuse leakage of dye. (**C**) Late phase of angiogram shows persistent diffuse leakage of dye. These findings are consistent with true optic disc swelling. (**D**) Appearance of optic disc thought to be swollen. (**E**) Arterial phase of angiogram shows no leakage of dye. (**F**) Late phase of angiogram shows staining of disc but no leakage of dye. These findings are consistent with pseudo-swelling of the optic disc.

- with marked hypermetropia or myopic astigmatism
- whereas true disc swelling due to papilledema is often seen in a patient who has:
  - headaches and sometimes nausea or vomiting
  - other neurologic manifestations

INVESTIGATIONS TO HELP DETERMINE IF PSEUDO-SWELLING OR TRUE SWELLING IS PRESENT

- ophthalmoscopic appearance
- autofluorescence (discs with pseudo-swelling often autofluoresce)
- fluorescein angiography (true swelling leaks; pseudo-swelling doesn't) (Fig. 4.6)
- ultrasonography
  - look for drusen (see Fig. 4.4B)
  - perform 30-degree test
- optical coherence tomography (Fig. 4.7)
  - look for drusen (lumpy, bumpy appearance) vs. evidence of subretinal fluid

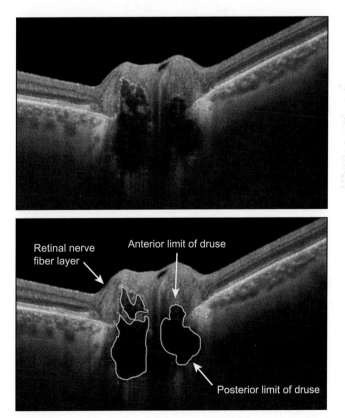

Fig. 4.7 Appearance of buried optic disc drusen on optical coherence tomography.

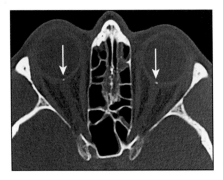

Fig. 4.8 Appearance of optic disc drusen *(arrows)* on axial computed tomography scan using bone window setting.

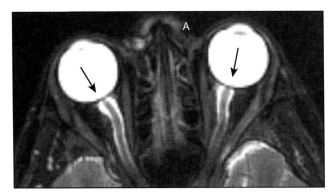

Fig. 4.9 Magnetic resonance imaging showing changes consistent with papilledema. Note widening of optic nerve sheaths and flattening of back of globes *(arrows)*.

- CT scan
  - look for buried drusen (bone windows) (Fig. 4.8)
  - look for intracranial mass
- MRI for one of the following suggesting true swelling: intracranial mass, flattening of globe, enlarged optic nerve sheaths (Fig. 4.9)
- LP if bilateral true swelling can't be excluded by the above

True Disc Swelling

SUGGESTED INVESTIGATIONS FOR SWOLLEN DISC/S WITH NORMAL VISION

(See summary box on p. 140.)

There are no clinically diagnosable causes of optic disc swelling with normal vision, so all these patients require thorough investigation. Because there are many possible causes for disc swelling, and many of these are life-threatening, it is ideal if the patient can be referred very urgently (same-day) to a neuro-ophthalmologist or neurologist for urgent investigation.

In some cases, there may be geographic or patient factors which make prompt referral difficult, or you may wish to perform the initial investigations yourself. In such circumstances, we recommend the following investigations as an initial basic work-up. However, given that there are many rare causes of disc swelling, if these initial investigations do not reveal a cause, we would recommend obtaining specialist neuro-ophthalmic advice.

1. Review History, Examination, and Perimetry

- Make sure it is true disc swelling, not pseudo-swelling: see earlier section for how to tell.
- Check the blood pressure:
  - Severe hypertension is a rare cause of unilateral or bilateral disc swelling and is usually accompanied by signs of severe hypertensive retinopathy such as hemorrhages, hard exudates, and cotton-wool spots.
  - However, finding elevated blood pressure does not indicate that this is the cause of the disc swelling:
    - The patient could have systemic hypertension as a coincidental finding, plus a brain tumor or dural venous sinus thrombosis.
    - Raised ICP can cause secondary raised blood pressure (Cushing's reflex).
  - Therefore, all the other investigations still need to be pursued even if severe systemic hypertension is present (don't just attribute the disc appearance to the blood pressure); however, the relevant specialists should also urgently investigate and (if necessary) treat the systemic hypertension.
- Check the temperature: patients with infectious optic neuritis, perineuritis or meningitis may have a fever.
- Urine analysis: glycosuria likely indicates diabetes; hematuria could indicate vasculitis.
- Are there other clues to the cause anywhere in the body?

2. Urgent (Same-Day) MRI of Optic Nerves and Brain With Contrast, Plus MRV Brain, or CT Brain and CTV

- Neuroimaging must be performed urgently: if a patient with disc swelling harbors a large intracranial tumor, brainstem herniation ("coning") can occur at any time and kill the patient; therefore, imaging should be performed the same day you see the patient.
- Request "urgent MRI optic nerves and brain with contrast, plus MRV brain" or "CT brain and orbits, with contrast, plus CTV"
  - This is the most appropriate initial investigation in all cases of disc swelling and ideally should be the first and only form of neuroimaging.
  - MRI will show optic nerve abnormalities, space-occupying lesions, hydrocephalus, and often abnormal meningeal enhancement in meningitis; subtle abnormalities can be missed if intravenous contrast is not given.
  - MRV or CTV will demonstrate dural venous sinus thrombosis (not an uncommon cause of papilledema, including in young obese women); it is essential to detect these cases urgently and administer anticoagulation because extension of the thrombus can kill the patient.

- CT brain scan
  - A normal CT brain scan alone is not adequate reassurance that serious intracranial disease is not present: CT alone will miss many smaller brain tumors and almost all cases of dural venous sinus thrombosis (unless CTV is used).
  - Hence, if a CT brain is to be performed, a CTV should be done at the same time.

3. LP if MRI and MRV or CT and CTV Are Normal

- Caution: LP must only ever be undertaken after neuroimaging has been performed and the result known:
  - LP may be contraindicated if the scan reveals a brain tumor or obstructive hydrocephalus (fatal post-LP brainstem herniation can occur).
- Serious disease can still be present even if MRI/MRV (or CT/CTV) is normal (e.g., communicating hydrocephalus or chronic meningitis); the only way to diagnose these conditions is to perform an LP.
- LP is also essential in the work-up of "suspected IIH" both to rule out abnormalities in the CSF constituents and to document the level of ICP (measured as the LP "opening pressure").
- Ask for opening pressure to be recorded:
  - The opening pressure is the CSF pressure measured with a manometer tube and provides a measure of the patient's ICP.
  - This should be measured with the patient lying on the side with legs bent (lateral decubitus).
  - CSF pressure measured with the patient prone gives readings similar to those measured in the lateral decubitus position.
  - CSF pressure should not be measured with the patient sitting upright as the readings do not reflect true ICP.
- Normal opening pressure is less than 25 cm H_2O in adults and less than 28 cm H_2O in children, but ICP may vary and one pressure reading alone may not be reflective of the "real" ICP:
  - Opening pressure can be falsely elevated if the patient is tense or straining or the LP is "difficult."
  - Opening pressure can be falsely low if repeated passes have already been made during that attempt, if a previous LP has been performed within the last few weeks, or if the patient is already on medical treatment to decrease ICP.
- You should also ask for the CSF to be sent urgently to:
  - biochemistry: for protein, glucose, and oligoclonal bands
  - microbiology: for microscopy, cell count, and culture
  - cytology: looking for malignant cells.
- Immediately after the LP is performed, blood should also be taken to send to biochemistry for blood glucose and oligoclonal bands (to allow comparison with the CSF results).
- Note: an LP may be difficult to perform in an obese patient; consider having it performed under fluoroscopy with the patient in the prone position (CSF pressure in this setting is similar to that with the patient in the lateral decubitus position; the CSF pressure should not be measured with the patient in the sitting position as that may give false readings).

4. Other Investigations in All Patients

Blood Tests

- These are necessary both to look for a cause for the disc swelling and as a baseline (before possible medical treatment is commenced).
- Basic
  - Full blood count
    - White cell count may be elevated in infections and leukemia.
    - Anemia may contribute to secondary PTCS.
  - Electrolytes and liver function tests
    - Severe electrolyte disturbance (e.g., that occurring in undiagnosed renal failure) can cause secondary PTCS.
    - Random glucose to check for undiagnosed diabetes.
    - Some potential treatments can cause electrolyte imbalance, so it is important to check that electrolytes are normal before commencing treatment.
  - ESR and CRP: elevated in infection, cancer, vasculitis
  - ACE: elevated in many cases of sarcoidosis (one cause of optic perineuritis and a rare cause of raised ICP)
  - ANA: elevated in systemic lupus erythematosus (SLE), an uncommon cause of raised ICP.
- Infectious serology, for causes of optic perineuritis if MRI/MRV, LP opening pressure, and CSF constituents are normal
  - Syphilis.
  - Less common causes of optic perineuritis are cat-scratch disease, toxoplasma, and Lyme disease (test only if history is suggestive, e.g., if rash, fever, and/or lymphadenopathy).
- Other tests if history or exam are suggestive or if results of MRI/MRV (or CTV) or LP are abnormal, e.g., blood tests for specific coagulopathies (such as anticardiolipin antibody syndrome) if dural venous sinus thrombosis is found on MRV or CTV.

Chest X-Ray and/or Chest CT Scan

- looking for signs of tuberculosis or sarcoidosis if perineuritis suspected

EYE DISEASE

- Many ocular diseases can cause optic disc swelling without optic nerve dysfunction, including:
  - Hypotony (often postsurgical or posttraumatic).
  - Central retinal vein occlusion (CRVO) (vision can remain normal if early or mild).
  - Intraocular inflammation of any cause: anterior, intermediate, posterior, or panuveitis can all result in secondary optic disc swelling without signs of optic neuropathy.

- In most cases, the diagnosis is obvious from ocular examination, but in cases where there is visible intraocular disease, optic disc swelling, and decreased vision, keep an open mind that the same process causing the intraocular disease could also be causing an optic neuropathy in its own right:
  - For example, a patient with uveitis, disc swelling, and reduced vision could have:
    - secondary disc swelling with no optic nerve dysfunction (the blurred vision being due to macular edema) or
    - some or all of the blurred vision could actually be due to optic nerve disease caused by the same process that is causing the uveitis (e.g., sarcoidosis).
- In unilateral or bilateral asymmetric cases, the presence of an RAPD (or visual field loss more extensive than that expected from the visible ocular disease) indicates that a true optic neuropathy is present, requiring investigation and treatment in its own right.

OPTIC NERVE DISEASE

In most cases, optic nerve disease causes decreased visual acuity and/or visual field loss. However, optic nerve disease may in rare cases present with unilateral or bilateral optic disc swelling with normal vision, if:

- The optic neuropathy is only early in its evolution or very mild.
- Inflammation affects only the optic nerve sheath, rather than the nerve itself: optic perineuritis.

Early or Mild Optic Neuropathy

- Many types of optic neuropathy can result in swollen disc/s with normal vision if mild or early in their course; vision often declines as the disease progresses. Remember that 20/20 vision may not be "normal." The patient with 20/20 vision who complains of decreased vision may have had 20/15 acuity previously!
- Optic nerve compression usually only results in optic disc swelling if the compressive lesion is in the orbit (e.g., an optic nerve sheath meningioma or an orbital tumor) (Fig. 4.10); optic nerve compression from intracranial tumors (such as pituitary tumors) rarely causes disc swelling, unless the lesion also causes raised ICP.

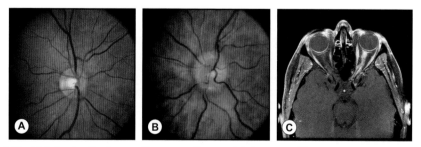

Fig. 4.10 Unilateral optic disc swelling caused by an orbital process. The patient was a 42-year-old woman with a 3-month history of slowly progressive visual loss in the left eye. (**A**) Normal right optic disc. (**B**) Swollen left optic disc. Note absence of peripapillary hemorrhages and exudates (i.e., "benign" swelling). (**C**) Axial magnetic resonance imaging shows diffuse enhancement of the left optic nerve sheath within the orbit, consistent with an optic nerve sheath meningioma.

Optic Perineuritis

- Inflammation affects the optic nerve sheath rather than the nerve itself, so vision and visual field are normal unless the nerve also is affected or becomes affected later.
- If the anterior nerve sheath is affected, disc swelling often occurs, making the condition difficult to distinguish from papilledema unless an LP is performed.
- Causes include:
  - infections, including syphilis, tuberculosis, and viruses (with or without meningitis in each case)
  - sarcoidosis
  - autoimmune.
- The optic nerve sheaths may be seen to be thickened and enhancing on MRI.

BLOOD DISEASE

Blood Pressure: Severe Hypertension

- Very severe hypertension (sometimes called "malignant" hypertension) can cause optic disc swelling; hence, every patient with disc swelling needs to have their blood pressure checked.
- Retinal changes of severe hypertensive retinopathy are usually also present: hemorrhages, cotton-wool spots, and/or hard exudates (Fig. 4.11).
- Even if severe hypertension is present, patients still require investigation as suggested in p. 140 to exclude coexistent or underlying intracranial pathology; the hypertension could be a coincidental finding or, in rare cases, high ICP can cause secondary systemic hypertension.
- If severe hypertension is found, inpatient treatment under the care of a physician expert in this condition is advisable; the blood pressure should be gradually reduced in a controlled fashion and an underlying cause sought.

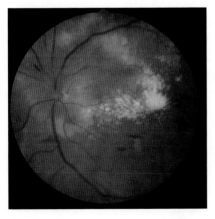

Fig. 4.11 Optic disc swelling in a patient with malignant hypertension. Note that florid hypertensive retinopathy is present in addition to the disc swelling; however, in some cases, disc swelling can be present without such changes.

Blood Glucose: Diabetic Papillopathy

- In "diabetic papillopathy," unilateral or bilateral disc swelling occurs in a patient with diabetes; vision usually remains normal, and with time, disc swelling resolves.
- In some cases, this is thought to be a "mild" form of anterior ischemic optic neuropathy (AION), but there may be a metabolic rather than ischemic etiology for the disc swelling.
- Signs of diabetic retinopathy are usually, but not always, present.
- However, it must be emphasized that just because a patient is diabetic, it doesn't mean that their disc swelling is due to diabetic papillopathy:
  - Diabetes is a common disease, and some patients with diabetes also develop (by chance) a brain tumor, dural venous sinus thrombosis, or IIH.
  - Patients with diabetes are also relatively immunosuppressed and are at risk of developing rare infectious causes of chronic meningitis (causing papilledema or optic perineuritis), e.g., fungal or tuberculous meningitis.
- Hence, diabetic papillopathy is a diagnosis of exclusion, after all the usual investigations for disc swelling (p. 140) have been pursued and found to be normal.
- Improving the patient's diabetic control and treating coexistent hypertension or renal dysfunction may accelerate the resolution of the condition.

Blood Electrolyte Disturbance

- Severe electrolyte disturbances are rare causes of disc swelling with normal or abnormal vision; examples include:
  - "uremic optic neuropathy" from renal failure
  - hypocalcemia
- Hence, electrolytes should be checked as part of the routine work-up for disc swelling.
- Improved metabolic control often results in resolution of disc swelling.

PAPILLEDEMA

Definition

- Papilledema is optic disc swelling due to proven raised ICP—proven by the presence of a large space-occupying lesion or hydrocephalus on neuroimaging, or by normal neuroimaging followed by an LP that shows a raised opening pressure.
- Papilledema is not a general name for optic disc swelling of all causes—it should only be used for disc swelling due to raised ICP; disc swelling of unknown cause should just be called "disc swelling."

Causes

(See pp. 159–176 for a more detailed discussion of these diseases.)

There are five main causes for papilledema:

1. Increased brain volume (common)
   - space-occupying lesions, such as a large brain tumor, hemorrhage, or abscess
   - cerebral edema from trauma or metabolic disease
2. Decreased skull volume (rare)
   - the craniosynostoses

3. Increased CSF production (rare)
   - choroid plexus tumors
4. Decreased CSF drainage (common)
   - Hydrocephalus
     - obstructive hydrocephalus: blockage of CSF flow through the ventricles (dilated ventricles on MRI)
     - communicating hydrocephalus: decreased absorption of CSF from the subarachnoid space by the arachnoid villi (normal ventricles on MRI).
   - Meningitis: bacterial, viral, fungal, leukemic, carcinomatous, causing a secondary obstructive or communicating hydrocephalus.
   - Subarachnoid hemorrhage: blood released into the CSF suddenly increases ICP and can cause a secondary communicating hydrocephalus.
   - Dural venous sinus thrombosis: thrombosis of one of the major dural venous sinuses causes decreased CSF resorption.
   - Extracranial venous outflow obstruction: blockage of an internal jugular vein in the neck or superior vena cava in the chest causes increased back-pressure into the venous sinuses and decreased CSF resorption.
5. PTCS (common)
   - Swollen disc/s, normal MRI/MRV or CT/CTV, normal CSF constituents, raised opening pressure on LP, no other neurologic disease
     - PTCS may be due to a known risk factor, e.g., tetracyclines, vitamin A, endocrine disease (e.g., hyper/hypothyroidism), sleep apnea, chronic respiratory disease (secondary PTCS).
     - PTCS associated with obesity (no other risk factors other than lateral venous sinus stenosis) is called primary PTCS or idiopathic intracranial hypertension (IIH).

Mechanism

- The optic nerves are surrounded by the optic nerve sheaths, an extension of the dura around the brain.
- The subarachnoid space of the optic nerve sheaths contains CSF that is in direct communication with the CSF flowing around the brain in the intracranial subarachnoid space.
- For this reason, if the CSF pressure around the brain is increased, high-pressure CSF in the optic nerve sheaths increases pressure on the optic nerves.
- Pressure on the optic nerve immediately behind the globe causes obstruction of orthograde axoplasmic flow in the optic nerve axons; a build-up of blocked axoplasm in the optic nerve head becomes visible as optic disc swelling.
- Early in the process, normal optic nerve function continues despite disc swelling; if the pressure is unrelieved or severe, optic nerve axon dysfunction and death can occur.

Incidence and Clinical Interpretation

Not all patients with raised intracranial pressure develop papilledema.
- Some patients with significantly raised ICP do not develop disc swelling at any time, particularly those in whom the pressure has increased slowly and those who have been shunted (e.g., for hydrocephalus) and who develop shunt failure.

- In addition, many brain tumors do not cause increased ICP in the first place.
- Hence, the absence of papilledema does not exclude serious intracranial pathology. The severity of disc swelling in papilledema does not necessarily correlate with the level of intracranial pressure.
  - Patients with severely raised ICP may only have mild disc swelling; conversely, fairly florid disc swelling can occur in patients with only modestly elevated ICP.
"Dead discs can't swell."
    - If extensive optic nerve axon death has already occurred, raised ICP will not cause disc swelling.
    - For example, in patients with preexisting optic atrophy of any cause (such as childhood hydrocephalus with untreated papilledema), the absence of disc swelling is NOT a reliable indication that ICP is not currently raised, as there are too few axons still alive for clinically visible swelling to occur.
    - Likewise, moderate or severe optic disc swelling will be seen to "resolve" as axon death occurs; this will be accompanied by worsening optic nerve function and increasing optic disc pallor as post-papilledema optic atrophy develops.
    - Optical coherence tomography can be used to show progressive neural damage by assessing the thickness of the retinal ganglion/inner plexiform layers.

Timecourse

- If changes in ICP are rapid and major, papilledema can both appear and disappear within hours of the pressure change; for example, papilledema can be visible within hours of a major subarachnoid hemorrhage.
- However, in cases of only mild or moderate IIH, it may take many weeks for disc swelling to appear, or to disappear if the raised pressure is relieved.

Symptoms

- Papilledema may be completely asymptomatic, with no headache and no visual symptoms, or any combination of the following symptoms may occur.

Neurologic Symptoms

- Headache with or without the following features suggestive of raised ICP:
  - new type of headache or unusually severe headaches
  - worse in the morning than the afternoon
  - worse on coughing, straining, bending over or lying down
- Note: many patients with raised ICP have very "benign"-sounding headaches (with none of these features) or no headache at all.
- Other neurologic symptoms:
  - pulsatile tinnitus (low-pitched "whooshing" noise in one or both ears in time with the pulse)
  - nonspecific paresthesias or weakness
  - symptoms related to the causative lesion (e.g., focal neurologic symptoms from a brain tumor or dural venous sinus thrombosis)

Ophthalmic Symptoms
- blurred vision due to:
  - optic nerve dysfunction
  - induced hypermetropia (the eyeball is shortened by pressure from the dilated optic nerve sheath); the patient may report difficulties reading despite intact distance vision
- transient visual obscurations (TVOs)
  - blurring or blacking out of the vision of one or both eyes, usually lasting seconds then resolving
  - often related to postural changes, coughing, or straining
  - probably caused by transient vascular insufficiency in the swollen disc
- photopsias (flashes or zig-zags of light)
- (sometimes) transient or persisting diplopia due to:
  - third, fourth, or sixth nerve palsy (or transient dysfunction of these) due to raised ICP
  - the causative brain lesion compressing one or more ocular motor nerves

Signs
- Unilateral or bilateral disc swelling
  - Although almost all cases of papilledema are bilateral, rare cases can be truly unilateral; this may be due to a congenital stenosis or adhesion of the optic nerve sheath to one nerve, so that increased CSF pressure is not transmitted to one optic nerve head.
  - However, in most cases of "unilateral" disc swelling due to proven raised ICP, the swelling is actually bilateral but highly asymmetric (subtle signs of swelling can be detected on the "normal" side with careful examination or fluorescein angiography).
- "Foster Kennedy syndrome"
  - This rare syndrome is the combination of unilateral papilledema with contralateral optic atrophy due to an intracranial tumor.
  - Classically caused by a large frontal olfactory groove meningioma that has caused compressive optic neuropathy on one side, plus papilledema due to its space-occupying effect in the brain (the atrophic disc does not swell, the other disc does).
  - A much more common cause of unilateral optic atrophy with contralateral disc swelling is a previous (sometimes unnoticed) optic neuropathy, with an anterior optic neuropathy of any cause on the contralateral side ("pseudo-Foster Kennedy syndrome").
- Visual acuity: normal or reduced
- Color vision: normal or reduced
- Visual fields: normal or any pattern of visual field defect, one or both eyes

Disc Appearance
Note: none of the following features is specific for papilledema rather than disc swelling of the many other possible causes, hence the need for thorough investigation.

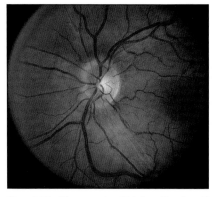

Fig. 4.12 Very early (Frisén Grade 1) papilledema. Note mild optic disc hyperemia and blurring of some but not all of the disc margin. There is no obscuration of the disc vessels.

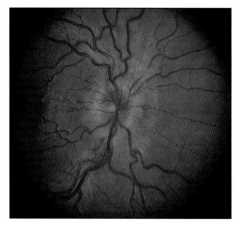

Fig. 4.13 Early (Frisén Grade 2) papilledema. The optic disc is definitely hyperemic and there is blurring of the entire disc margin. The vessels are not obscured.

Nevertheless, the Frisén grading scale often is used to describe the severity of papilledema (and other types of optic disc swelling).

- VERY EARLY papilledema (Frisén Grade 1; Fig. 4.12):
  - mild disc hyperemia
  - mild blurring of some but not all disc margin
- EARLY papilledema (Frisén Grade 2; Fig. 4.13):
  - disc hyperemia
  - blurring of entire disc margin
- MODERATE papilledema (Frisén Grade 3; Fig. 4.14):
  - disc hyperemia
  - obvious disc elevation
  - blurring of all disc margins
  - obscuration of some (but not all) of the major vessels as they cross the border of the disc
- MARKED papilledema (Frisén Grade 4; Fig. 4.15):
  - obvious disc elevation
  - disc hyperemia
  - blurring of entire disc margin
  - obscuration of some vessels overlying the disc
  - pseudo-drusen (bright yellow bodies resembling disc drusen) may be present on disc surface
- SEVERE papilledema (Frisén Grade 5; Fig. 4.16):
  - obvious disc elevation
  - disc margin appears blurred and rounded
  - ALL major vessels crossing disc obscured
  - pseudo-drusen often present

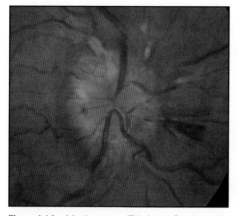

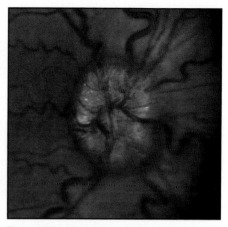

Fig. 4.14 Moderate (Frisén Grade 3) papilledema. There is obvious disc hyperemia and elevation, blurring of all disc margin, and obscuration of some (but not all) of the major vessels as they cross the border of the disc.

Fig. 4.15 Marked (Frisén Grade 4) papilledema. There is obvious disc hyperemia and elevation, blurring of the entire disc margin, obscuration of some vessels overlying the optic disc, and pseudo-drusen (bright yellow bodies resembling disc drusen).

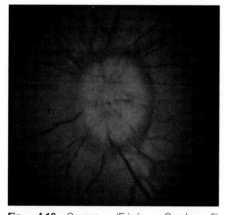

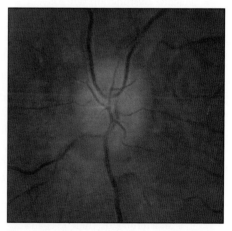

Fig. 4.16 Severe (Frisén Grade 5) papilledema. There is obvious disc elevation. The disc margin is blurred and rounded. All major vessels crossing the disc are obscured.

Fig. 4.17 Postpapilledema optic atrophy. The disc is diffusely pale and has a "fuzzy" appearance.

- Postpapilledema optic atrophy (no Frisén grade; Fig. 4.17):
    - disc minimally or no longer elevated; disc pale
    - "fuzzy" (gliotic) appearance; halo around disc
    - no hemorrhages or exudates (but may have exudates in macula if papilledema was previously severe)
    - remnants of retinal folds or striae may be visible

Complications

Neurologic
- complications of the cause, e.g., the brain tumor, meningitis, etc.
- complications of raised ICP itself, e.g., a unilateral or bilateral sixth nerve palsy

Ophthalmic
- Optic nerve dysfunction:
  - Persistent papilledema of ANY cause, if acute and severe or moderate and prolonged, can cause permanent optic nerve dysfunction or even blindness.
  - Decreased color vision and midperipheral visual field loss on perimetry are usually the earliest indicators of optic nerve damage; these may sometimes be reversed if ICP is normalized with treatment.
  - Later on, central acuity can be lost; irreversible bilateral blindness can eventually occur from unrelieved papilledema.
  - Acute severe papilledema can cause sudden severe irreversible visual loss within days if untreated; the mechanism may be secondary acute infarction of the swollen discs.
  - Less severe papilledema can cause slowly progressive visual field loss (and, as in glaucoma, eventually acuity loss) over weeks or months.
- Macular dysfunction due to:
  - Serous fluid or hard exudates in the macula or subretinal fluid under the macula.
  - Retinal or choroidal folds crossing the macula.
- CRVO: compression of the central retinal vein by a swollen optic nerve head can cause a secondary CRVO.
- Hemorrhage:
  - Peripapillary hemorrhages (often splinter or flame-shaped disc margin hemorrhages).
  - In rare cases, a peripapillary choroidal neovascular membrane can develop and leak fluid or bleed.
  - Preretinal ± vitreous hemorrhage can occur when there is a sudden severe rise in ICP, as in subarachnoid hemorrhage (Terson syndrome).
- Refractive change:
  - Patients with significant disc swelling may have induced hypermetropia from a shortening of their eyeball's axial length as the swollen optic nerve sheath indents the posterior sclera.
  - Patients with this problem often benefit greatly from the appropriate refractive correction, if their distance or near vision improves significantly with pinhole.

Differential Diagnosis
- Pseudo-disc swelling.
- True disc swelling from other causes (anterior optic neuropathy of any cause)
  - There are no specific signs that can tell you that disc swelling is papilledema rather than disc swelling from other causes.
  - Because of this, all cases of bilateral disc swelling (with normal or reduced vision) must be urgently investigated to exclude brain tumors and other causes of raised ICP.

Investigations

- Investigations to confirm that the discs are truly swollen (and not "pseudo-swelling"): see p. 145 earlier.
- If true disc swelling is present: refer to a neuro-ophthalmologist or neurologist, or investigate urgently as suggested on p. 140.

Treatment

- All patients with papilledema require regular ophthalmic follow-up, including visual acuity, color vision, perimetry, and disc examination at each visit.
- It is a tragedy if the brain tumor or dural venous sinus thrombosis is eventually "cured" but the patient is left blind with optic atrophy from persistent neglected papilledema.
- In some cases, decreasing optic nerve function may be the only indication to operate or treat.
- See treatment sections for specific diseases later.

DISEASES THAT CAN CAUSE PAPILLEDEMA

- brain tumors
- hydrocephalus
- meningitis
- dural venous sinus thrombosis
- extracranial venous outflow obstruction
- PTCS of known cause (secondary PTCS)
- PTCS associated with obesity and venous sinus stenosis (primary PTCS, aka IIH)

BRAIN TUMORS

Demographic

- any age, male or female.

Mechanism

There are three possible mechanisms by which tumors cause papilledema:
- as large space-occupying lesions (Fig. 4.18)
- by causing obstructive hydrocephalus (Fig. 4.19)
- by producing excessive CSF (rare).

Symptoms

- The patient may or may not have any visual symptoms related to the papilledema.
- In some cases, there is also persisting or transient diplopia.
- Headaches may be "suspicious" sounding, sound like "migraine" or "common tension headache," or the patient may not have headaches at all.
- There may or may not be other neurologic symptoms, such as personality change, memory difficulties, seizures, problems with walking or coordination, focal weakness, focal numbness/pins and needles.

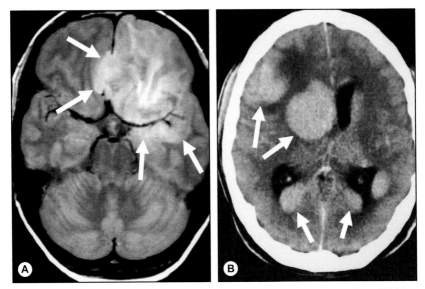

Fig. 4.18 Examples of brain tumors causing papilledema from their mass effect. (**A**) Magnetic resonance imaging shows a large oligodendroglioma *(arrows)* causing swelling of the left frontal and temporal lobes. (**B**) Computed tomography scan shows multicentric lymphoma causing both a mass effect and hydrocephalus *(arrows)*.

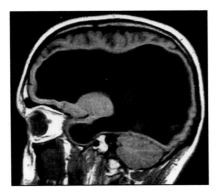

Fig. 4.19 Magnetic resonance imaging shows marked obstructive hydrocephalus. The patient had severe postpapilledema optic atrophy by the time of the evaluation.

Signs

- Papilledema may be unilateral or bilateral and, if bilateral, may be symmetric or highly asymmetric.
- There may in some cases also be a homonymous visual field defect on confrontation testing or perimetry due to compression of the retrochiasmal visual pathways.
- Motility may be abnormal if the tumor is directly compressing an ocular motor center in the brain or ocular motor nerve/s, or if raised ICP itself is exerting pressure on one or more of the third, fourth, or sixth nerves (unilateral or bilateral).

Investigations

- MRI brain with contrast will detect almost all brain tumors (see Fig. 4.18A) (CT may miss small tumors, but should detect tumors that cause papilledema; see Fig. 4.18B).
- Further investigations may include biopsy of the mass and extracranial imaging looking for a primary tumor (in the case of a suspected metastasis).

Treatment

- Treatment options include observation, surgery, radiotherapy, chemotherapy, or a combination of these.
- Whatever the specific therapy, it is essential that any patient with a brain tumor causing papilledema is also followed closely by an ophthalmologist with serial examinations including visual field testing.

HYDROCEPHALUS

Definition

- There is obstruction to the normal flow of CSF within the cranial cavity or a decrease in its resorption into the venous system.

Demographic

- any age, male or female

Mechanism and Types

- Congenital or acquired: expansion of skull diameter occurs in infants with congenital or early acquired hydrocephalus (this does not occur in older children or adults).
- Communicating or obstructive
  - Communicating hydrocephalus
    - CSF flows freely through the ventricles and out into the subarachnoid space but has impaired absorption into the dural venous sinuses.
    - An MRI scan of the brain shows normal-sized ventricles.
    - Causes include meningitis and subarachnoid hemorrhage.
  - Obstructive hydrocephalus
    - CSF flow is obstructed at some point within the brain.
    - MRI scan shows dilation of one or more ventricles (see Fig. 4.19).
    - Causes include compressive tumor, infection, hemorrhage, idiopathic.

Symptoms

- The patient may or may not have headaches, and if headaches are present, they may or may not sound "suspicious."
- There may or may not be visual symptoms related to papilledema.
- Diplopia may also sometimes occur.

Signs

- Papilledema may be mild to severe.
- Note: "dead discs don't swell"
  - Many patients with long-standing hydrocephalus have postpapilledema optic atrophy from earlier neglected papilledema.
  - If both discs are moderately or severely pale and there is substantial acuity and/or field loss, it is important to realize that the lack of disc swelling is not a reliable indicator that ICP is normal.
- Pressure from hydrocephalus can sometimes cause abnormal ocular motility, including unilateral or bilateral third, fourth, or sixth nerve palsies or dorsal midbrain syndrome.

Investigations

- In cases of obstructive hydrocephalus, MRI brain scan with contrast demonstrates both the dilated ventricles and the causative lesion if present.
- However, a normal MRI scan does not exclude the possibility of communicating hydrocephalus: hence, the need to always obtain an LP if an MRI and MRV (or CTV) are normal in a patient with papilledema.

Treatment

- Communicating hydrocephalus: treatment is often medical (e.g., for chronic meningitis).
- Obstructive hydrocephalus: treatment is usually surgical. An obstructing tumor may be excised; the obstructed foramen can be surgically enlarged or a ventriculoperitoneal CSF shunt can be placed in the obstructed ventricle to drain the high-pressure fluid.

MENINGITIS

Causes

- Infectious meningitis
  - acute bacterial
  - chronic bacterial, including tuberculosis
  - viral.
  - fungal (e.g., cryptococcal)
- Carcinomatous meningitis: the meninges are diffusely seeded by malignant cells, from leukemia, lymphoma, or metastasis from an extracranial solid tumor (e.g., breast cancer).
- sarcoid meningitis

Mechanism

- Papilledema can occur from raised ICP due to secondary hydrocephalus (often communicating, less commonly obstructive).

Symptoms

- There may be persistent or intermittent blurred vision or diplopia: this can be a result of raised ICP or the causative organisms or cancer cells can directly invade and destroy the optic nerves and/or the ocular motor nerves.

- It should be noted that in chronic meningitis (tuberculous, fungal, carcinomatous, or sarcoid), there are often none of the "meningitic" warning symptoms of acute meningitis; often headaches are nonspecific and there is no neck stiffness, photophobia, or rash.

Signs

- There may be visual acuity or field defects from severe or prolonged papilledema or direct optic nerve invasion.
- ± Abnormal ocular motility.
- There may also be dysfunction of any of the other cranial nerves.

Investigations

- MRI plus MRV (or CTV) should always be performed before LP; sometimes the MRI shows meningeal enhancement with contrast in meningitis.
- The only way to diagnose meningitis is by analysis of CSF from LP
  - Opening pressure is often elevated.
  - Microbiologic study may reveal the infectious organism or a raised white cell count, suggesting infection.
  - Cytology may show malignant cells in carcinomatous meningitis.
  - Often in chronic meningitis, CSF protein is increased and glucose is decreased.

Treatment

- infectious meningitis: high-dose intravenous antibiotics ± surgical procedures to relieve ICP
- carcinomatous meningitis: often whole-brain radiotherapy and/or chemotherapy

DURAL VENOUS SINUS THROMBOSIS

Demographic

- male or female, any age

Mechanism

- The superior sagittal sinus and/or one of the transverse sinuses become obstructed with clot and ceases to drain CSF from the subarachnoid space (Fig. 4.20).
- This leads to a rise in ICP, causing headaches and papilledema.
- The venous sinuses also drain the cerebral veins; sinus obstruction can cause back-pressure in these veins, resulting in cerebral venous infarction leading to a stroke.

Causes

- factors increasing venous blood clotting (coagulopathy)
  - anticardiolipin antibody/lupus anticoagulant (LA) syndrome
  - infection adjacent to a sinus (e.g., infectious mastoiditis from a middle ear infection)
  - others, e.g., dehydration, pregnancy, cancer
- factors interrupting venous sinus blood flow: compression of a sinus by a tumor is a rare cause
- idiopathic

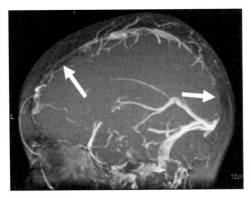

Fig. 4.20 Magnetic resonance venography showing thrombosis of the superior sagittal sinus. Thrombi are indicated by *arrows*.

Symptoms

- Visual symptoms
  - There may or may not be transient or persistent blurred vision from papilledema.
  - Diplopia may also occur.
- Neurologic symptoms
  - Headache
    - Often of sudden onset and severe; however, may be less acute.
    - Often has features suggestive of raised ICP (p. 154).
  - Other neurologic symptoms
    - The patient may be "otherwise well" apart from headache or
    - There may be neurologic symptoms due to brain dysfunction from venous congestion or stroke (drowsiness, confusion, arm or leg numbness or weakness, sometimes coma).

Signs

- Papilledema ranges from mild to very severe.
- Ocular motility may be disturbed, e.g., unilateral or bilateral sixth nerve palsy.
- Other neurologic signs may be absent or, if present, of any severity.

Investigations

- Urgent MRI plus MRV or CTV
  - Dural venous sinus thrombosis is often visible on MRI scan alone, but MRV or CTV will sometimes detect a thrombosis that MRI alone will miss.
  - CT scan is not appropriate, as it will miss most cases of venous sinus thrombosis.
- Investigations to determine the underlying cause, e.g., a coagulopathy (LA panels, activated protein C resistance, protein C and protein S activity, antithrombin activity, and specific factor activity levels).

Treatment

- Most patients are admitted to an acute neurology unit for supportive care and anticoagulation to prevent extension of the clot and to possibly open the lumen of the vessel.

- Anticoagulation alone, however, may not result in rapid resolution of papilledema: if severe papilledema is present and permanent visual loss is likely, urgent CSF diversion surgery (shunt) or optic nerve sheath fenestration may be required to save sight; obtain an urgent neuro-ophthalmic opinion if possible.
- If moderate papilledema is present, medical treatment may be sufficient to protect vision.
- The underlying cause of the thrombosis should be treated.

EXTRACRANIAL VENOUS OUTFLOW OBSTRUCTION

Mechanism

- All venous blood from the brain drains back to the heart via the internal jugular veins in the neck and the superior vena cava in the chest.
- Obstruction of these veins in the neck or chest can therefore cause venous back-pressure in the head, reducing CSF drainage and causing headaches and/or papilledema (Fig. 4.21A and B).

Causes

- Compression of the veins: skull base, neck, or superior mediastinal tumors, e.g., glomus tumors, large thyroid goiters or thyroid tumors, mediastinal lymphoma.
- Severe chronic respiratory disease: can cause obstructed venous return from the head by effects on intrathoracic pressure.

Symptoms and Signs

- Headaches and/or visual symptoms, plus in some cases:
  - The external jugular venous pressure may be elevated on examination (dilated external jugular vein visible with the patient sitting up) (see Fig. 4.21C).
  - A neck or sternal notch mass may be palpable.

Investigations

- If the condition is suspected and MRI plus MRV (or CTV) brain are normal, request MRI neck and upper thorax as well, looking for a compressive lesion.

Treatment

- Surgery or chemotherapy for the compressive neck or chest mass often causes complete resolution of both headaches and papilledema.

SECONDARY PSEUDOTUMOR CEREBRI SYNDROME (PSEUDOTUMOR CEREBRI OF KNOWN CAUSE OTHER THAN OBESITY AND VENOUS SINUS STENOSIS)

Definition

- Swollen optic disc/s ± headaches.
- No neurologic signs other than a unilateral or bilateral sixth nerve palsy in some cases.

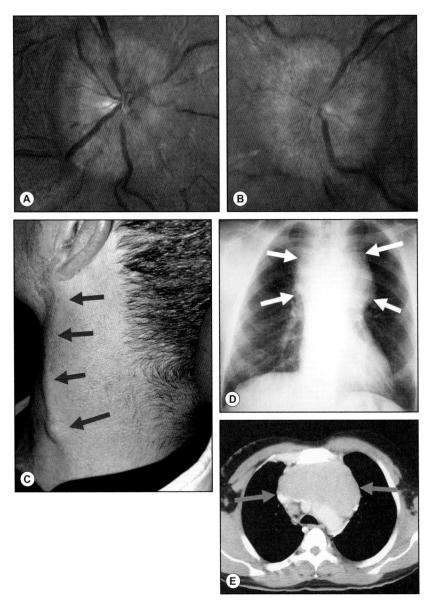

Fig. 4.21 Papilledema due to extracranial venous outflow obstruction. (**A, B**) This 37-year-old man was noticed by his optometrist on a routine examination to have bilateral disc swelling. (**C**) Examination of the patient's neck revealed elevated external jugular venous pressure *(arrows)*. (**D**) Chest x-ray showed a widened mediastinum. (**E**) Chest computed tomography revealed a large mediastinal tumor compressing the superior vena cava. Papilledema resolved as tumor size decreased with chemotherapy.

- Normal MRI and MRV or CTV brain (other than dilated optic nerve sheaths or slightly narrowed ventricles in some cases) (CT brain is not adequate). (Please note that this does not necessarily differentiate secondary pseudotumor cerebri from primary pseudotumor cerebri.)
- LP shows raised opening pressure and absolutely normal CSF constituents (normal microbiology, biochemistry, and cytology).
- Normal full blood count, glucose, electrolytes, liver function tests, ESR, CRP, ACE, ANA; normal blood pressure, temperature, chest x-ray, and urine analysis.
- On specific questioning, there is a history of one or more systemic diseases, therapeutic drugs, vitamins, or toxins that can cause secondary PTCS (see list below), other than obesity and venous sinus stenosis.

Demographic

- any age, male or female

Mechanism

- The specific mechanism is unknown, but it is thought that resorption of CSF by the dural venous sinuses is impaired (without evidence of dural venous sinus thrombosis on imaging).

Possible Causes

- Medications and foods, including:
    - vitamin A, vitamin A–containing compounds (e.g., some acne treatment creams or tablets such as isotretinoin) and excessive intake of vitamin A–containing foods (e.g., carrots or liver)
    - tetracycline antibiotics (often used long term as acne treatment)
    - steroids (or steroid withdrawal)
    - some nonsteroidal anti-inflammatory drugs
    - cyclosporin
    - oral contraceptive pill or contraceptive implants
    - others (see "Suggested reading," p. 341)
- Diseases:
    - severe chronic respiratory disease, including obstructive sleep apnea syndrome (suspect if history of severe snoring with headache and drowsiness in the morning)
    - renal failure
    - severe anemia
    - endocrine disease, e.g., hypo/hyperthyroidism, Addison disease
- Toxins, e.g., lead poisoning
- In addition, there are many reports of other possible, but as yet unproven, risk factors.

Symptoms and Signs

- identical with those of IIH (see later)

Investigations

- As suggested on p. 140.
- Take a careful medication history; ask especially about acne treatment (creams or tablets) and contraception.
- If system review questions reveal a possible undiagnosed disease (e.g., symptoms of hyper- or hypothyroidism), add the appropriate tests to your investigations.
- Sleep studies may help to confirm possible obstructive sleep apnea syndrome.

Treatment

- Treat or eliminate the risk factor if possible, for example:
  - Cease a possibly causative medication (e.g., vitamin A-based acne cream or tetracycline tablets) or food (excessive intake of carrots).
  - Treat a possibly causative underlying disease, e.g., dialysis for renal failure, blood transfusion for severe anemia, treatment of obstructive sleep apnea syndrome with a positive pressure mask during sleep.
- It is essential to look for and treat these possible risk factors if at all possible, as this may result in partial or complete resolution of the IIH.
- However, moderate or severe papilledema also requires treatment in its own right, even if a known risk factor has been identified; for example, acetazolamide treatment or CSF diversion surgery may be necessary to save vision (don't just wait for treatment of a possible cause to result in improvement). See the IIH section next for treatment options.

IDIOPATHIC INTRACRANIAL HYPERTENSION (IIH; ALSO KNOWN AS PRIMARY PSEUDOTUMOR CEREBRI SYNDROME) ASSOCIATED WITH OBESITY AND VENOUS SINUS STENOSIS

Definition

- Swollen optic disc/s ± headaches.
- No neurologic signs other than a unilateral or bilateral sixth nerve palsy in some cases.
- Normal MRI and MRV (or CTV) brain (other than dilated optic nerve sheaths, flattening of the posterior globe, slightly narrowed ventricles in some cases, and lateral [transverse] stenosis in most cases; Fig. 4.22) (CT brain is not adequate).
- LP shows raised opening pressure and absolutely normal CSF constituents (normal microbiology, biochemistry, and cytology).
- Normal full blood count, glucose, electrolytes, liver function tests, ESR, CRP, ACE, ANA; normal blood pressure, temperature, chest x-ray, and urine analysis.
- On specific questioning, no history of systemic disease, therapeutic drugs, vitamins, or toxins that can cause secondary pseudotumor cerebri syndrome (see list in p. 167), other than obesity.

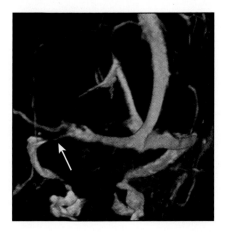

Fig. 4.22 Computed tomographic venography showing severe stenosis of the right lateral (transverse) sinus *(arrow)* in a patient with intracranial hypertension.

Terminology

- Previously called "benign intracranial hypertension" (BIH).
- However, this is not a "benign" disease: many patients lose vision despite treatment, complete bilateral blindness is possible, and many patients have severe disabling headaches.
- Hence, the preferred term is "idiopathic intracranial hypertension" or "primary pseudotumor cerebri syndrome."

Demographic

- Peak incidence in overweight young and middle-aged women (Fig. 4.23).
- Overweight men can also develop the condition.
- Caution: just because a patient with papilledema is an obese young woman does NOT mean that the diagnosis is primary IIH! We have seen many overweight female patients "clinically diagnosed" as IIH, when further investigation in fact reveals dural venous sinus thrombosis or a brain tumor.

Mechanism

- The mechanism is unknown but CSF absorption into the dural venous sinuses seems to be impaired.

Symptoms

- Visual
  - Vision may be normal or constantly blurred or the patient may complain of TVOs (blurred vision usually lasting seconds, one or both eyes, often precipitated by a change in posture).
  - In some cases there are flashes of light (photopsias).
  - There may also be transient or constant diplopia from a unilateral or bilateral sixth nerve palsy.

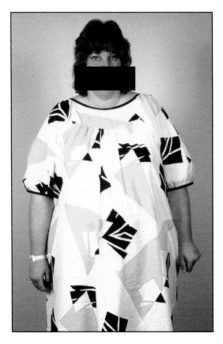

Fig. 4.23 Appearance of a young with idiopathic intracranial hypertension.

- Neurologic
  - Headache
    - Constant or intermittent.
    - Often described as throbbing or pounding but patients may also have intermittent "sharp pains."
    - Often, but not always, suggestive of raised ICP: worse in the morning or with coughing, straining, bending over or lying down.
    - However, some patients have no headache at all or only minor headache, despite prominent visual symptoms.
  - Pulsatile tinnitus
    - Low-pitched "whooshing" noise heard in one or both ears in time with the pulse.
    - Often intermittent; may be precipitated by coughing, straining, or lying down.
    - There should be no other significant neurologic symptoms.

Signs

- ophthalmic
  - papilledema (usually bilateral but may be highly asymmetric)
  - otherwise normal ocular examination
  - in some patients, unilateral or bilateral sixth nerve palsy
- neurologic: no other systemic neurologic signs

Complications

- It is essential that ophthalmologists retain contact with patients with IIH because, although headaches can be very troubling, visual loss is the only permanent disability that can result (Fig. 4.24).

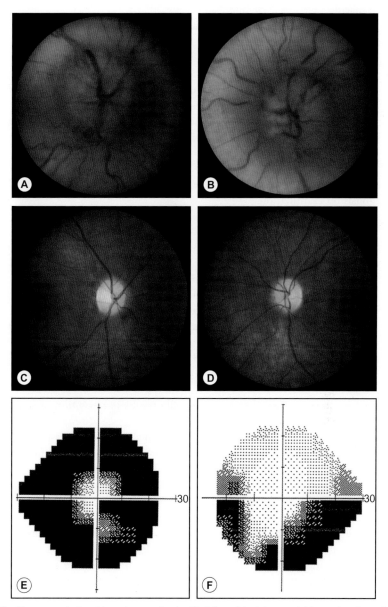

Fig. 4.24 Permanent visual loss in a patient with idiopathic intracranial hypertension who was not treated in a timely manner. (**A, B**) Marked/severe papilledema at time of initial examination. (**C, D**) Postpapilledema optic atrophy. (**E, F**) Visual fields show significant defects, worse in the right eye (**E**) than in the left (**F**).

- Acuity loss
  - A worrying sign indicating severe involvement.
  - Can occur early and suddenly (secondary to acute disc infarction) in acute severe IIH or as a gradual late change in patients with moderate but neglected IIH.
  - Often irreversible unless caused by hemorrhage, exudate, and/or subretinal fluid in macula.
- Color vision loss: usually occurs late but sometimes reversible.
- Field loss
  - Usually the earliest detectable change.
  - Midperipheral scotomas, arcuate scotomas, and nasal steps are common early findings. There is generalized field constriction in some patients; in addition, the blind spots are usually enlarged.
  - As with glaucoma, visual field is almost always lost before visual acuity decreases; unlike glaucoma, some of this field loss may be reversible if ICP is normalized.

Differential Diagnosis

- All other causes of disc swelling; there are no clinical features specific for IIH as a diagnosis on examination.

Investigations

- IIH must never be diagnosed unless ALL the following have been performed and found to be completely normal:
  - MRI optic nerves and brain with contrast, plus MRV (or CTV) brain.
  - CSF microbiology, biochemistry, and cytology.
  - Blood pressure, temperature, chest x-ray, and urine analysis.
  - Blood test for full blood count, electrolytes, glucose, liver function tests, ESR, CRP, ACE, ANA.
- The only abnormality should be raised opening pressure on LP.

Treatment

- Timely and appropriate treatment generally results in resolution of symptoms of increased ICP and papilledema (Fig. 4.25).
- The only permanent "cure" is weight loss, which should be aggressively pursued.
- While the patient loses weight, safeguard their vision and alleviate their headaches with medical and/or surgical control of their ICP
  - In cases of acute severe IIH, early surgical intervention using shunt insertion or optic nerve sheath fenestration is advisable as medical treatment alone may not avert acute visual loss.
  - In mild or moderate cases, treat with oral acetazolamide initially, progressing to surgery if visual loss develops or progresses despite this.
- Refer to a neuro-ophthalmologist early if you are unsure of the appropriate treatment; once visual loss has occurred in IIH, it is usually irreversible.
- Treatment options include the following.

Observation Without Treatment Other Than Weight Loss

- Is appropriate in mild cases without significant headache and with only mild papilledema, with no visual symptoms and normal visual acuity, color acuity, and perimetry.

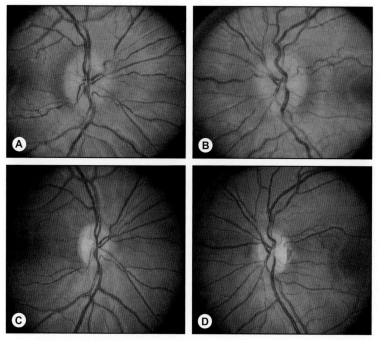

Fig. 4.25 Resolution of papilledema with preservation of normal vision in a patient with idiopathic intracranial hypertension. (**A, B**) Appearance of the optic discs when patient was first examined. Note early (Frisén Grade 2) papilledema. The patient was treated with acetazolamide (500 mg bid) with rapid and complete resolution of papilledema (**C, D**).

Weight Loss

- First check that there are no other underlying causes other than obesity (see list p. 167), e.g., that the patient is not also using a vitamin A–containing acne cream that could be exacerbating the disease.
- All patients with confirmed primary IIH should have their diagnosis carefully explained to them, along with the fact that the only permanent "cure" for their condition is weight loss (medication and surgery for their raised ICP is only a temporizing measure).
- Substantial weight loss almost always improves both headaches and papilledema.
- Enlisting the help of the patient's family physician early on is essential; referral to a dietitian may also help.
- There is evidence that bariatric surgery, especially gastric bypass, is more likely to be effective in achieving weight loss than a weight loss program, both short-term and long-term.

Medical Treatment

Oral Acetazolamide (Diamox)

- Usually the first-line medical treatment for IIH.
- Mechanism: decreases the production of CSF by the choroid plexus; also aids in weight loss.

- Contraindications
  - pregnancy (warn women not to become pregnant while taking the drug and for 6 months after ceasing it)
  - liver or renal failure

**Sulfa allergy is NOT a contraindication to using acetazolamide; it is a different form of sulfa!

- Side effects
  - common (warn the patient to avoid undue concern and increase compliance)
    - fatigue, depression
    - numbness or "pins and needles" around the mouth and in the fingers and toes
    - nausea
    - metallic taste of carbonated drinks
  - Rare
    - electrolyte disturbance; liver or renal compromise
    - side effects of sulfa drugs, including allergic rash, aplastic anemia, and Stevens-Johnson syndrome
- Dose
  - Usually begin with 500 mg sustained-release bid (the sustained-release capsules have a more powerful clinical effect than the standard tablets) or 250 mg tid or qid nonsustained release.
  - If visual function improves or stabilizes and papilledema resolves, the dose can be slowly decreased as the patient loses weight.
  - If visual function, headaches, and/or papilledema worsen, the dose can be increased up to 4 g/day depending on patient's tolerance of side effects.

Note that many patients with IIH have headaches unrelated to increased ICP. In such patients, the headaches often respond to antimigraine medications.

- Monitoring: may be appropriate to perform blood test at each visit (or at least before and just after starting the drug) for full blood count, electrolytes, renal and liver function tests.

Oral Diuretics

- Second-line treatment, usually reserved for patients who cannot tolerate acetazolamide.
- Because of the risk of hypokalemia with a single diuretic, the use of a combined "potassium-sparing" diuretic (e.g., amiloride plus furosemide: co-amilofruse) is safest.
- May cause electrolyte disturbance, hence the need for regular blood monitoring.

Oral Topiramate (Topamax)

- Theoretically reduces CSF production, decreases appetite, and treats headache.
- Unproven efficacy.
- Side effects are common, including tiredness, drowsiness, dizziness, loss of coordination, tingling of the hands/feet, loss of appetite, bad taste in the mouth, diarrhea, and weight loss—similar to side effects of acetazolamide!
- Should never be used in pregnant women as may cause oral clefts in infants of mothers who use drug during pregnancy.
- May cause choroidal effusions leading to shallowing of the anterior chamber angle and secondary angle-closure glaucoma.

Surgical Treatment

- Although all techniques have a high failure rate in the long term, they are good temporizing measures to save vision and/or relieve severe headaches while the patient loses weight.
- The right time to consider these treatments is before irreversible visual loss occurs.
- An urgent neuro-ophthalmic opinion is advisable before referring patients for surgical treatment.
- There are three principal techniques available: optic nerve sheath fenestration, neurosurgical shunt insertion, and stenting of a stenosed cerebral venous sinus (usually the transverse).
  - Optic nerve sheath fenestration:
    - Indication: IIH where vision is threatened and headache is not severe.
    - Mechanism: a window is cut in the immediately retrobulbar part of the distended optic nerve sheath, allowing high-pressure CSF to escape into the orbit (where it is absorbed by the orbital tissues).
    - Complications:
      - damage to the optic nerve or retinal vasculature (e.g., central retinal artery or vein occlusion), which can result in blindness
      - diplopia
      - persistent anisocoria
    - As with shunt insertion, there is usually only a temporary benefit from this procedure: the majority will stop working within a year or two so it is essential that the patient attempts to "cure themselves" with weight loss before the fenestration stops working.
    - It is not safe to repeat sheath fenestration once it fails; this is a "once-only" procedure.
  - Neurosurgical shunt insertion:
    - Indication: IIH where vision is threatened and/or headaches are severe and not controlled by medical treatment.
    - Mechanism:
      - CSF is drained by an implanted tube (from the lateral ventricle or lumbar subarachnoid space) into the peritoneal cavity in the abdomen or the atrium of the heart, where it is absorbed.
      - As opposed to optic nerve sheath fenestration, shunt insertion usually substantially relieves headache and safeguards vision.
    - Complications:
      - meningitis
      - hemorrhage
      - peritonitis
      - overdrainage causing low-pressure headaches
      - moderate failure rate (i.e., shunt obstruction) in the short term
    - Efficacy:
      - As with optic nerve sheath fenestration, some shunts will stop working within a year or two, so it is essential that the patient attempts to "cure themselves" with weight loss before this occurs.
      - However, as opposed to sheath fenestration, shunts can be revised or replaced as many times as necessary.

- Stenting:
  - Indication: IIH where vision is threatened and/or headaches are severe and not controlled by medical management AND there is unilateral or bilateral cerebral venous sinus stenosis (usually transverse sinus).
  - Mechanism: eliminates the gradient across the stenosed sinus, allowing normal venous drainage.
  - Complications:
    - recurrent stenosis proximal to the stent
    - bleeding
    - infection.
  - Efficacy:
    - immediately lowers intracranial pressure
    - almost always rapidly improves papilledema, headache, and vision

Note: "serial LPs"
- One or more LPs performed in the acute phase for severe acute IIH may be a useful temporizing measure; as well as acutely decreasing ICP, some CSF usually continues to leak from the perforated spinal dura for up to several weeks after the LP.
- However, LPs repeated many times over several months as "treatment" are often very uncomfortable for the patient and this is not a substitute for surgical intervention if medical treatment is failing to control the disease.

Follow-up

- The follow-up of patients with stable chronic IIH is similar to that for patients with chronic glaucoma: regular clinic visits over many years, with perimetry at every visit, and changes in medication based on changes in the visual field and disc examination.
- The exception is in acute severe IIH, where frequent (even daily) monitoring, often as an inpatient in an acute neurology unit, is required to detect rapid changes that may mandate urgent surgical intervention.
- It is essential that every patient with IIH undergoes serial perimetry until the disease has completely resolved
  - As with glaucoma, the visual loss of severe or prolonged papilledema usually affects the peripheral visual field first, with central visual acuity only declining as a late change (after severe irreversible field loss has occurred).
- Some general neurologists don't appreciate the importance of this, so if you have handed over the treatment of your patient to a neurologist, it is important that you also continue ophthalmic follow-up of the patient; advise the neurologist of changes in the perimetry that may indicate the need for additional treatment to save vision.

Transient Visual Loss

Introduction

Transient visual loss can be caused by disease of the:

- eye
- optic nerve
- orbit
- brain
- neck
- heart

A careful history and examination can often localize the disease. The most critical distinction is whether transient visual loss is monocular or binocular, but this is often very difficult to establish on history as patients may believe that because they have transiently lost vision to the left or right, the loss has been in the left or right eye!

Overall, the most common cause of monocular transient visual loss seen by ophthalmologists is amaurosis fugax due to carotid stenosis; the most common cause of transient binocular visual disturbance is migraine. However, there are many other causes, including giant cell arteritis (GCA), compressive optic nerve tumor, and papilledema.

Nonmigraine transient visual loss is often the first warning sign of serious systemic vascular disease. Rather than just reassuring the patient that "there is nothing wrong with your eyes," it is important to refer or investigate them appropriately. A few minutes of your time may add many years to their life.

As eye care professionals, we all need to know the following four things about transient visual loss:

1. How to make a clinical diagnosis of amaurosis fugax and how patients with this symptom should be investigated (p. 180).
2. How to make a clinical diagnosis of the visual prodrome of migraine (with or without headache) (p. 181).
3. How to make a clinical diagnosis of vertebrobasilar insufficiency (VBI) and how patients with this condition should be investigated (p. 182).
4. And what to do for all other patients with transient visual loss. We recommend that these patients be referred to a neuro-ophthalmologist for further assessment.

MONOCULAR TRANSIENT VISUAL LOSS

Transient visual loss in one eye can be caused by disease in the:
- eye: transient angle-closure glaucoma, tear film disturbance, incipient retinal vascular occlusion, retinal vasospasm (previously called "ocular migraine")
- optic nerve: compressive orbital tumor, Uhthoff phenomenon, GCA
- brain: papilledema, pituitary tumor compressing one intracranial optic nerve
- neck: amaurosis fugax (transient monocular embolic visual loss) or ocular ischemic syndrome due to carotid artery atherosclerosis or internal carotid dissecting aneurysm
- heart: valve disease releasing emboli that cause amaurosis fugax

BINOCULAR TRANSIENT VISUAL LOSS

Transient visual loss in both eyes can be caused by disease in:
- both eyes or optic nerves at the same time (rare)
- the brain: migraine (with or without headache), transient visual obscurations (TVOs) due to papilledema, bilateral optic nerve, or chiasmal compression by pituitary tumor
- the neck or heart: transient homonymous or global visual field loss due to embolism in the carotid or vertebrobasilar arterial systems, VBI due to atherosclerosis or dissecting aneurysm, postural hypotension/presyncope

Examination Checklist

TRANSIENT VISUAL LOSS

Have you asked about, and looked for, all the following key features?

History

- ☐ Ophthalmic symptoms?
- ☐ Related to changes in posture (e.g., changing from lying to sitting position)?
- ☐ The episode/s of transient visual loss
  - ☐ One or both eyes affected? How do you know? Did you cover one eye and then the other to see if one or both eyes were affected?
  - ☐ Activities at onset/precipitating factors?
  - ☐ Speed of onset?
  - ☐ Exact nature of visual symptoms? Positive phenomena (e.g., flashing lights, zigzag lines), negative phenomena (blacking or blanking out), or both?
  - ☐ Development over time?
  - ☐ How long did it last?
  - ☐ Speed and nature of recovery of vision?
  - ☐ Any residual symptoms or is everything back to normal now?
- ☐ Any neurologic symptoms before, during, or after the episode?
  - ☐ Any headache? If so, describe nature; did it occur before, during, or after the visual loss?
  - ☐ Nausea, vomiting, photophobia, or sonophobia?

      ☐ Transient numbness, weakness, collapse, problems walking, or talking during the episode of blurred vision?

      ☐ If neurologic symptoms present, have they completely resolved?

   ☐ Any other ophthalmic symptoms?

      ☐ Haloes around lights and/or red painful eye during episode: suspect angle-closure glaucoma.

      ☐ Transient diplopia?

   ☐ Previous medical and surgical history

      ☐ True migraine? (caution: some patients call every headache "migraine").

      ☐ Somnambulism in childhood, cyclic vomiting in childhood, or previous or current motion sickness? (all migraine equivalents).

      ☐ Transient ischemic attacks or stroke?

      ☐ Atherosclerotic risk factors?

      ☐ Recent neck trauma, car accident, chiropractic manipulation, roller-coaster ride? (internal carotid artery [ICA] dissection).

   ☐ Social history: smoker?

   ☐ Family history of true migraine? (caution: some patients call every headache "migraine").

   ☐ If patient over 50: symptoms of GCA?

   ☐ System review questions

      ☐ Neck or face pain? (ICA dissection).

      ☐ Any clues to the cause anywhere in the body?

EXAMINATION

   ☐ Visual acuity testing.

   ☐ Color vision testing.

   ☐ Visual field testing to confrontation.

   ☐ Eye movement testing.

   ☐ Pupils

      ☐ Relative afferent pupillary defect (RAPD)?

      ☐ Anisocoria?

   ☐ Eyelids: ptosis?

   ☐ Orbits: proptosis, injection, chemosis?

   ☐ Decreased corneal and/or facial sensation to light touch?

   ☐ If patient over 50: palpate temporal arteries.

   ☐ Measure blood pressure in all cases.

   ☐ Carotid bruit audible with stethoscope?

   ☐ Full neurologic examination: in all cases of unexplained transient visual loss.

Plus: Perform Perimetry

   ☐ IN ALL CASES

Management Flowchart
TRANSIENT VISUAL LOSS

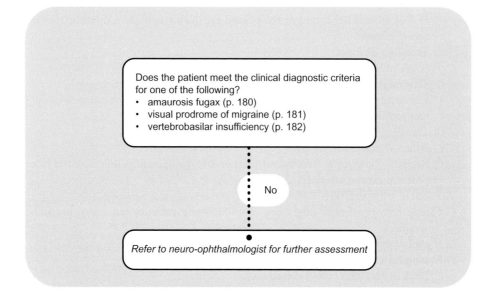

Does the patient meet the clinical diagnostic criteria for one of the following?
- amaurosis fugax (p. 180)
- visual prodrome of migraine (p. 181)
- vertebrobasilar insufficiency (p. 182)

No

Refer to neuro-ophthalmologist for further assessment

CLINICAL DIAGNOSTIC CRITERIA FOR AMAUROSIS FUGAX—TRANSIENT MONOCULAR EMBOLIC VISUAL LOSS

The patient must have ALL of the following:

HISTORY
- age over 50 and vasculopathic risk factors
- sudden onset of severe visual loss in one eye (usually at least several minutes, most often >5 minutes)
- visual loss over part or all of the monocular visual field ("a curtain came over my vision")
- visual loss completely resolves within 1 hour (usually resolves within 10 minutes)
- normal vision in the other eye throughout
- no other neurologic symptoms
- no neck pain, no history of neck injury (possible carotid dissecting aneurysm)
- no symptoms of GCA (p. 85)

EXAMINATION
- normal ocular examination in both eyes, with the exception that retinal emboli may or may not be seen in one or both eyes
- normal neuro-ophthalmic examination; specifically no Horner syndrome (possible carotid dissecting aneurysm)
- no signs of GCA (p. 85)

PERIMETRY
- normal in both eyes

IF THE PATIENT MEETS ALL THESE CRITERIA, SEE P. 186 FOR INVESTIGATIONS AND MANAGEMENT.

CLINICAL DIAGNOSTIC CRITERIA FOR VISUAL PRODROME OF MIGRAINE

The patient must have ALL of the following:

HISTORY

- Known history of true migraine headaches or migraine equivalents (e.g., motion sickness, somnambulism, cyclic vomiting) commencing before age 40.
- History of expanding scintillating scotoma
  - Area of blurred vision in both eyes (seen with both eyes open).
  - Begins as a small area of blurred vision that then expands slowly over 10–30 minutes before resolving; this may or may not be hemianopic.
  - The scotoma is surrounded by one or more of the following: zig-zags, flashing or sparkling lights, or wavy/"watery" vision.
- Vision returns completely to normal in both eyes.
- If headache is present, it begins after the start of visual symptoms (headache starting before or at the same time as the onset of visual symptoms could be a mass lesion).
- The visual loss may or may not be followed by a transient period with one or more of nausea, vomiting, photophobia, sonophobia, or malaise.
- No other neurologic symptoms (migraine can cause other neurologic symptoms but the presence of other symptoms indicates the patient should be seen by a neurologist).
- (If older than 50) no symptoms of GCA (p. 85)

EXAMINATION

- normal ocular examination in both eyes
- normal neuro-ophthalmic examination
- (if older than 50) no signs of GCA (p. 85)

PERIMETRY

- normal in both eyes

IF THE PATIENT MEETS ALL THESE CRITERIA, SEE P. 188 FOR INVESTIGATIONS AND MANAGEMENT.

CLINICAL DIAGNOSTIC CRITERIA FOR VERTEBROBASILAR INSUFFICIENCY

The patient must have ALL of the following:

HISTORY

- over 50 and vasculopathic risk factors
- sudden onset of visual loss in both eyes; this may or may not be hemianopic
- visual loss completely resolves within 1 hour (more often within minutes)
- often one or more other transient neurologic symptoms are present (lasting minutes usually, then completely resolving)
  - loss of balance/vertigo
  - problems walking, talking, or swallowing
  - numbness around the mouth
  - numbness or weakness on one or both sides of the body
  - collapse
- no neck pain, no history of neck injury (possible vertebrobasilar dissecting aneurysm)
- no symptoms of GCA (p. 85)

EXAMINATION

- normal ocular examination in both eyes
- normal neuro-ophthalmic examination
- no signs of GCA (p. 85)

PERIMETRY

- normal in both eyes

IF THE PATIENT MEETS ALL THESE CRITERIA, SEE P. 191 FOR INVESTIGATIONS AND MANAGEMENT.

Monocular Transient Visual Loss

This can be due to:

- binocular visual loss mistakenly attributed to one eye
- eye disease
- optic nerve disease
  - papilledema
  - compressive tumor
  - Uhthoff phenomenon
- vascular disease
  - GCA
  - ocular ischemic syndrome
  - embolic monocular transient visual loss ("amaurosis fugax")
  - vasospastic monocular transient visual loss ("retinal migraine")

BINOCULAR VISUAL LOSS MISTAKENLY ATTRIBUTED TO ONE EYE

Patients often wrongly attribute binocular homonymous hemianopic field loss to the eye that has lost the temporal field. For example, a patient who has had a transient right homonymous hemianopia may complain that "my right eye went blind" because they lost the right side of their vision.

EYE DISEASE

- Intermittent angle-closure glaucoma can present as monocular transient visual loss, with or without pain, redness, or "haloes" in the affected eye. For this reason, all patients with monocular visual loss require intraocular pressure (IOP) measurement and gonioscopy.
- Tear film or corneal disease can sometimes cause patients to complain that their vision went "blurry" in one eye for hours or minutes; the clues to this diagnosis are:
  - The visual loss was only mild (compared with the severe visual loss of vascular events).
  - There is usually a history of dryness or foreign body sensation at the same time.
  - The blurring got better with eye closure, blinking, or eyedrop use.
- Incipient retinal vascular occlusions (arterial or venous) can present as transient visual loss:
  - "Warning signs" are usually visible in the form of arterial narrowing or visible emboli, or venous engorgement or hemorrhages.
  - It is essential to rule out GCA in the case of incipient arterial occlusion and to treat factors that may prevent the occlusion (e.g., check for raised IOP, start aspirin, etc.).

OPTIC NERVE DISEASE

- Papilledema often causes "TVOs": transient visual loss in one or both eyes that usually lasts seconds and is described as blacking, graying, or blanking out of vision ("as if water were splashed in my eyes").
  - These obscurations are often precipitated by bending over, straining, coughing, or arising from a lying to a sitting or standing position.
  - For this reason, it is important to examine the optic discs of all patients with transient visual loss.
- Optic nerve, orbital, or pituitary region tumors are rare causes of transient monocular visual loss.
  - Compression can cause transient visual loss by compromising the blood supply to the optic nerve: when posture or blood pressure changes, the nerve can undergo temporary ischemia.
  - In some cases, the patient may also complain of positive visual phenomena such as flashes or sparkles.
  - If a patient complains of transient monocular visual loss only when looking in a certain direction, you should suspect an orbital tumor compressing the optic nerve (with the tumor compressing the nerve more in one direction of gaze).
- Uhthoff phenomenon is fading or dimming of vision in one or both eyes when the body temperature increases or the patient exercises due to slowed conduction in the optic nerve/s.
  - The most common cause of this is optic nerve demyelination from multiple sclerosis; in some cases, this is the first symptom of the disease.
  - However, optic nerve disease of almost any cause can result in this phenomenon.

VASCULAR DISEASE

Giant Cell Arteritis (GCA)

- GCA (Fig. 5.1) is an uncommon but important cause of transient visual loss in one or both eyes:
  - It is essential to detect GCA at this stage because often urgent high-dose steroid treatment can prevent permanent visual loss.
  - Therefore GCA must be considered and ruled out in all patients over age 50 with transient visual loss.
- The mechanism by which GCA causes monocular transient visual loss can be:
  - Embolism from an involved carotid arterial system.
  - Early involvement of the posterior ciliary arteries (prior to the visual loss of anterior ischemic optic neuropathy [AION], with a normal or swollen disc).
  - By causing ocular or orbital ischemic syndrome.

Ocular Ischemic Syndrome

- In this syndrome, the whole eyeball suffers from hypoperfusion.
- Causes include:
  - ICA occlusion or severe stenosis
  - GCA

Symptoms

One or more of:

- transient monocular visual loss or blurred vision improved on lying down
- eye or orbital ache or pain improved on lying down
- transient neurologic symptoms such as contralateral numbness or weakness

Signs

One or more of:

- decreased acuity
- low IOP
- cataract
- anterior or panuveitis
- retinal venous engorgement and tortuosity
- retinal hemorrhages (especially midperipheral blot hemorrhages)
- retinal or iris neovascularization
- optic disc swelling

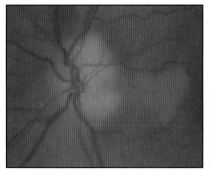

Fig. 5.1 This patient with giant cell arteritis (GCA) noticed intermittent "blacking out" of the vision in her left eye the day before the eye became permanently blind due to arteritic anterior ischemic optic neuropathy. GCA must always be considered as a cause of transient visual loss in any patient over age 50.

Investigations
- rule out GCA
- duplex Doppler carotid ultrasound

Treatment
- Treatment of GCA.
- If severe ICA stenosis is present, carotid endarterectomy may result in decreased pain and improved vision, but florid retinal and iris neovascularization may still occur after the procedure and require photocoagulation.

Embolic Monocular Transient Visual Loss—Amaurosis Fugax

(See clinical diagnostic criteria, p. 180.)

Causes
- ICA atherosclerosis
  - The ICA becomes stenosed and its endothelium irregular because of atherosclerotic change.
  - Small platelet-fibrin thrombi or cholesterol plaques form and embolize upward; some of these may flow through the ophthalmic artery to the central retinal artery, temporarily blocking off retinal arterial supply (sudden loss of vision) before dissolving or moving peripherally (return of vision).
- ICA dissecting aneurysm
  - A tear develops in the ICA and blood dissects along the interior of the arterial wall.
  - This can cause both stenosis of the artery and a roughened lumen that causes thrombosis and embolization.
  - Can occur in all ages.
  - Causes include neck trauma (e.g., motor vehicle accident "whiplash"), connective tissue diseases, chiropractic manipulation, roller coaster rides or idiopathic.
  - Patients often complain of neck and/or facial pain and may have signs of Horner syndrome ipsilateral to the dissection.
- GCA
- Cardiac disease (e.g., heart valve disease, patent foramen ovale)

Symptoms
- sudden onset of severe visual loss in one eye (over seconds to a minute)
- visual loss over the whole monocular visual field ("a curtain came over my vision")
- visual loss completely resolves within 1 hour (usually resolves within 10 minutes)
- normal vision in the other eye throughout
- no other neurologic symptoms

Signs
- normal ocular examination in both eyes, with the exception that retinal emboli (Fig. 5.2) may or may not be seen in one or both eyes
- normal neuro-ophthalmic examination

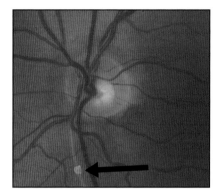

Fig. 5.2 Amaurosis fugax due to calcific embolus from a heart valve *(arrow)*. The complete monocular blindness resolved subjectively but the embolus has moved on to cause a branch retinal artery occlusion.

Investigations
- It is important that these patients be fully investigated as soon as possible, just as you would in a patient with any type of transient ischemic attack; the following investigations thus should be urgently pursued by yourself, the patient's internist or family physician, a vascular specialist or a neurologist:
  - Urgent full blood count, erythrocyte sedimentation rate (ESR), c-reactive protein (CRP) to assess likelihood of GCA.
  - If ICA dissecting aneurysm suspected (history of neck trauma, Horner syndrome, or neck pain): magnetic resonance imaging (MRI) plus MR angiogram (or computerized tomographic [CT] scan plus CT angiography) of neck vessels, specifically looking for this.
  - If no suspicion of dissecting aneurysm:
    - duplex Doppler carotids looking for ICA stenosis
    - cardiac assessment and ECG ± echocardiogram
    - MRI with diffusion weighted imaging (DWI) looking for silent infarcts.

Treatment
- GCA: urgent high-dose steroid treatment
- ICA dissection: anticoagulation for at least 6 months (seek specialist advice)
- severe ICA stenosis: commence platelet inhibitor treatment; urgent referral to vascular surgeon to consider carotid endarterectomy or angioplasty and stenting

Vasospastic Monocular Transient Visual Loss ("Retinal Migraine")
- It is thought that the retinal circulation transiently goes into spasm.
- This should not be confused with the much more common binocular transient visual loss prodrome of migraine (scintillating scotoma).
- Causes include:
  - idiopathic (in otherwise well, young adults)
  - history of migraine
  - vasospastic syndromes, e.g., Raynaud

Symptoms
- usually an otherwise well, young adult; the same eye is affected every time
- stereotyped pattern of "patchy" fading of vision in the affected eye over about 1 minute, followed by poor vision for 1–5 minutes; then return of vision in the reverse pattern to which visual loss occurred
- no positive visual phenomena
- no neurologic symptoms

Signs
- entirely normal ocular and neuro-ophthalmic examinations (unless the patient is examined during an episode, in which case arteriolar spasm may be observed)

Investigations and Treatment
- It is ideal if these patients can be seen by a neuro-ophthalmologist.
- A calcium channel blocker such as nifedipine may be successful in reducing the frequency of spasm.

Binocular Transient Visual Loss

This can be due to:
- monocular visual loss mistakenly attributed to both eyes
- bilateral simultaneous eye or optic nerve disease
- retrochiasmal disease
- vascular disease
  - GCA
  - VBI

MONOCULAR VISUAL LOSS MISTAKENLY ATTRIBUTED TO BOTH EYES

- Rarely, a patient with transient visual loss in one eye may say that both eyes were affected (however, this is much less common than patients attributing bilateral loss, especially homonymous loss to one side, to one eye).

BILATERAL SIMULTANEOUS EYE OR OPTIC NERVE DISEASE

- Uhthoff phenomenon (p. 160) can occur in both optic nerves simultaneously, as can TVOs from papilledema.
- Bilateral transient acute angle-closure glaucoma is rare but can occur.

RETROCHIASMAL DISEASE

Seizure Activity From a Tumor or Arteriovenous Malformation (AVM)

- An uncommon cause of transient binocular visual loss is focal epilepsy induced by an occipital AVM or tumor.
- The patient may see positive visual phenomena (colored and small circular flashing patterns) at the time of blurred vision.

- However, in contrast to the visual phenomena of migraine:
  - A slowly expanding then resolving scintillating scotoma is rare.
  - If headache is present, the blurred vision often occurs after or at the same time as the headache (rather than before the headache as in migraine).

Migraine

(See clinical diagnostic criteria, p. 181.)

- Migraine is a specific diagnosis based on a careful history from the patient and lack of abnormal findings on a detailed neuro-ophthalmic examination, including visual field testing.
- Patients with transient visual loss due to migraine often present to ophthalmologists because:
  - The migrainous visual loss may occur without headache ("acephalgic" migraine).
  - The patient may have a history of migraine but never previously experienced a visual prodrome.
- It is important to note that many patients (and some physicians) call almost every headache "migraine"; therefore do not assume patients have a past history of true migraine just because they say they "get migraines" (Fig. 5.3).

Mechanism

- The visual prodrome of migraine is caused by a wave of spreading neuronal depression which starts at the tip of the occipital lobe and radiates forward through the visual cortex.
- This is then followed by a headache phase which is associated with vascular dilation and the release of inflammatory mediators.

Symptoms

- Patients may experience the visual phase alone, headache alone or the visual phase preceding the headache.
- Visual phase:
  - Expanding scintillating scotoma.
  - Area of blurred vision in both eyes (seen with both eyes open).
  - Begins as a small area of blurred vision which then expands slowly over 10–30 minutes before resolving; this may or may not be hemianopic.

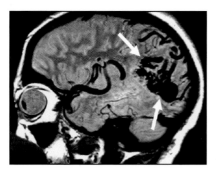

Fig. 5.3 This 45-year-old woman complained of "migraines" in which headaches were accompanied by flashing lights and blurred vision. Perimetry showed a homonymous hemianopic defect, so magnetic resonance imaging was performed; a large occipital arteriovenous malformation *(arrows)* was identified.

- The scotoma is surrounded by one or more of the following: zig-zags, achromatic flashing or sparkling lights or wavy/"watery" vision.
- Vision returns completely to normal in both eyes.
- Headache:
  - Often, but not always, hemicranial (but recurrent episodes not always on the same side).
  - Mild to severe, lasting 1–24 hours.
  - Often associated with one or more of the following, all of which resolve completely within hours:
    - photophobia (the patient lies in a dark room)
    - sonophobia (sensitivity to noise)
    - nausea, sometimes vomiting
    - sometimes numbness or weakness of a limb.
- At the end of the episode the vision, headache, and any other neurologic symptoms should have completely resolved, although the patient often feels fatigued; persisting symptoms of any kind suggest a more serious cause.

Signs
- It is rare for ophthalmologists to see patients during the visual phase; almost always the ophthalmologist is consulted after all symptoms have resolved.
- A full neuro-ophthalmic examination, including perimetry, must be entirely normal before the patient is diagnosed with migraine.

Investigations
- No investigations are necessary if there is a clear previous history.
- However, it is wise to seek the opinion of a neurologist or neuro-ophthalmologist if you are unsure whether or not the patient's visual symptoms are due to migraine.

Treatment
- Effective antimigraine treatments exist that reduce the frequency and/or severity of migraine headache (consult the patient's physician or a neurologist).
- Patients suffering migraine have an increased risk of stroke; this is greatly increased if they smoke, so any smoker with migraine should be strongly counseled to cease.

Note: "retinal migraine"/"ocular migraine"
- This is monocular transient visual loss due to retinal vasospasm (p. 186 above); often the patient has no history of true migraine.
- This is not the same as acephalgic migraine (binocular expanding scintillating scotoma occurring without headache).

VASCULAR DISEASE

Giant Cell Arteritis

GCA (p. 184) is a rare cause of binocular transient global or hemianopic visual loss from vertebrobasilar embolism.

Vertebrobasilar Insufficiency

(See clinical diagnostic criteria, p. 182.)

VBI is relatively common among elderly patients; if transient visual loss is the only or most prominent symptom, these patients are often referred to ophthalmologists.

Mechanism

- The vertebrobasilar arterial system supplies the brainstem, cerebellum, and (via the posterior cerebral arteries) the occipital visual cortex.
- Therefore insufficient blood flow in this arterial system can cause one or more of:
  - Transient brainstem or cerebellar symptoms.
  - Binocular transient loss of vision that may be global (loss of all vision in both eyes due to loss of arterial flow to both occipital lobes) or hemianopic (transient ischemia of one occipital lobe).

Causes

- Vertebrobasilar arterial disease
  - Arterial stenosis due to atherosclerosis (with hypoperfusion often triggered by kinking of a stenosed vessel on looking up or postural hypotension on suddenly standing up).
  - Embolism due to atherosclerotic plaque.
  - Dissecting aneurysm (rare).
  - GCA (rare).
- Postural hypotension/presyncope
  - On suddenly standing up, arterial blood pressure may drop and cause transient vertebrobasilar ischemia.
  - "Blacking out" or "graying out" of vision is also common immediately before a patient faints.
- Heart disease
  - Cardiac thromboembolism, e.g., due to heart valve disease or a patent foramen ovale.
  - Transient arrhythmia may cause transient hypotension.

Symptoms

- As opposed to the transient visual loss of migraine, that caused by VBI is characterized by blurred vision or complete loss of vision in both eyes with no positive visual phenomena (that is, no flashing lights, sparkles, or zig-zags).
- Visual loss is usually very sudden (over seconds), then recovers in seconds or minutes.
- One or more of the following symptoms indicating brainstem or cerebellar dysfunction is usually present:
  - Problems walking, talking, or swallowing.
  - Face or limb numbness or weakness.
  - Vertigo, disorientation, or collapse.
- All symptoms (visual and neurologic) resolve completely within 1 hour (usually within minutes).

Signs
- Usually the patient sees an ophthalmologist long after the episode; thus, a full neuro-ophthalmic examination, including perimetry, should be entirely normal.

Investigations
- It is important that these patients be investigated urgently by yourself, their physician, a vascular specialist or neurologist.
- The patient requires a full systemic neurologic exam, cardiac assessment, and evaluation of lying and standing blood pressure.

Treatment
- If vertebrobasilar stenosis is suspected in the absence of other problems, the patient is often started on a platelet inhibitor; if episodes are frequent, the patient may need to be anticoagulated to prevent a stroke.

Double Vision

Introduction

Double vision can be caused by disease of the:
- eye
- orbit
- extraocular muscles
- neuromuscular junction
- ocular motor nerves
- brain

A careful history and detailed examination will often give clues to the likely location of the disease in your patient.

The most common causes of double vision in adults are the presumed ischemic ocular motor nerve palsies. However, just because a patient is elderly or a vasculopath does not mean that atherosclerosis is the cause of their diplopia: aneurysms, brain tumors, and giant cell arteritis (GCA) are not uncommonly the cause of double vision, and patients with these life-threatening conditions often present first to an ophthalmologist.

As eye care professionals, we all need to know the following four things about double vision:

1. How to make a safe clinical diagnosis of ischemic third nerve palsy (p. 199).
2. How to make a safe clinical diagnosis of ischemic or congenital fourth nerve palsy (pp. 200–201).
3. How to make a safe clinical diagnosis of ischemic sixth nerve palsy (p. 202).
4. And what to do for all other patients with unexplained double vision. We recommend that these patients be referred to a neuro-ophthalmologist for further assessment (urgently if the diplopia is of acute onset). If prompt referral is difficult due to geographic or patient factors, or if you wish to work the patient up yourself, the recommended further clinical assessment and initial basic investigations are outlined on p. 203.

EYE DISEASE

Ocular media disease is an uncommon cause of diplopia and results in monocular diplopia. Examples include high astigmatism, iridectomy, decentered intraocular lens, incorrect spectacles, corneal disease, or cataract. The three clues that monocular diplopia is present are:

- The two images are not equal; one is a clear image and the other is a ghost.
- The two images are almost always touching each other.
- Double vision persists despite covering one eye.

ORBIT OR EXTRAOCULAR MUSCLE DISEASE

Thyroid orbitopathy causing restriction of one or more muscles is a common cause of diplopia and is usually easily diagnosed from the attendant orbital signs. Other causes of muscle disease, such as mitochondrial myopathy, can occur in the absence of any visible indicators of orbital disease.

NEUROMUSCULAR JUNCTION DISEASE

Myasthenia is one of the "great mimickers" causing diplopia and can simulate a fourth, sixth or pupil-sparing third nerve palsy.

OCULAR MOTOR NERVE DISEASE

Third, fourth, and sixth nerve palsies are potentially the most dangerous causes of double vision because they are often caused by an intracranial aneurysm or brain tumor compressing the nerve. Up to one-third of third nerve palsies are caused by aneurysmal compression, and identification of these cases is a matter of great urgency because the aneurysm can rupture and kill the patient within hours to days of the onset of double vision; many patients with undiagnosed brain aneurysms first present to ophthalmologists with diplopia. Partial third nerve palsies can be very difficult to diagnose as they can present with many different patterns of motility disturbance (p. 222). The "rule of the pupil" is not a safe guide to whether or not an aneurysm is present (p. 225). However, the majority of third, fourth, and sixth nerve palsies are caused by ischemia from atherosclerosis, diabetes, or GCA (or are congenital, in the case of fourth nerve palsy).

BRAIN DISEASE

A stroke, tumor, or degenerative disease within the brain can present with double vision by causing an ocular motor nerve palsy, an internuclear ophthalmoplegia (INO), a skew deviation, or a supranuclear palsy. The clue that a supranuclear palsy is present is that different types of eye movement (pursuit, saccadic, vestibulo-ocular, convergence) are affected to different extents.

Examination Checklist

DIPLOPIA

Have you asked about, and looked for, all the following key features?

History

- ☐ The double vision
    - ☐ Does it disappear if either eye is covered? (if it does, it is binocular diplopia; if diplopia persists despite covering one eye, it is monocular diplopia).
    - ☐ Are both images the same or is one image a "ghost?" (if one is a ghost, it probably is monocular diplopia).
    - ☐ Are the images side by side, one on top of another, or obliquely displaced?
    - ☐ Does it change with distance versus near viewing?
    - ☐ Does it change with direction of gaze?
    - ☐ When did it start? How quickly did it start? (very sudden onset: possible ischemic palsy or pituitary apoplexy).
    - ☐ Development over time?
    - ☐ Is it getting better or worse or staying the same?
    - ☐ Does the severity or direction of the double vision change at different times of the day or vary from day to day? (possible myasthenia).
- ☐ Any other ophthalmic symptoms?
    - ☐ Pain in or behind the eye? (ischemia, tumor, aneurysm).
    - ☐ Blurred vision or field loss?
- ☐ Any neurologic symptoms: headache? Numbness, weakness, problems walking or talking?
- ☐ Previous medical and surgical history: cancer? Atherosclerotic risk factors?
- ☐ Social history: smoker?
- ☐ If patient over 50: symptoms of GCA?
- ☐ System review questions: any clues to the cause anywhere in the body?

Examination

- ☐ Visual acuity. (Regardlesss of the level of visual acuity, in patients with monocular diplopia, viewing with the affected eye(s) through a pinhole may eliminate the diplopia).
- ☐ Color vision testing.
- ☐ Visual field testing to confrontation.
- ☐ Eye movement testing
    - ☐ Are the eyes aligned in primary position? Cover test or red-glass test, with and without glasses, distance and near.
    - ☐ Smooth pursuit testing of range of eye movement: both eyes open, then one eye at a time.
    - ☐ Are the eyes aligned differently in right gaze, left gaze, upgaze, and downgaze?
    - ☐ Saccades: horizontal, then vertical.
    - ☐ Convergence.
    - ☐ Vestibulo-ocular reflex (VOR) ("doll's-head") if a bilateral motility disturbance is found.

☐ Pupils
  ☐ Relative afferent pupillary defect (RAPD)? (possible orbital apex syndrome from tumor).
  ☐ Anisocoria? (possible partial third nerve palsy or Horner syndrome from tumor, aneurysm, or dissection).
  ☐ Aberrant regeneration? (miosis on eye adduction or depression: possible tumor or aneurysm).
☐ Eyelids
  ☐ Ptosis? (possible myasthenia; possible partial third nerve palsy or Horner syndrome from tumor or aneurysm).
  ☐ Aberrant regeneration? (lid retraction on eye depression or adduction: possible tumor or aneurysm).
☐ Orbits: proptosis or enophthalmos, injection, chemosis?
☐ Decreased corneal or facial sensation to light touch? (possible tumor).
☐ Orbicularis or facial weakness? (possible myasthenia or myopathy).
☐ If patient over 50: palpate temporal arteries.
☐ Measure blood pressure in all cases.
☐ Full neurologic examination: in all cases of unexplained diplopia.

Plus: Perform Perimetry If

☐ field defect to confrontation
☐ decreased visual acuity, color vision or RAPD

Management Flowchart

DOUBLE VISION

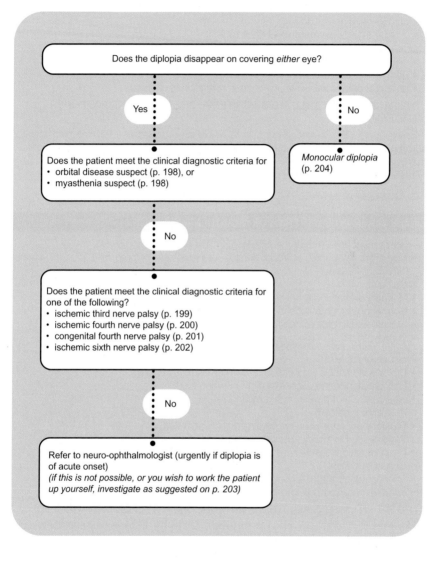

Does the diplopia disappear on covering *either* eye?

Yes

No

Does the patient meet the clinical diagnostic criteria for
• orbital disease suspect (p. 198), or
• myasthenia suspect (p. 198)

Monocular diplopia (p. 204)

No

Does the patient meet the clinical diagnostic criteria for one of the following?
• ischemic third nerve palsy (p. 199)
• ischemic fourth nerve palsy (p. 200)
• congenital fourth nerve palsy (p. 201)
• ischemic sixth nerve palsy (p. 202)

No

Refer to neuro-ophthalmologist (urgently if diplopia is of acute onset)
(if this is not possible, or you wish to work the patient up yourself, investigate as suggested on p. 203)

CLINICAL DIAGNOSTIC CRITERIA FOR ORBITAL DISEASE SUSPECT

The patient must have NONE of the following:
- severe headache, pulsatile tinnitus, or neurologic symptoms (if present, suspect primary intracranial disease with orbital signs, e.g., cavernous sinus thrombosis [CST] or carotid-cavernous fistula [CCF])
- (if older than 50) symptoms of GCA (p. 85)

plus, one or more of:
- pain on (or increased on) eye movement
- unilateral or bilateral proptosis
- unilateral or bilateral ocular injection ± conjunctival chemosis

IF THE PATIENT MEETS ALL THESE CRITERIA, SEE PP. 205 AND 208 FOR MANAGEMENT.

However, if further investigation fails to reveal an orbital cause for diplopia, refer to a neuro-ophthalmologist or investigate further for possible neuromuscular junction, nerve, or brain disease.

CLINICAL DIAGNOSTIC CRITERIA FOR MYASTHENIA SUSPECT

The patient must have ALL of the following:
- No severe headache, pulsatile tinnitus, or neurologic symptoms (if present, suspect intracranial disease).
- No pain.
- Normal corneal and facial sensation.
- Normal pupils: no anisocoria, no RAPD.
- Normal visual fields to confrontation.
- (If over 50) no symptoms of GCA (p. 85).

Plus one or more of:
- Diplopia is variable in direction or severity from day to day.
- Diplopia significantly worse at night or when tired.
- Hoarse voice or problems swallowing.
- Problems breathing.
- Ptosis appears or worsens on upgaze for 2 minutes.
- Weakness of eyelid closure on testing.
- Facial muscle weakness on testing.
- Cogan lid twitch.
- Enhancement of ptosis on manual elevation of contralateral eyelid.
- Improvement in ptosis and/or strabismus with ice test.

IF THE PATIENT MEETS ALL THESE CRITERIA, SEE P. 212 FOR MANAGEMENT.

However, if further investigation fails to reveal myasthenia, refer to a neuro-ophthalmologist or investigate further for possible nerve or brain disease.

CLINICAL DIAGNOSTIC CRITERIA FOR ISCHEMIC THIRD NERVE PALSY

The patient must have ALL of the following:

HISTORY
- AGE: 40 or over
- MEDICAL HISTORY:
  - One or more vasculopathic risk factors (e.g., hypertension, diabetes, smoking).
  - No history of cancer, vasculitis, or autoimmune disease.
- TIME COURSE:
  - SUDDEN onset of diplopia and unilateral ptosis while awake or first noted upon waking (with no ptosis and single vision the night before).
  - Ptosis becomes complete within 24 hours of onset.
- No persisting orbital, hemifacial, or hemicranial pain; no numbness or "pins and needles."
- No other systemic neurologic symptoms.
- (If older than 50) no symptoms of GCA (p. 85).

EXAMINATION
- On the affected side
  - The palsy must be COMPLETE: complete ptosis, no movement on attempted elevation, depression, or adduction.
  - Entirely NORMAL PUPIL (same size as the other side, constricts briskly to light).
  - Fourth nerve function normal (intorsion of the eye is seen on attempted depression in abduction).
  - Sixth nerve function normal (full abduction present).
  - No signs of aberrant regeneration (no changes in pupil size and no lifting of the ptosis on attempted elevation, depression, or adduction).
- On the other side
  - No ptosis.
  - Entirely normal motility.
  - Normal-sized pupil that constricts briskly to light.
- On both sides: normal:
  - Visual acuity (unless unrelated intraocular disease present).
  - Visual fields to confrontation.
  - Swinging light test (no RAPD present).
  - Eye appearance (no redness, proptosis or chemosis).
  - Corneal and facial sensation.
  - Orbicularis and facial strength.
  - Intraocular examination (no iritis, vitritis or optic disc abnormalities).
  - (If older than 50) temporal arteries and no scalp tenderness.

AND ON FOLLOW-UP
- No other abnormalities develop.
- The ptosis begins to lift and motility begins to improve within 3 months.

If the patient meets all the other diagnostic criteria at the first visit, you can make a provisional diagnosis of ischemic third nerve palsy, but this can only be confirmed as the definite diagnosis retrospectively, once spontaneous recovery begins.

IF THE PATIENT MEETS ALL THESE CRITERIA, SEE P. 226 FOR MANAGEMENT.

CLINICAL DIAGNOSTIC CRITERIA FOR ISCHEMIC FOURTH NERVE PALSY

The patient must have ALL of the following:

HISTORY

- AGE: 40 or over
- MEDICAL HISTORY:
  - One or more vasculopathic risk factors (e.g., hypertension, diabetes, smoking).
  - No history of cancer, vasculitis, or autoimmune disease.
- TIME COURSE:
  - SUDDEN onset of diplopia while awake or first noted upon waking (with single vision the night before).
  - The type and severity of diplopia then remain stable until spontaneous improvement begins; the diplopia does not vary during each day or from day to day.
- Subjective torsion is often noticed (the second image is "tilted").
- No persisting orbital, hemifacial or hemicranial pain, numbness, or "pins and needles."
- No other systemic neurologic symptoms.
- (If older than 50) no symptoms of GCA (p. 85).

EXAMINATION

- Vertical or oblique deviation in the primary position on cover test.
- Motility testing:
  - Hypertropia in the primary position that increases on gaze toward the side of the lower eye and on tilting of the head to the side of the higher eye.
  - Hypertropic eye (sometimes) has a visible motility disturbance: one or both of:
    - Inferior oblique overaction (upshoot of the affected eye on adduction).
    - Superior oblique underaction (limitation of depression in adduction).
  - Hypotropic eye: entirely normal motility.
  - No difference in deviation when patient assessed in sitting vs supine position (Wong's Upright-Supine Test to distinguish fourth nerve palsy from skew deviation).
- Both sides: normal:
  - Visual acuity (unless unrelated intraocular disease present).
  - Visual fields to confrontation.
  - Pupils (equal size, both briskly reactive to light, no RAPD).
  - Eyelids (no ptosis).
  - Eye appearance (no redness, proptosis or chemosis).
  - Corneal and facial sensation.
  - Orbicularis and facial power.
  - Intraocular examination (no iritis, vitritis or optic disc abnormalities).
  - (If older than 50) temporal arteries and no scalp tenderness.
- Vertical prism fusional amplitude testing (p. 40): less than 5 prism diopters.
- Torsion testing (p. 42)
  - Fundoscopy shows extorsion of the affected eye.
  - Double Maddox rod: subjective extorsion of less than 10 degrees.

AND ON FOLLOW-UP

- No other abnormalities develop.
- The diplopia begins to resolve within 3 months.

If the patient meets all the other diagnostic criteria at the first visit, you can make a provisional diagnosis of ischemic fourth nerve palsy, but this can only be confirmed as the definite diagnosis retrospectively, once spontaneous recovery begins.

IF THE PATIENT MEETS ALL THESE CRITERIA, SEE P. 232 FOR MANAGEMENT.

CLINICAL DIAGNOSTIC CRITERIA FOR CONGENITAL FOURTH NERVE PALSY

The patient must have ALL of the following:

HISTORY

- Any age.
- MEDICAL HISTORY: otherwise well; no history of cancer, vasculitis or autoimmune disease.
- TIME COURSE
  - Evidence from relatives or old photographs of head tilt from early childhood.
  - Diplopia may have any time course (sudden or gradual onset, intermittent or persisting).
- No subjective torsion (the second image is not "tilted").
- No orbital, hemifacial, or hemicranial pain; no numbness or "pins and needles."
- No other systemic neurologic symptoms.
- (If older than 50) no symptoms of GCA (p. 85).

EXAMINATION

- Vertical or oblique deviation in the primary position on cover test.
- Patient prefers to hold his or her head tilted to the side of the lower (hypotropic) eye.
- Motility testing:
  - Hypertropia in the primary position that increases on gaze to the side of the lower eye and tilt to the side of the higher (hypertropic) eye.
  - Hypertropic eye sometimes has a visible motility disturbance: one or both of:
    - Inferior oblique overaction (upshoot on adduction).
    - Superior oblique underaction (limitation of depression in adduction).
  - Hypotropic eye: entirely normal range of movement.
- Often mild facial asymmetry.
- Both sides: normal:
  - Visual acuity (unless unrelated intraocular disease present).
  - Visual fields to confrontation.
  - Pupils (equal size, both briskly reactive to light, no RAPD).
  - Eyelids (no ptosis).
  - Eye appearance (no redness, proptosis or chemosis).
  - Corneal and facial sensation.
  - Orbicularis and facial power.
  - Intraocular examination (no iritis, vitritis or optic disc abnormalities).
  - (If older than 50) normal temporal arteries and no scalp tenderness.
- Vertical prism fusional amplitude testing (p. 40): greater than 5 prism diopters.
- Torsion testing (p. 42):
  - Fundoscopy shows extorsion of the affected eye.
  - Double Maddox rod: no torsion or less than 10 degrees of extorsion.
- Check old photographs for evidence of a head tilt toward the side of the lower eye.

AND ON FOLLOW-UP

- No other abnormalities develop.

IF THE PATIENT MEETS ALL THESE CRITERIA, SEE P. 232 FOR MANAGEMENT.

CLINICAL DIAGNOSTIC CRITERIA FOR ISCHEMIC SIXTH NERVE PALSY

The patient must have ALL of the following:

HISTORY

- AGE: 40 or over
- MEDICAL HISTORY:
  - One or more vasculopathic risk factors (e.g., hypertension, diabetes, smoking).
  - No history of cancer, vasculitis, or autoimmune disease.
- TIME COURSE:
  - SUDDEN onset of diplopia while awake or first noted upon waking (with single vision the night before).
  - The type and severity of diplopia then remain stable until spontaneous improvement begins; the diplopia does not vary during each day or from day to day.
- No persisting orbital, hemifacial, or hemicranial pain; no numbness or "pins and needles."
- No unexplained deafness, tinnitus, or facial weakness on the side of the sixth nerve palsy.
- No other systemic neurologic symptoms.
- (If older than 50) no symptoms of GCA (p. 85).

EXAMINATION

- esotropia in the primary position on observation and cover test
- motility testing: UNILATERAL restriction of abduction with slow abducting saccades
- other motility testing entirely normal (no limitation of elevation, depression, or adduction on the affected side; normal motility on the other side)
- both sides: NORMAL:
  - visual acuity (unless unrelated intraocular disease present)
  - visual fields to confrontation
  - pupils (equal size, both briskly reactive to light, no RAPD)
  - eyelids (no ptosis)
  - eye appearance (no redness, proptosis or chemosis)
  - corneal and facial sensation
  - orbicularis and facial power
  - intraocular examination (no iritis, vitritis, or optic disc abnormalities)
  - (if older than 50) normal temporal arteries and no scalp tenderness

AND ON FOLLOW-UP

- No other abnormalities develop.
- The diplopia begins to resolve within 3 months.

If the patient meets all the other diagnostic criteria at the first visit, you can make a provisional diagnosis of ischemic sixth nerve palsy, but this can only be confirmed as the definite diagnosis retrospectively, once spontaneous recovery begins.

IF THE PATIENT MEETS ALL THESE CRITERIA, SEE P. 237 FOR MANAGEMENT.

SUGGESTED INVESTIGATIONS FOR DIPLOPIA THAT CANNOT BE CLINICALLY DIAGNOSED

We recommend that patients with diplopia who do not meet the previously mentioned clinical diagnostic criteria for orbital disease, myasthenia, ischemic third nerve palsy, ischemic or congenital fourth nerve palsy, or ischemic sixth nerve palsy be referred to a neuro-ophthalmologist (urgently, if the diplopia is of acute onset).

However, if, due to geographic or patient factors, neuro-ophthalmic referral is not possible, or if you choose to investigate the patient yourself, the following approach is suggested.

In the case of ACUTE onset of diplopia, all the following should be pursued URGENTLY.

1. Careful ocular motility assessment including:
   - Prism measurement of deviation in primary position and in all directions of gaze, distance and near.
   - Smooth pursuit (quality? is there limitation of movement in any direction?).
   - Saccades (speed? accuracy?).
   - (If diplopia is long-standing) assessment of fusional ability and identification of suppression if present.

2. Full neuro-ophthalmic assessment including looking specifically for:
   - Anisocoria.
   - Ptosis (including if it is possible to produce a ptosis on sustained upgaze) or lid retraction.
   - Corneal and facial sensation, orbicularis strength.
   - Optic disc appearance.
   - Perimetry.

If there is strong suspicion of orbital disease, myasthenia, or any other specific disease on the previously mentioned assessments, investigate further as suggested in the relevant section of this chapter. If not, proceed with:

3. Magnetic resonance imaging (MRI) orbits and brain, with contrast, plus MR angiography (MRA) (or computed tomographic angiography [CTA]) brain if there is any possibility that this could be a partial third nerve palsy (i.e., the patient has new-onset diplopia and an esotropia, hypertropia, hypotropia, or oblique deviation, with or without ptosis, with or without anisocoria). If the diplopia is of recent onset, the scan should be performed urgently (the same day you first see the patient).

If this shows a cause for the diplopia, refer or investigate further as appropriate. If not, refer to neuro-ophthalmologist or proceed with:

4. Advanced assessment tailored to the patient's particular case, that may include one or more of:
   - Detailed orthoptic testing of the patient's sensory status and fusional abilities.
   - Full systemic clinical history and neurologic examination, including asking about symptoms of myasthenia or (if patient over 50) GCA; blood pressure, temperature, and urine analysis.
   - Blood tests for possible causes (e.g., erythrocyte sedimentation rate [ESR], C-reactive protein [CRP], angiotensin converting enzyme [ACE], antinuclear antibody [ANA]).
   - Chest x-ray or CT or positron emission tomography (PET) scan.
   - Lumbar puncture.

Monocular Diplopia

CAUSES

- ocular (common)
  - cataract (most common)
  - corneal disease (Fig. 6.1)
  - high astigmatism
  - iridotomy or iridodialysis
  - decentered intraocular lens
  - ill-fitting or decentered spectacles
  - macular edema
- brain ("cortical" diplopia), very rare: visual association cortex lesions
- nonorganic ("functional")–rare

SYMPTOMS

- Ocular causes
  - Usually only one eye is affected; the diplopia disappears when this eye is covered but persists when the other eye is covered.
  - The second image is often seen as a faint and blurred "ghost" of the real image.
  - Images are touching each other.
  - Symptoms of the cause, e.g., glare from cataract.
- Brain lesion: each eye sees an identical double image; diplopia persists on covering either eye.

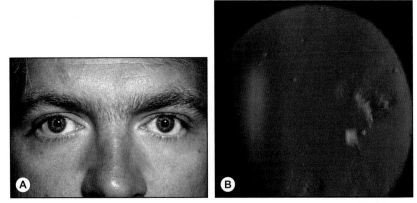

Fig. 6.1 This 32-year-old man was referred for complaints of double vision; however, his eyes were straight. (**A**) The double vision persisted when he covered his right eye; the double images were actually a main image and a ghost image that was touching the main image, and slit-lamp examination revealed a unilateral corneal epithelial dystrophy (map-dot-fingerprint dystrophy). (**B**) The double vision improved with treatment of the corneal dystrophy.

SIGNS

- Ocular causes
  - If a refractive or ocular media cause is present, the diplopia usually disappears when the patient views through a pinhole.
  - Signs of the cause on slit-lamp examination.
- Brain lesion: the diplopia does not disappear with pinhole.

INVESTIGATIONS AND TREATMENT

- ocular causes: no investigation needed, treat the cause if possible (e.g., cataract extraction, contact lens, new glasses)
- in the very rare instance of suspected "cortical" diplopia, MRI brain with contrast

Binocular Diplopia

Binocular diplopia is much more common than monocular diplopia and occurs because the visual axes of the two eyes are misaligned. The double vision of binocular diplopia disappears when either of the eyes is covered. It can be caused by diseases affecting the orbit, extraocular muscles, neuromuscular junction, ocular motor nerves, or brain.

Muscle or Orbit Disease

RESTRICTIVE MYOPATHY

- One or more of the extraocular muscles are tight (enlarged, fibrosed, or entrapped), causing limitation of movement when the eye tries to look in the opposite direction.
- For example, right medial rectus restriction causes a right esotropia in primary position, with limitation of abduction of the right eye.

Causes

- Muscle disease
  - Thyroid orbitopathy (most commonly affecting the medial or inferior recti, causing a restrictive esotropia and/or hypotropia).
  - Orbital myositis can cause any pattern of strabismus (it can also cause a paretic myopathy due to weakness of the involved muscle/s or a combined pattern).
  - Myotoxicity after retrobulbar or peribulbar anesthetic injection.
- Other orbital inflammation, e.g., orbital cellulitis, autoimmune inflammation.
- Orbital trauma: muscle entrapment in orbital fractures, orbital hemorrhage.
- Orbital tumors.

Symptoms

- Diplopia worse in a particular direction of gaze (e.g., to the right with right medial rectus restriction).
- Myositis is often painful (with pain increased on eye movement).

Signs

- Almost always "orbital" signs are present: one or more of:
  - Eyelid retraction (very suggestive of thyroid orbitopathy).
  - Proptosis (due to inflammation or tumor) or enophthalmos (due to tight muscle/s, orbital fracture or sclerosing tumor).
  - Conjunctival injection or chemosis (may be over muscle insertion in thyroid orbitopathy or orbital myositis).
- Smooth pursuit:
  - Limitation of movement of the eye in the direction opposite to the field of action of the involved muscle/s (e.g., limited abduction due to medial rectus restriction).
  - Globe retraction may occur at the limit of movement, due to the tight restricting muscle pulling the eyeball backwards in the orbit.
- Saccades: normal (fast) up to the point of restriction, then an abrupt stop (Fig. 6.2, Video 6.1).
- Forced duction test (pp. 42–43):
  - Restriction to manual movement of the eye in the direction of limitation.
  - Strong tug felt on active force generation testing.

Investigations

- CT scan of the orbits with contrast is usually satisfactory and has the advantage in posttraumatic cases of clearly showing orbital fractures (MRI is not good at imaging bone).
- Ultrasound may be helpful in distinguishing thyroid from other myopathies as it may show enlarged, hyperreflexic extraocular muscles with normal-appearing tendons or increased orbital fat content.

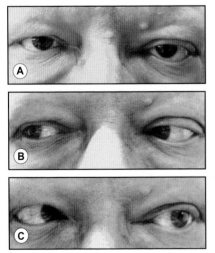

Fig. 6.2 (A–C) Restrictive left esotropia due to thyroid orbitopathy. The left eye cannot abduct fully due to a "tight" left medial rectus. However, the lateral rectus is still working normally, so abducting saccades are fast (not slow as in sixth nerve palsy). Note swelling of upper eyelids and lower lid retraction, left more than right.

Treatment

- Treat the underlying disease if possible.
- For thyroid eye disease, perform orbital decompression (if necessary) before strabismus surgery, then wait for stability.
- Strabismus surgery: recess one or more muscles (never resect).

PARETIC MYOPATHY

- One or more of the extraocular muscles are weak.
- This can be due to disease within the muscle itself or to any disease that breaks the "chain of command" between the brain and the muscle (brain, ocular motor nerve, neuromuscular junction).

Causes

- brain, nerve, neuromuscular junction disease: see the relevant sections in this chapter
- trauma
- orbital myositis (specific cause or idiopathic)
- genetic myopathies, e.g., mitochondrial myopathy causing chronic progressive external ophthalmoplegia (CPEO) (Fig. 6.3, Video 6.2)

Symptoms

- Myositis is painful (with pain increased on attempting to look in the direction of action of the inflamed muscle).
- Others are usually painless.

Signs

- Smooth pursuit: limitation of movement of the eye in the direction of action of the involved muscles (e.g., limited adduction due to a paretic medial rectus).
- Saccades are slow and hypometric in the direction of action of the involved muscle, with the eye coming to a gradual stop (see Video 6.13).
- Forced duction test (pp. 42–43)
  - No restriction to manual movement of the eye in the direction of limitation.
  - Weak "tug" felt on active force generation testing.

Investigations

- specific investigations as indicated for the diseases you suspect, for example:
  - MRI brain for suspected brain disease or unexplained ocular motor nerve palsies
  - acetylcholine receptor antibody blood test and ice or Prostigmin (neostigmine) test for myasthenia
  - genetic tests for possible inherited myopathies

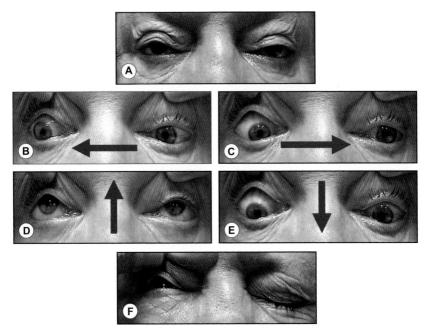

Fig. 6.3 (A–F) Chronic progressive external ophthalmoplegia due to a mitochondrial myopathy. This patient has bilateral ptosis (**A**) and reduction of the movements of both eyes in all directions (**B–E**; *arrows* indicate attempted directions of gaze). Saccades were slow in all directions. There was orbicularis weakness on attempted eye closure against resistance (**F**). The range of extraocular movements did not improve with "doll's-head" vestibulo-ocular reflex stimulation (compared with progressive supranuclear palsy, in which doll's-head testing does elicit greater movements than pursuit or saccades).

Treatment

- Treat the underlying disease if possible.
- Strabismus surgery for paretic myopathy:
  - Wait for recovery (at least 6 months) and for the deviation to be stable on serial prism measurements of the strabismus.
  - Partial paralysis: consider resecting the paretic muscle and recessing the antagonist muscle.
  - Complete permanent paralysis, other muscles healthy: consider transposition strabismus surgery.

ACUTE ORBITOPATHY

- Acute onset of unilateral or bilateral ocular injection and proptosis, often with associated diplopia.
- Remember that primary intracranial disease (such as a carotid-cavernous sinus fistula [CCF] or cavernous sinus thrombosis [CST]) can present with diplopia and an "orbital" clinical picture.

Causes

- Infectious: herpes zoster ophthalmicus, fungal orbital or cavernous sinus infection (e.g., mucormycosis invading from an infected paranasal sinus).
- Neoplastic: lymphoma in particular can present acutely with red proptosed eye/s; metastases.
- Vascular:
  - CCF (low or high flow) (Fig. 6.4).
  - CST (septic or sterile).
  - GCA.
  - Orbital ischemic syndrome from internal carotid artery (ICA) stenosis or occlusion.
- Autoimmune inflammatory:
  - Specific orbital inflammation (e.g., Wegener granulomatosis, sarcoid).
  - Nonspecific (idiopathic) orbital inflammation ("orbital pseudotumor").

Symptoms

- change in appearance (often marked): red eye/s, proptosis
- often pain, "pressure" sensation, or headache (may be severe)
- ± symptoms of ophthalmic complications including:
  - diplopia
  - blurred vision due to optic neuropathy
- ± symptoms specific to particular causes, for example:
  - pulsatile tinnitus ("whooshing" noise heard by the patient in time with their pulse) in CCF
  - fevers in infection
  - fatigue and weight loss in chronic infection, vasculitis or cancer
  - symptoms of GCA

Signs

- unilateral or bilateral red eye ± proptosis (mild to severe)
- ± conjunctival chemosis
- ± acquired strabismus with limitation of motility in one or more (sometimes all) directions
- ± signs specific to particular causes, such as:
  - increased temperature and pulse rate in orbital cellulitis or septic CST
  - bruit audible with stethoscope, palpable pulsatile proptosis, increased ocular pulse pressure on tonometry, and/or dilated tortuous conjunctival vessels in high-flow CCF
  - necrotic black periorbital skin or nasal tissue in fungal orbital apex or cavernous sinus infection
  - retinal venous dilation or retinal hemorrhage (or frank central retinal vein occlusion) may occur in all but is more likely in CCF and CST
  - confusion, headache, loss of consciousness in high-flow CCF, CST, or brain infection secondary to orbital cellulitis
  - decreased vision ± sluggish pupils or RAPD due to:

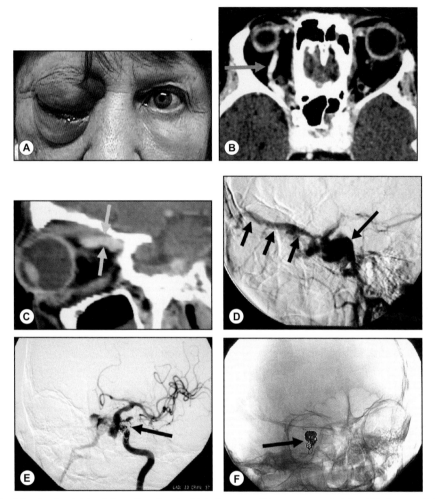

Fig. 6.4 Acute right orbitopathy due to high-flow carotid-cavernous fistula. (**A**) Severe right proptosis, ptosis and lid swelling. (**B, C**) Computed tomography shows dilated right superior ophthalmic vein *(arrows)*. (**D**) Angiogram shows high-velocity arterial blood flowing from the carotid fistula into the cavernous sinus *(long arrow)* and then forward through the superior ophthalmic vein into the orbit *(short arrows)*. (**E**) The fistula was closed by injection of platinum coils *(arrow)* through a catheter inserted into the femoral artery; the fistula is seen to have closed and the anterior flow through the superior ophthalmic vein has ceased. (**F**) The coils on a plain skull x-ray *(arrow)*.

- central retinal vein or artery occlusion (caused by increased intraocular pressure or venous drainage obstruction)
- ischemic, compressive, inflammatory, or infiltrative optic neuropathy
- keratopathy, corneal ulcer, or perforation (due to exposure from proptosis, neurotrophic ulcer secondary to loss of corneal sensation or from anterior segment ischemia)
- intraocular inflammation (anterior, posterior or panuveitis): infectious, inflammatory, neoplastic, or ischemic

Investigations

- Urgent (same-day) orbit and brain imaging:
    - CT is often more readily available than MRI and is a reasonable first option as long as dedicated high-resolution orbital and cavernous sinus views are obtained, with contrast ("CT brain" alone is of little value). Ask for: magnified axial and coronal fine-cut CT orbits, plus CT brain with cavernous sinus views, with contrast.
    - This will identify most orbital tumors and collections that can present with acute orbitopathy and shows bone erosion (from cancer) better than MRI.
    - MRI provides better resolution of the orbital apex and cavernous sinus.
    - Ultrasound may be helpful in distinguishing some types of orbital lesions.
    - However, many diffuse orbital processes (infection of any cause, lymphoma, autoimmune inflammation) all look the same on imaging (diffuse increase in signal in the orbital soft tissue) so other investigations are needed to determine the underlying cause.
    - Whichever scan you get, look specifically to see whether there is a:
        - Solid tumor mass.
        - Drainable orbital pus collection.
        - Opacification of one or more of the ethmoid, maxillary, or sphenoid sinuses (possible primary infection or cancer which has then spread into the orbit).
        - Dilated superior ophthalmic vein: this is the most reliable CT or MRI sign of a CCF—MRA and MR venography (MRV) may be of value in the diagnosis of this condition.
        - Enlargement of one or more of the extraocular muscles.
        - Enlargement or enhancement of the optic nerve.
- Other investigations required may include:
    - Blood tests for thyroid function, infectious and autoimmune causes.
    - Chest x-ray looking for primary or secondary cancer, tuberculosis, or sarcoidosis.
    - Transnasal endoscopic aspiration and biopsy of a potentially infected or cancerous ethmoid or sphenoid sinus (specimen to microbiology, histology, cytology).
    - Direct orbital biopsy.
    - Lumbar puncture.
    - Chest and abdomen CT or MRI and/or bone scan, looking for primary or secondary neoplastic lesions.
    - Catheter angiography for diagnosis (± treatment) of CCF.

Treatment

- treat the underlying cause, for example:
    - intravenous antibiotic treatment ± surgical drainage or debridement of infection
    - endovascular occlusion of a CCF
    - anticoagulation for CST
    - chemotherapy and radiotherapy for lymphoma
    - immunosuppression for specific or non-specific autoimmune inflammation
- protect the eye
    - lower intraocular pressure if necessary (medically or with orbital decompression)
    - protect the cornea if exposed (especially if the cornea is also anesthetic)

Neuromuscular Junction Disease

MYASTHENIA GRAVIS

Summary of clinical features suggestive of myasthenia: see p. 198.

- Myasthenia is one of the "great mimickers" and can simulate almost any ocular motility disorder.
- Its ophthalmic clinical hallmarks are ptosis and/or diplopia that are usually fatigable and variable.
- If limited to one or more of the extraocular muscles (without ptosis), it can be very difficult to diagnose.

Mechanism

- Autoantibodies directed against the acetylcholine receptors are produced, circulate in the blood and destroy or block many of the receptors.
- The decreased number of functioning acetylcholine receptors results in the fatigability that is so often seen clinically: on repeated or sustained contraction, fewer receptors are available for activation and the strength of the muscle fades.

Causes

- idiopathic myasthenia (in most cases)
- medications: "drug-induced" myasthenia (penicillamine, aminoglycosides, beta-blockers, chlorpromazine, etc.)

Symptoms

- These usually have a gradual onset and are usually initially mild or intermittent. However, in some cases there is the acute onset of severe ophthalmic and/or systemic symptoms.

Diplopia

- Horizontal, vertical, or oblique (but usually not torsional).
- The nature of the diplopia may be variable, e.g., sometimes vertical, sometimes horizontal.
- The severity of the diplopia may also vary:
  - From day to day ("good days and bad days").
  - During each day (diurnal variation): usually myasthenic diplopia is least on waking in the morning and worst at night or when the patient is tired (but diplopia caused by nerve or muscle disease can also sometimes worsen when the patient is tired).
  - It may improve or resolve with rest (if the patient closes the eyes for a few minutes).

Ptosis

- unilateral, bilateral, or alternating sides
- when bilateral, may be symmetric or asymmetric
- often:
  - has a gradual or intermittent onset
  - varies from day to day

- worsens during the day (being worst at night; however, age-related "aponeurotic" ptosis is also sometimes reported as being worst at night)
- may improve or resolve with rest

Systemic Symptoms
- Dyspnea, dysphagia (problems with swallowing), or dysphonia (hoarse voice): these are all very worrying symptoms as they indicate severe generalized myasthenia; these patients require urgent neurologic assessment.
- Weakness of arm or leg muscles: ask the patient "Are there any things you used to be able to do that you now have trouble with?," e.g., getting up out of chairs, walking up stairs, taking the tops off jars.
- Fatigue, lack of energy.

Signs

Abnormal Ocular Motility (Figs 6.5 and 6.6, Videos 6.3 and 6.4)
- Myasthenia can:
  - Mimic any other cause of strabismus, including unilateral or bilateral pupil-sparing partial or complete third nerve palsy, fourth nerve palsy, or sixth nerve palsy or INO.

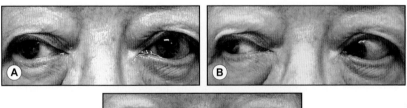

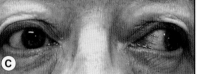

Fig. 6.5 (A–C) Right exotropia due to myasthenic weakness of the right medial rectus muscle; there is defective adduction of the right eye. Adducting saccades were of normal velocity (as opposed to the slow adducting saccades seen with partial third nerve palsy or internuclear ophthalmoplegia).

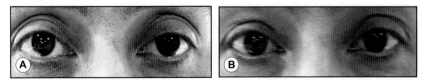

Fig. 6.6 This patient had vertical diplopia due to a small right hypertropia, without ptosis. She reported that the diplopia was worse at night or when tired. Acetylcholine receptor antibodies were negative and Tensilon testing was performed. (A) Before Tensilon injection, showing a small right hypertropia. (B) 30 seconds after injection of Tensilon, the patient reported that her diplopia had resolved and the vertical deviation was seen to resolve on observation and prism cover measurement. Note also elevation of both eyelids, right more than left.

- (Usually) cause an incomitant strabismus, with any pattern of limitation of movement of one or both eyes (including underaction of a single muscle on one side).
- (Rarely) present as a gradual or acute-onset comitant strabismus, with no obvious limitation of movement in any direction.
- Cause intermittent diplopia, with an entirely normal motility examination when you see the patient.
- Present as a horizontal or vertical gaze palsy without diplopia.

- The principal examination clue that myasthenia is present is demonstrating "clinical fatigability":
  - Make the patient hold their gaze in the direction of the worst limitation of motility.
  - As the affected muscle fatigues, the eye may slowly drift back toward the primary position.
  - This is not completely specific for myasthenia (partial nerve palsies can also show fatigability) and neither does the absence of demonstrable fatigability rule out myasthenia.
  - An alternative is to make repetitive saccades in the direction of action of the affected muscle/s; it should be noted that, as opposed to the slow saccades of myopathy or neuropathy, saccades may be of normal velocity or slow in myasthenia but (especially with fatigue) become hypometric: smaller than they should be, with the eye "undershooting" the target.
- "Gaze-paretic nystagmus":
  - This can be seen in extraocular muscle weakness of any cause (nerve palsy, myasthenia or paretic myopathy).
  - It occurs due to increased innervation to the agonist muscle of the other eye, if a patient with a paretic muscle is asked to look in the direction of action of the weak muscle.
  - The importance of this is that myasthenia can very closely mimic INO if it affects mainly the medial rectus muscle, with gaze-paretic nystagmus being seen in the other (abducting) eye on attempted adduction of the affected eye.
  - For example, if myasthenia is affecting only the left medial rectus, on attempted right gaze, the patient may show decreased adduction of the left eye and jerk nystagmus of the abducting right eye.

Ptosis (See Chapter 11, p. 305)
- Very mild ptosis to complete lid closure, unilateral or bilateral.
- Bilateral ptosis may be symmetric or asymmetric.
- Mild to severe decrease in levator function.
- Skin crease: some unlucky patients have both age-related (aponeurotic) and myasthenic ptosis, so the finding of a high skin crease or a thin upper lid does not rule out myasthenia.
- Demonstrating "clinical fatigability" of ptosis
  - Measure the palpebral aperture and levator function.
  - Have the patient look up to a target on the ceiling.

- Ask the patient to keep looking there without moving the eyes for 2 minutes (make sure the patient does not progressively lean their head back to compensate).
- Then ask the patient to look back to a target in the primary position; remeasure palpebral aperture and then levator function.
- If fatigability is present, the ptosis will be significantly worse after prolonged upgaze, then recover back to its normal level with rest.

Other Ophthalmic Signs of Myasthenia
- Orbicularis weakness (weak lid closure against resistance) or facial weakness: this is an important sign to find, as it indicates that the diplopia is likely due to neuromuscular junction or muscle disease (not a nerve palsy).
- "Cogan lid twitch" test:
  - Ask the patient to look down at a target for 15–30 seconds.
  - Then ask the patient to look straight at your nose.
  - A "lid twitch" is said to be present if the upper lid shows a series of small rapid retractions before settling into position or if the lid goes up normally but then descends again.
  - The finding of a lid twitch is suggestive of myasthenia but it is not diagnostic and its absence does not exclude myasthenia.
- Enhancement of ptosis:
  - Elevate one eyelid and observe the contralateral eyelid position.
  - Enhancement is said to be present if the contralateral eyelid descends.
  - However, this sign is not specific for myasthenia.
- Pupils:
  - The pupils are never involved clinically in myasthenia gravis.
  - If a patient with ptosis and diplopia has a poorly reactive dilated pupil, the diagnosis is not myasthenia!

Systemic Signs
- Systemic weakness, dysphonia, or dyspnea may be evident on casual observation of the patient during your consultation.
- You can also test for clinical fatigability of systemic muscles (e.g., on repeated hand grip).

Clinical Tests

Sleep/Rest Test
- Because myasthenic weakness worsens with muscle use and improves with rest, both myasthenic ptosis and diplopia lessen with prolonged rest or sleep.
- Measure the ptosis and motility defect, have the patient close the eyes and rest for 30 minutes (preferably in a dark room), then remeasure; a significant improvement after rest is suggestive of myasthenia.
- This test is time-consuming in a busy clinic and overall is not as sensitive or specific as the other tests.

Ice Test

- This is a great test for possible myasthenic ptosis but is not as useful if the patient has diplopia without ptosis.
- How to test
  - Put a small amount of crushed ice in a surgical glove or use a cold pack.
  - Measure (and ideally photograph) the ptosis in the primary position.
  - Ask the patient to close both eyes.
  - After 2 minutes, have the patient open eyes and remeasure the ptosis.
  - Next, ask the patient to close both eyes again; place the ice-filled glove or ice pack directly on one closed eye; don't touch the other eye.
  - Leave the ice there for 2 minutes.
  - After 2 minutes, remove the ice, ask the patient to open their eyes, and immediately remeasure (and ideally photograph) the ptosis again in the primary position.
  - A significant improvement of the ptosis (2 mm or more) on the "iced" side is highly suggestive of myasthenia.
  - In many cases of bilateral ptosis from myasthenia, the ice test will result in improvement in ptosis on both sides.

Prostigmin Test

- Prostigmin (neostigmine bromide) is a long-acting acetylcholinesterase inhibitor; it is given intramuscularly and lasts 45–60 minutes.
- This is an excellent and sensitive test for myasthenia in children or in adults with poor or no venous access who have diplopia associated with limitation of eye movement without associated ptosis.
- It may "miss" some cases of true myasthenia (false-negative result); false-positive results are rare but do occur.
- Because Prostigmin can cause significant gastrointestinal (GI) and other side effects, the medication is always given mixed with atropine. Usually 1.5 mg neostigmine is mixed with 0.6 mg atropine for adults; 0.04 mg/kg (not to exceed 1.5 mg) neostigmine is mixed with an appropriate dose of atropine for children. Consult a pediatric neuro-opthalmologist if you are considering performing this test on a child.

Investigations

- Blood test for acetylcholine receptor blocking and binding antibodies:
  - Detectable in 90% of patients with generalized myasthenia but only about 50% of patients who only have ophthalmic symptoms; hence, a negative blood test does not exclude myasthenia.
  - However, if the test is positive, it is extremely likely that the patient has myasthenia (false-positives are rare).
  - The level of the antibody does not correlate with the severity of the disease.

- Other blood tests:
  - Other myasthenic antibodies (e.g., antiskeletal muscle antibodies) are occasionally present when acetylcholine receptor antibodies are not, but routine testing for these is usually not indicated.
  - Tests for other autoimmune diseases: myasthenic patients are more likely to have or develop other autoimmune diseases so it is appropriate to also perform:
    - Thyroid function tests: a significant number of myasthenics also have Graves' disease (and rarely can have diplopia from restrictive thyroid myopathy rather than or in addition to paretic myasthenic myopathy).
    - ANA assay for systemic lupus erythematosus (SLE).
- Electrophysiologic testing:
  - Electromyography (EMG) and (ideally) single-fiber electromyography (sf-EMG) can detect myasthenia in most cases, but the testing is most accurate if performed on a "clinically weak" muscle (making this difficult in isolated "ocular" myasthenia).
  - False-negatives and false-positives occur.
- CT chest should be performed in all patients with diagnosed myasthenia, as 10% of patients have a potentially malignant thymus gland tumor (thymoma).

Natural History

- Three-quarters of myasthenics first present with ptosis and/or diplopia without other significant symptoms.
- 80% of these patients go on to develop systemic muscle weakness ("generalize") within 2 years.
- Some patients gradually worsen for several years, remain severe for some time, then slowly improve; other patients have a relapsing and remitting course.
- Whatever the course, most patients will eventually improve and may be able to cease some or all treatment (although this may take many years).

Treatment

- Myasthenia is a potentially life-threatening disease.
  - It is advisable for the patient to be managed by a neuro-ophthalmologist, neurologist, or neuromuscular specialist.
  - Warn the patient to present to a hospital general emergency department immediately at any stage if they become short of breath, has problems swallowing, develops a hoarse voice or severe arm or leg weakness (possible myasthenic crisis).
- In general, treatment is given to keep the patient as comfortable and safe as possible until the disease "burns itself out."

Optical Treatment

- Because myasthenic diplopia is usually variable, prism spectacles are often of little benefit.
- Occlusion of one spectacle lens is often well tolerated.

Medical Treatment

- In general, ophthalmic manifestations of myasthenia respond less well to pyridostigmine than systemic weakness, and often, oral prednisone or other immunosuppression is required for symptomatic improvement of diplopia.
- However, in all cases, the risk of treatment should be weighed against the potential benefit; for instance, it is not wise to treat a patient with high-dose steroids for years (giving them diabetes and osteoporosis) purely for mild or intermittent diplopia, when occluding one spectacle lens would be a much safer alternative.
- Pyridostigmine (Mestinon)
  - Usually the first treatment used once myasthenia has been diagnosed.
  - An anticholinesterase (as is Prostigmin): it stops the breakdown of acetylcholine molecules in the neuromuscular junction, increasing their concentration and effect (leading to stronger activation of the surviving acetylcholine receptors).
- Prednisone
  - Commencing prednisone treatment can precipitate a myasthenic crisis; consult a neurologist first (the patient may need to be admitted for safety).
  - Prednisone treatment directly suppresses the autoimmune process causing the disease and may possibly prevent conversion of ocular myasthenia to generalized myasthenia.
- Other immunosuppressive treatment: patients who benefit from steroid treatment can often be treated with a "steroid-sparing" agent (e.g., azathioprine, mycophenolate mofetil) that allows reduction or withdrawal of the steroids over time.

Surgical Treatment

- Thymectomy
  - Necessary in all cases of thymoma found on chest CT.
  - May also benefit patients with severe generalized myasthenia without thymoma and even patients with severe refractory ocular myasthenia.
- Ptosis surgery
  - This should be considered only if the ptosis is severe, stable, and unresponsive to maximum medical treatment; however, there is some risk involved, specifically:
    - If the orbicularis is also weak there is a risk of causing corneal exposure.
    - If the myasthenia resolves with time, the patient may be left with lid retraction.
- Strabismus surgery
  - This is rarely appropriate in myasthenia, due to the highly variable nature of the disease and the fact that usually it is a self-limited condition that will resolve with time, with eventual return of normal motility.
  - Nevertheless, it may be appropriate in selected patients on maximum medical therapy with a long-standing, stable strabismus.

Nerve Disease

THIRD NERVE PALSY

Check that your patient meets ALL the clinical diagnostic criteria on p. 199 before you diagnose "ischemic" third nerve palsy!

Causes

- Compression
  - Aneurysm (most often at junction of internal carotid and posterior communicating arteries) (see Fig. 6.6)
    - This causes up to a third of all third nerve palsies.
    - An expanding aneurysm can rupture and kill the patient within hours to days of the onset of diplopia; hence, the assessment of possible third nerve palsy is the most urgent of all ophthalmic emergencies.
  - Brain tumors (e.g., pituitary tumors that have extended into the cavernous sinus; sphenoid wing meningiomas).
  - Raised intracranial pressure (ICP) with uncal herniation (causing "fixed dilated pupil/s" in an unconscious patient).
- Ischemia: this is the most common cause of third nerve palsy
  - Atherosclerosis.
  - Diabetes.
  - Hypertension.
  - GCA.
- Inflammation
  - Multiple sclerosis (MS) can rarely cause a fascicular third nerve palsy.
  - Infection (viral or postviral).
- Trauma (severe open or closed head injuries).

Symptoms

One or more of:
- Diplopia:
  - A partial third nerve palsy may cause horizontal, vertical, and/or oblique diplopia.
  - Patients with complete third nerve palsies don't notice diplopia as they have a complete ipsilateral ptosis.
- Ptosis: may sometimes be the earliest change noticed by the patient or may commence at the same time as or after diplopia.
- Pupil changes:
  - Some patients (or their relatives/friends) notice an increase in pupil size in the affected eye.
  - However, partial third nerve palsies rarely present as an isolated pupil change (usually diplopia or ptosis is also present).
- Pain:
  - Both compressive and ischemic third nerve palsies may be painful.
  - Persisting severe pain is more likely to be due to an aneurysm than ischemia.
  - Orbital, hemifacial, or hemicranial pain that was present for days or weeks before the onset of diplopia is likely to be due to aneurysm or tumor.

- Symptoms of the underlying disease, for example:
    - Symptoms of GCA (GCA can cause ischemic third nerve palsy).
    - Headaches or hormonal changes due to a pituitary tumor.
    - Headaches, meningism, and photophobia due to subarachnoid hemorrhage if a posterior communicating artery aneurysm has started to rupture.

Signs

- localizing signs: see Table 6.1 and Fig. 6.7

TABLE 6.1 ■ Clinical Localization of the Lesion Causing Third Nerve Palsy

SIGNS; Partial or Complete Third Nerve Palsy With	Localizes the Lesion to	Why?	What Lesions Can Cause This?
Bilateral symmetric ptosis and/or contralateral SR weakness and/or other neurologic signs	Third nerve nucleus in midbrain	In the third nerve nucleus, a single midline subnucleus supplies the levator on both sides and the superior rectus subnucleus on each side supplies the SR on the opposite side	Stroke, MS, tumor
Contralateral arm or leg tremor	Third nerve fascicle in midbrain from the third nerve nucleus through the red nucleus (damage here causes both a third nerve palsy and contralateral tremor—Benedikt syndrome)	The third nerve fibers pass through the red nucleus	Stroke, MS, tumor
Contralateral arm or leg weakness	Third nerve fascicle in midbrain or third nerve at exit from brainstem	The third nerve fibers pass through the cerebral peduncle before exiting from the brainstem; both intrinsic and extrinsic lesions can cause this syndrome (Weber syndrome)	Stroke, MS, tumor

SIGNS; Partial or Complete Third Nerve Palsy With	Localizes the Lesion to	Why?	What Lesions Can Cause This?
One or more of fourth, fifth,[a] or sixth nerve palsy or Horner syndrome	Cavernous sinus	The third nerve runs in the lateral wall of the cavernous sinus superior to the fourth nerve, ophthalmic and maxillary divisions of the fifth nerve, and lateral to the sixth nerve and sympathetic fibers (which run through the sinus itself); in the anterior sinus it divides into superior and inferior divisions[b]	Tumor, CST or fistula,[a] infection, inflammation
Optic nerve dysfunction ± fourth, fifth,[a] or sixth nerve palsy	Orbital apex	The third nerve divisions and other ocular motor nerves lie close to the optic nerve in the orbital apex	Tumor, infection, inflammation
Proptosis and/or eye injection; any muscles involved	Orbit	The third nerve divisions split into fine branches to the supplied muscles; these can be damaged by orbital disease	Inflammation, infection, tumor
NO signs other than the third nerve palsy	"Isolated" third nerve palsy—site unknown	This is often due to a lesion of the third nerve in its subarachnoid course (between the fascicle and the cavernous sinus) OR (rarely) at ANY OTHER PART of its course	Compression (aneurysm, tumor); ischemic; raised ICP

CST, Cavernous sinus thrombosis; *ICP*, intracranial pressure; *MS*, multiple sclerosis; *SR*, superior rectus.

[a]Fifth (trigeminal) nerve palsy (often from a tumor) can present with persistent eye, orbital, hemifacial, or hemicranial pain; numbness; or "pins and needles" sensation, with or without decreased corneal or facial sensation on testing.

[b]"Divisional" partial third nerve palsy: most often due to cavernous sinus or orbital apex disease (the nerve divides into superior and inferior divisions in the lateral wall of the cavernous sinus) but can also occur at any other site throughout the course of the nerve (including nuclear and fascicular lesions in the midbrain). Superior division: only superior rectus and levator affected; inferior division: medial and inferior rectus, inferior oblique, pupil affected.

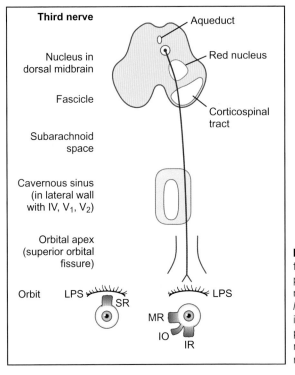

Fig. 6.7 Schematic anatomy of the third nerve. Ciliary ganglion and pupil fibres aren't shown; Left III nucleus control muscles are shown. *IO*, Inferior oblique muscle; *IR*, inferior rectus muscle; *LPS*, levator palpebrae superioris muscle; *MR*, medial rectus muscle; *SR*, superior rectus muscle.

Partial Third Nerve Palsy (Figs 6.8 and 6.9, Videos 6.5–6.8)

- Aneurysmal partial third nerve palsy is one of the "great mimickers" and can present with ANY type of ocular deviation except esotropia.
- One or more of the muscles that the third nerve innervates can be affected, to any degree (mild to severe), in any combination, causing one or more of:
  - Exotropia due to medial rectus weakness.
  - Hypertropia due to inferior rectus weakness.
  - Hypotropia due to superior rectus and/or inferior oblique weakness.
  - Ptosis due to levator palpebrae superioris weakness.
  - Enlarged pupil (in some cases) that is poorly responsive to both light and near, due to sphincter pupillae weakness.
- "Aberrant regeneration."
  - Signs: upper lid retraction, pupil constriction, and/or inappropriate eye movements on attempted adduction, elevation, or depression of the eye.
  - Explanation: because the third nerve supplies so many different muscles (four extraocular muscles, a lid muscle and a pupil muscle), if it is damaged by compression along its course, axons often grow back along the wrong routes, to the "wrong muscles." By this mechanism:
    - Nerve fibers that "should" have gone to the medial rectus may instead go to the sphincter pupillae (causing the pupil to become smaller on attempted adduction of the eye).

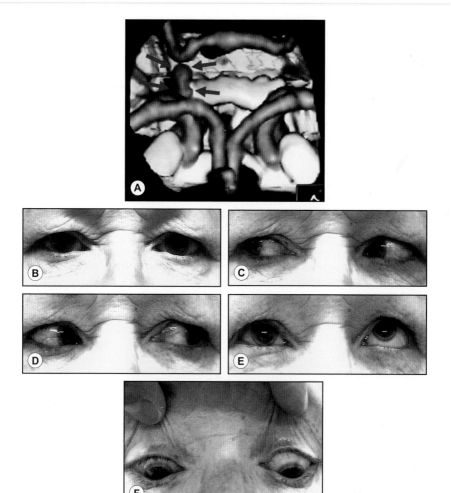

Fig. 6.8 Partial right third nerve palsy due to posterior communicating artery aneurysm (**A**) *(arrows)*, as seen on computed tomographic angiography. The patient presented with vertical diplopia and a small vertical strabismus. All eye movements were normal (**B–D, F**), with the exception of slightly reduced right eye elevation (**E**). There was no ptosis and the pupils were equal in size and both briskly reactive to light.

- ▪ The inferior rectus nerve fibers may have misrouted to the levator muscle (causing lid retraction on attempted downgaze).
- ▪ Fibers that used to supply one rectus muscle instead now innervate a different rectus muscle (causing, for example, an inward movement of the eye in attempted upward gaze).
- ▪ Significance: if you see aberrant regeneration, the nerve palsy is NOT ISCHEMIC.
- ▪ If there is aberrant regeneration without a preceding history of acute nerve palsy (i.e., it has just gradually developed—"primary aberrant regeneration"), it is very likely that there is a slow-growing lesion, usually an aneurysm or meningioma compressing the third nerve, often in the cavernous sinus.

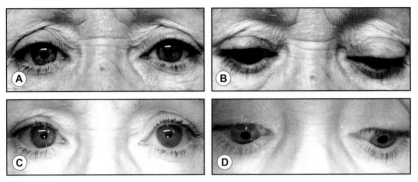

Fig. 6.9 Primary aberrant regeneration in a patient with a slowly progressive right partial third nerve palsy due to cavernous sinus meningioma. (**A**) The upper lid level is symmetric in primary position, but in downgaze (**B**), right upper lid retraction is apparent (aberrant regenerating fibers that should have gone to the inferior rectus are now innervating the levator muscle). (**C**) The pupils are equal in size in primary position, but in downgaze (**D**), the right pupil constricts relative to the left (aberrant regenerating fibers that should have gone to the inferior rectus are now innervating the sphincter pupillae).

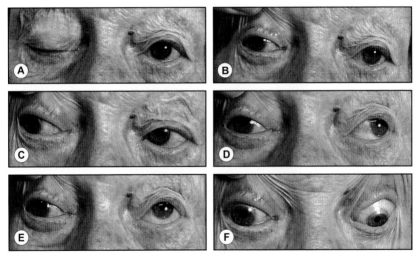

Fig. 6.10 (**A–F**) Complete right third nerve palsy with pupil involvement. There is a complete right ptosis and the right eye has complete lack of adduction, elevation, and depression. The right pupil is larger than the left.

Complete Third Nerve Palsy (Fig. 6.10, Video 6.9)

- complete ptosis
- pupil normal or enlarged
- complete external ophthalmoplegia (no elevation, depression or adduction), with intact:
    - intorsion on attempted downgaze in abduction (superior oblique—fourth nerve)
    - abduction (lateral rectus—sixth nerve)

"Pupil-Sparing" Third Nerve Palsy (Fig. 6.11, Video 6.10)

- A common and dangerous misperception is that if the pupil is normal, the third nerve palsy is ischemic and the patient doesn't need imaging.
- However, this only applies if the palsy is otherwise complete and meets all the clinical diagnostic criteria for ischemic third nerve palsy on p. 199.
- All patients with partial third nerve palsies, or complete nerve palsies not meeting these criteria, must be urgently imaged with MRI plus MRA or CTA to rule out an aneurysm.
- This is because aneurysmal partial third nerve palsies may be "pupil sparing" early in their evolution.

Differential Diagnosis

- of partial third nerve palsy with pupil spared:
  - myasthenia
  - skew deviation
  - INO
- of complete third nerve palsy with pupil spared: myasthenia

Investigations

- All patients not meeting the clinical diagnostic criteria for ischemic third nerve palsy on p. 199: urgent MRI brain with contrast, plus magnetic resonance angiogram (MRA) or CTA; MRI alone may miss some aneurysms.
- Patients meeting the clinical diagnostic criteria for ischemic third nerve palsy:
  - If the patient is over age 50 and has symptoms or signs suspicious for GCA, take blood for an urgent ESR, CRP, and complete blood count.
  - If no suggestion of GCA: investigate (or have the patient's physician investigate) atherosclerotic risk factors.
  - Obtain MRI plus MRA or CTA of brain if:
    - The palsy has not started to resolve by 3 months after onset.
    - New neurologic symptoms or signs develop at any stage.

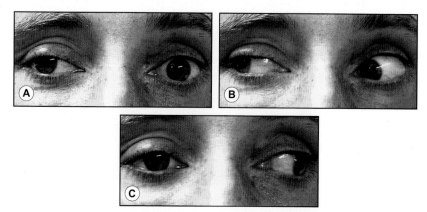

Fig. 6.11 Despite this right partial third nerve palsy being "pupil sparing" (the pupils were equal in size and both briskly reactive to light) (**A–C**), imaging revealed the cause to be a posterior communicating artery aneurysm.

Treatment

- Aneurysm
  - Treatment options include surgery to clip the aneurysm and endovascular coiling (catheter angiography with the injection of coils into the aneurysm) (Fig. 6.12).
  - Urgent treatment often saves the patient's life.
  - Partial or complete recovery of the third nerve palsy may occur after successful treatment.
- Ischemic third nerve palsy
  - The patient's physician should treat specific vascular risk factors identified (stop smoking, reduce cholesterol, monitor blood pressure, improve diabetic control); this could prevent a heart attack or stroke in the future.
  - Many neuro-ophthalmologists would recommend treatment with long-term low-dose aspirin (unless contraindicated) to decrease future vascular risk.
  - "Ischemic" third nerve palsy usually starts to recover within 3 months and motility may spontaneously return to normal.
- Prism spectacles may be helpful for small residual deviations; otherwise occlusion of one eye for symptomatic relief.
- If after 12 months some motility deficit remains, no further recovery is occurring and the deviation is stable, strabismus surgery may be helpful based on the residual function of the muscles; ptosis surgery may also be beneficial.

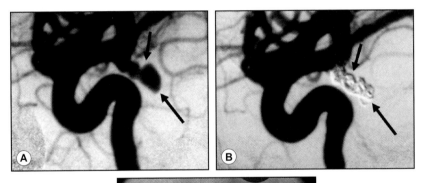

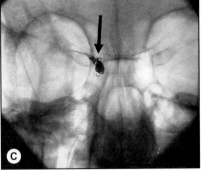

Fig. 6.12 Treatment of a posterior communicating artery aneurysm by endovascular placement of coils. Platinum coils are injected via a catheter fed upward from a femoral artery incision; this technique can avoid the need for open neurosurgery in some patients. (**A**) Angiogram showing aneurysm before treatment. (**B**) Aneurysm obliterated by coils. (**C**) Coils in position.

FOURTH NERVE PALSY

Check that your patient meets ALL the clinical diagnostic criteria on:
- (p. 200) before you diagnose "ischemic" fourth nerve palsy
- (p. 201) before you diagnose "congenital" fourth nerve palsy

Causes

- congenital, unilateral
  - common
- acquired
  - traumatic, unilateral or bilateral
    - common
    - usually due to severe closed head injury
  - ischemic, unilateral
    - common
    - due to atherosclerosis, diabetes, hypertension, GCA
  - compressive, unilateral, or bilateral
    - rare
    - due to midbrain, pineal region, or cavernous sinus tumors
  - inflammatory, usually unilateral
    - rare
    - e.g., infectious or postinfectious neuritis

Symptoms and Signs

- Localizing signs: see Table 6.2 and Fig. 6.13.
- Note: you may need to use the following examination techniques:
  - Measuring vertical fusional amplitude—p. 40.
  - Measuring extorsion with double Maddox rod—p. 42.
  - Observing for fundus extorsion.
  - Look at old photographs for head tilt to side of lower eye.

Acquired Unilateral Fourth Nerve Palsy (Fig. 6.14, Video 6.11)

- symptoms: vertical or oblique ± torsional diplopia
- signs
  - often a head tilt away from the side of the palsy
  - eye movements
    - hypertropia or oblique deviation of one eye
    - secondary overaction of the ipsilateral inferior oblique (causing upshoot of the eye in adduction)
    - (sometimes) visible underaction of the ipsilateral superior oblique (underaction visible when the eye looks down and to the opposite side)
  - vertical prism fusional amplitude testing: less than 5 prism diopters
  - torsion testing
    - double Maddox rod: extorsion of less than 10 degrees
    - fundus observation: extorsion of the fundus on the affected side

TABLE 6.2 ■ Clinical Localization of the Lesion Causing Fourth Nerve Palsy

SIGNS; Fourth Nerve Palsy With	Localizes the Lesion to	Why?	What Lesions Can Cause This?
Other brainstem signs (e.g., those of dorsal midbrain syndrome, p. 246)	Fourth nerve nucleus or fascicle the midbrain	The paired fourth nerve nuclei lie in the dorsal midbrain near the aqueduct, at the level of the inferior colliculus; damage here will often cause damage to nearby brainstem areas (note: because the fourth nerves cross after emerging from the brainstem, fibers from the right fourth nerve nucleus travel through the right fourth nerve fascicle, then cross and exit the brain to become the left fourth nerve to the left superior oblique)	Stroke, MS, tumor (e.g., pinealoma)
One or more of third, fifth,[a] or sixth nerve palsy or Horner syndrome	Cavernous sinus	The fourth nerve runs in the lateral wall of the cavernous sinus inferior to the third nerve, superior to the ophthalmic and maxillary divisions of the fifth nerve and lateral to the sixth nerve and sympathetic fibers (that run through the sinus itself)	Tumor, CST or fistula, infection, inflammation
Optic nerve dysfunction ± third, fifth,[a] or sixth nerve palsy	Orbital apex	The fourth and other nerves lie close to the optic nerve in the orbital apex	Tumor, infection, inflammation
Proptosis and/ or eye injection; any muscles involved	Orbit	The orbital fourth nerve branches can be damaged by orbital disease (usually other nerves or muscles affected too)	Inflammation, infection, tumor
NO signs other than the fourth nerve palsy	"Isolated" fourth nerve palsy—site unknown	This is often due to a lesion of the fourth nerve in its subarachnoid course (between the fascicle and the cavernous sinus) OR (rarely) at ANY OTHER PART of its course	Congenital, trauma, ischemia, tumor

CST, Cavernous sinus thrombosis; *MS,* multiple sclerosis.
[a]Fifth (trigeminal) nerve palsy (often from a tumor) can present with persistent eye, orbital, hemifacial, or hemicranial pain; numbness; or "pins and needles" sensation, with or without decreased corneal or facial sensation on testing.

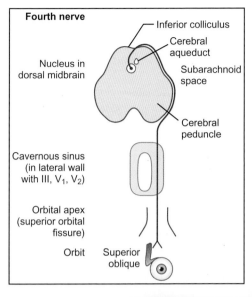

Fourth nerve

Inferior colliculus

Cerebral aqueduct

Nucleus in dorsal midbrain

Subarachnoid space

Cerebral peduncle

Cavernous sinus (in lateral wall with III, V$_1$, V$_2$)

Orbital apex (superior orbital fissure)

Orbit

Superior oblique

Fig. 6.13 Schematic anatomy of the fourth nerve.

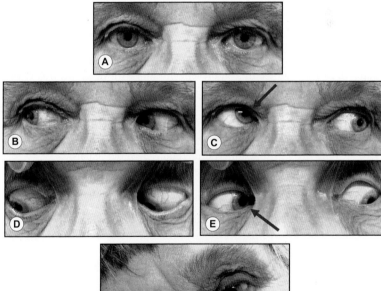
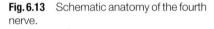
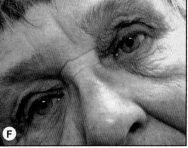

Fig. 6.14 Right ischemic fourth nerve palsy. (**A**) There is a small right hypertropia (not easily visible but can be measured on prism cover test) in primary position. Note that the right hypertropia increases in left gaze *(arrow)* (**B, C**) and that there is underaction of the right superior oblique visible as decreased depression in adduction (when the patient looks down and left—*arrow*) (**D, E**). (**F**) The right hypertropia measured on prism cover test increased when the patient tilted his head to the right.

Acquired Bilateral Fourth Nerve Palsy
- Symptoms: torsional ± vertical or oblique diplopia.
- Signs
  - There may be a head tilt; often the head is tilted downward.
  - Eye movements
    - Relative hypertropia of one eye or no vertical deviation.
    - If hypertropia is present, this often reverses with gaze side-to-side (e.g., left hypertropia in right gaze, right hypertropia in left gaze).
    - Secondary overaction of both inferior obliques (causing upshoot of each eye on adduction), leading to a "V" pattern exotropia in upgaze.
    - (Sometimes) visible underaction of the both superior obliques (underaction visible when each eye looks down and to the opposite side).
  - Vertical prism fusional amplitude testing: less than 5 prism diopters.
  - Torsion testing
    - Double Maddox rod: often extorsion of 10 degrees or more.
    - Fundus observation: extorsion of the fundus on both sides.

Congenital Unilateral Fourth Nerve Palsy (Fig. 6.15, Video 6.12)
- Symptoms: no sensation of torsion:
  - The images are double but neither is "tilted."
  - Vertical or oblique diplopia only, often intermittent.
- Signs (Fig. 6.15):
  - Head tilt away from the side of the palsy (often visible on old family photographs). In fact, some children present initially with head tilt; this is why every child with a head tilt should have an ophthalmic examination.
  - Chronic head tilt sometimes causes the side of the face opposite the palsy to grow less than the ipsilateral side (causing hemifacial hypoplasia); if you look carefully, many children and adults with congenital fourths have this sign.
  - Eye movements: as for acquired unilateral fourth nerve palsy.
  - Vertical prism fusional amplitude testing:
- Greater than 5 prism diopters.
  - Torsion testing:
    - Double Maddox rod: often no subjective torsion but some patients with congenital fourth nerve palsy do have extorsion measurable on double Maddox rod testing, despite not having torsional diplopia.
    - Fundus observation: extorsion of the fundus on the affected side.

Differential Diagnosis

- Skew deviation:
  - This is a comitant or incomitant vertical or oblique deviation, usually caused by brainstem stroke, MS, or tumor.
  - A skew deviation can closely mimic a fourth nerve palsy; however, the following two tests may help differentiate the two:
  - Torsion: in a skew deviation the hypertropic eye is usually intorted, not extorted (hence, the importance of measuring torsion and looking for fundus torsion in all patients with a vertical deviation).

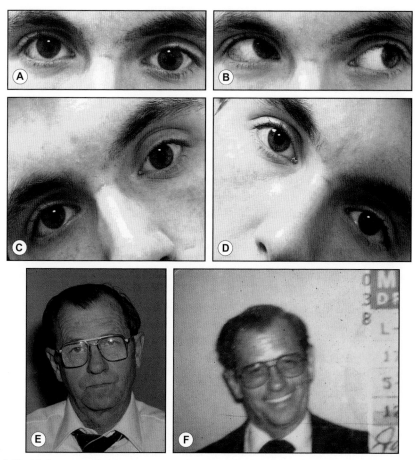

Fig. 6.15 Right congenital fourth nerve palsy. Note the moderate right hypertropia in primary position (**A**), increased on left gaze (**B**) and right head tilt (**C**); improved on left head tilt (**D**). (**E**) Another patient who presents with a decompenated congenital fourth nerve palsy later in life; his old driver's license photo (**F**) shows that his head tilt has been long-standing.

- The "upright-supine test":
  - A patient with a vertical skew deviation will usually show a significant (>50%) decrease in the deviation, measured by prism cover test, when they lie down.
  - By comparison, there is no difference in the measured vertical deviation of a fourth nerve palsy between the sitting and lying positions.
- Partial third nerve palsy (isolated partial inferior rectus palsy, causing hypertropia).
- Myasthenia gravis.
- Orbital disease limiting vertical eye movement.

Investigations

- It is rare for tumors (and very rare for aneurysms) to cause an isolated unilateral fourth nerve palsy.
- However, to exclude this possibility, any patient with a nontraumatic unilateral fourth nerve palsy who does not meet the diagnostic criteria for a congenital or ischemic fourth should have an MRI brain. This may also pick up brainstem disease causing a skew deviation that is "masquerading" as a fourth nerve palsy.
- Any patient with a nontraumatic bilateral fourth requires MRI, as there is a significant risk of pineal region tumor.
- Patients with traumatic fourths usually have already had neuroimaging early in the management of their head injury; if not, they also require MRI (rarely tumors present with fourths from "minimal trauma").
- If a patient with fourth nerve palsy meets the clinical diagnostic criteria for ischemic palsy:
  - If over 50, ask and look for features of GCA; investigate and treat appropriately if suspicious.
  - If no suggestion of GCA: investigate (or have their physician investigate) their atherosclerotic risk factors.
  - MRI brain with contrast if no improvement by 3 months.

Treatment

- Treat the underlying disease if identified.
- Traumatic fourth: observe for at least 6 months; many resolve completely.
- Ischemic fourth
  - Almost all begin to resolve within 3 months and almost all eventually resolve completely.
  - Many neuro-ophthalmologists would recommend the patient be treated with long-term low-dose aspirin (unless contraindicated) to decrease future vascular risk.
- Strabismus surgery is often highly successful for congenital or nonresolving acquired fourth nerve palsy
  - For the correction of hypertropia in congenital or acquired unilateral fourth, inferior oblique weakening procedures (myectomy or recession) are usually very successful.
  - The correction of excyclotorsion in an acquired unilateral or bilateral fourth is more difficult; however, superior oblique tendon repositioning procedures such as the Harada-Ito procedure may help.

SIXTH NERVE PALSY

Check that your patient meets ALL the clinical diagnostic criteria on p. 202 before you diagnose "ischemic" sixth nerve palsy! In particular, make sure it is truly isolated—no other cranial neuropathies (e.g., trigeminal), no anisocoria, no ptosis.

Remember that a patient with acute horizontal diplopia associated with an esotropia and abduction weakness may have a mechanical/myopathic (e.g., thyroid eye disease) or neuromuscular (e.g., myasthenia gravis) cause, rather than a sixth nerve paresis.

Causes

- ischemic—common, unilateral
  - atherosclerosis
  - diabetes
  - GCA (if over 50)
- compressive—common, unilateral, or bilateral
  - sphenoid wing meningioma
  - cavernous internal carotid aneurysm
  - others, e.g., pituitary tumor, nasopharyngeal carcinoma, metastatic carcinoma invading the cavernous sinus
- inflammatory—rare, unilateral
  - sarcoidosis
  - infectious: viral infection, meningitis, mastoiditis, sphenoid sinusitis
- raised ICP of any cause—unilateral or bilateral
- traumatic—unilateral or bilateral
  - severe blunt head injury (particularly those causing base of skull fractures)

Symptoms

- Horizontal diplopia: if mild, sixth nerve palsy may produce diplopia that is only noticed for distance (with single vision for near) or only on side gaze to the side of the lesion (with single vision in primary position).
- Symptoms suggestive of tumor
  - Gradual or intermittent onset of horizontal diplopia: rather than the very sudden onset of diplopia over seconds or minutes that is characteristic of ischemic sixth nerve palsy.
  - Progression: the patient says the image separation increased further over days or weeks after onset (rather than the usual "ischemic" pattern of sudden onset, then no change in the amount of diplopia for several weeks, then gradual resolution)
  - Pain: both ischemic and compressive sixths may be painful or painless but severe persisting orbital, hemifacial, or hemicranial pain increases the likelihood of an underlying tumor or aneurysm.
  - Numbness or "pins and needles": of the ipsilateral orbital region or face.
  - New-onset facial weakness, deafness, tinnitus, or vertigo: on the same side as a sixth nerve palsy are highly suggestive of a vestibular schwannoma (sometimes called "acoustic neuroma") in the cerebello-pontine angle (CPA).

Signs

- localizing signs: see Table 6.3 and Fig. 6.16
  - decreased abduction of one eye with slow abducting saccades (Fig. 6.17, Video 6.13)
  - signs suggestive of tumor
    - decreased corneal or facial sensation: likely middle cranial fossa tumor
    - facial weakness, deafness, nystagmus: likely vestibular schwannoma
    - limitation of eye movements in other directions, ptosis, anisocoria: cavernous sinus tumor (causing partial third or fourth nerve palsies or Horner syndrome)
    - bitemporal field defect on confrontation testing: pituitary tumor enlarging into the cavernous sinus
    - abduction deficit of the other eye (bilateral sixth nerve palsy): base of skull tumor; or tumor causing raised ICP (look for papilledema).

TABLE 6.3 ■ Clinical Localization of the Lesion Causing Sixth Nerve Palsy

SIGNS; Sixth Nerve Palsy With	Localizes the Lesion to	Why?	What Lesions Can Cause This?
Conjugate horizontal gaze palsy, e.g., right gaze palsy: right eye can't abduct (as you would expect with right sixth nerve palsy) but also left eye can't adduct ± seventh nerve palsy (on the side of the abduction weakness) ± any of the features of fascicle damage below	Sixth nerve nucleus in the pons	Each sixth nerve nucleus in the pons contains both neurons to the ipsilateral lateral rectus and interneurons that drive the contralateral medial rectus subnucleus of the third nerve nucleus (these cross to ascend the contralateral MLF). Hence, damage to one sixth nerve nucleus causes paresis of both the ipsilateral lateral rectus and the contralateral medial rectus. The seventh nerve fascicle runs very close to the sixth nerve nucleus and is often also damaged.	Stroke, MS, tumor
One or more of: ipsilateral fifth nerve palsy,[a] seventh nerve palsy, Horner syndrome; contralateral arm or leg weakness	Sixth nerve fascicle in the pons	The sixth fibers run anteriorly through the pontine tegmentum, passing close to: part of the trigeminal nerve nucleus (that supplies sensation to the face); the facial nerve fascicles and nucleus; descending sympathetic fibers (damage to these causes a "central" Horner syndrome); and, further anteriorly, damage to the pyramidal tract can cause a contralateral hemiplegia	Stroke, MS, tumor
Ipsilateral deafness, tinnitus or vertigo ± ipsilateral fifth[a] or seventh nerve palsy	Sixth nerve root in the CPA	The fifth, sixth, seventh, and eighth nerves all emerge from the anterior aspect of the pons near its junction with the medulla and the cerebellum (the CPA) and some or all of these nerves can be compressed by tumors in this region	Compression by vestibular schwannoma, CPA meningioma, other tumors

SIGNS; Sixth Nerve Palsy With	Localizes the Lesion to	Why?	What Lesions Can Cause This?
Ipsilateral ear pain and signs of otitis media with mastoiditis ± seventh nerve palsy	Sixth nerve as it crosses the apex of the petrous temporal bone	As it crosses the apex of the petrous temporal bone, the nerve can be affected by infection spreading from the middle ear into the mastoid bone	Infectious mastoiditis (now rare)
One or more of third, fourth or fifth[a] nerve palsy or ipsilateral Horner syndrome	Cavernous sinus	The sixth nerve runs in the body of the cavernous sinus near the ICA and sympathetic fibers; the lateral wall of the sinus contains the third and fourth nerves and the ophthalmic and maxillary divisions of the fifth nerve	Tumor, CST or fistula, infection, inflammation, intracavernous ICA aneurysm
Optic nerve dysfunction ± third, fourth, or fifth[a] nerve palsy	Orbital apex	The sixth and other nerves lie close to the optic nerve in the orbital apex	Tumor, infection, inflammation
Proptosis and/or eye injection; any muscles involved	Orbit	The orbital sixth nerve branches can be damaged by orbital disease (usually other nerves or muscles affected too)	Inflammation, infection, tumor
NO signs other than the sixth nerve palsy	"Isolated" sixth nerve palsy—site unknown	This is often due to a lesion of the sixth nerve in its subarachnoid course (between the fascicle and the apex of the petrous temporal bone) OR (rarely) at ANY OTHER PART of its course	Ischemia, tumor, raised ICP

CPA, Cerebello-pontine angle; *CST*, cavernous sinus thrombosis; *ICA*, internal carotid artery; *ICP*, intracranial pressure; *MLF*, medial longitudinal fasciculus; *MS*, multiple sclerosis.
[a]Fifth (trigeminal) nerve palsy (often from a tumor) can present with persistent eye, orbital, hemifacial, or hemicranial pain; numbness; or "pins and needles" sensation, with or without decreased corneal or facial sensation on testing.

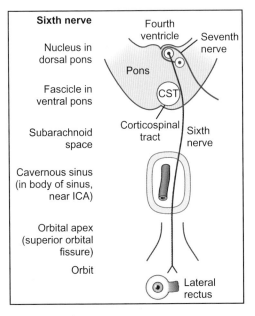

Fig. 6.16 Schematic anatomy of the sixth nerve. *CST*, cavernous sinus thrombosis.

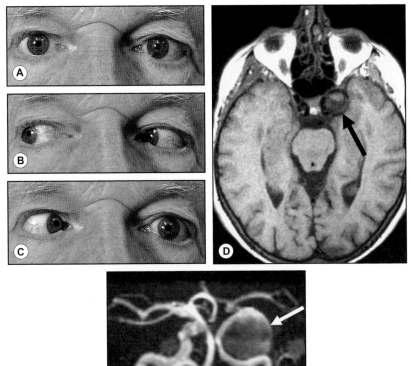

Fig. 6.17 (A–E) Slowly progressive left sixth nerve palsy due to an internal carotid artery aneurysm.

Differential Diagnosis

- Myasthenia gravis.
- Restrictive esotropia from a "tight" medial rectus (e.g., in thyroid eye disease).
- Congenital Duane retraction syndrome
  - Patients with this usually do not experience diplopia and usually know that they have the problem but confusion may arise if the patient's optometrist or doctor "incidentally notices" the motility problem.
  - Brain MRI shows absent sixth nerve in cases of Duane syndrome.

Investigations

- Patients who do not meet all the clinical diagnostic criteria for ischemic sixth nerve palsy on p. 202:
  - MRI brain with contrast (to determine if a tumor is present).
- Patients who do meet the criteria for ischemic sixth:
  - If over 50, ask and look for features of GCA; investigate and treat appropriately if suspicious.
  - If no suggestion of GCA: investigate (or have their physician investigate) atherosclerotic risk factors.
  - MRI brain with contrast if no improvement by 3 months.
- Traumatic sixth: MRI brain (if neuroimaging not already performed); tumors can sometimes present with a sixth after "minimal" trauma.

Treatment

- Ischemic sixth:
  - Observe for 3 months; if improving, continue to observe (good chance of full recovery).
  - Many neuro-ophthalmologists would recommend treatment with long-term low-dose aspirin (unless contraindicated) to decrease future vascular risk.
- Botulinum toxin injections to the medial rectus: some neuro-ophthalmologists recommend injecting the ipsilateral medial rectus muscle 3 months after onset of the palsy (of any cause) if there has been no significant improvement, to:
  - Test if there is any lateral rectus function at all (if the eye can abduct past the midline after toxin injection to the ipsilateral medial rectus, some sixth nerve function is present).
  - (Possibly) decrease permanent medial rectus fibrosis.
- Surgical treatment: wait at least 6 months; if no continuing recovery:
  - If some lateral rectus function is present, consider medial rectus recession/lateral rectus resection surgery.
  - If no lateral rectus function at all, consider transposition strabismus surgery (the superior and inferior rectus insertions are moved adjacent to the lateral rectus insertion, ± botulinum toxin to the medial rectus).

UNILATERAL MULTIPLE NERVE PALSIES

Causes include:
- cavernous sinus syndrome
- orbital apex syndrome
- (uncommonly) any of the causes of bilateral multiple nerve palsies (see p. 239)

Cavernous Sinus Syndrome

- multiple palsies of the nerves that run through the cavernous sinus on each side (Fig. 6.18): two or more of III, IV, V1, V2, VI, Horner syndrome, all on one side; normal optic nerve function
  - V1 = ophthalmic division of trigeminal nerve, supplying sensation to the eye, orbit, and forehead
  - V2 = maxillary division of trigeminal nerve, supplying sensation to the cheek and upper teeth

Causes

- acute
  - pituitary apoplexy (bleed into an undiagnosed pituitary tumor)
  - CST (sterile or septic)
  - CCF
  - sudden enlargement of cavernous sinus ICA aneurysm
  - acute infection (e.g., fungal from sphenoid sinus—mucormycosis)
  - acute idiopathic inflammation
- slowly progressive
  - cavernous sinus ICA aneurysm or tumor
  - chronic infection (e.g., tuberculosis)
  - chronic idiopathic inflammation

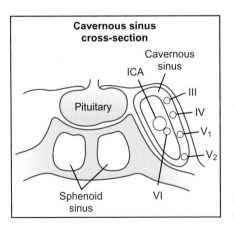

Fig. 6.18 Schematic anatomy of the cavernous sinus.

Symptoms

- diplopia
- trigeminal nerve irritation or palsy: persisting unilateral eye, orbital, forehead, cheek, hemifacial or hemicranial pain, numbness, or "pins and needles"
- other symptoms depending on cause (e.g., severe headache and lethargy in pituitary apoplexy)

Signs (Video 6.14)

- two or more of (ipsilateral):
  - partial or complete third nerve palsy (± primary aberrant regeneration if long-standing compressive lesion)
  - fourth nerve palsy
  - sixth nerve palsy
  - reduced sensation in V1 or V2
  - Horner syndrome (mild ptosis and miosis)
- ± signs of specific cause (e.g., pulsatile proptosis due to CCF)
- ± "orbital" signs (red eye, chemosis, proptosis) may or may not be present

Investigations

- urgent MRI brain with contrast, with special views of the orbits and cavernous sinus
- bloods, chest x-ray, bone scan, etc. looking for infection or a primary tumor site (if suspected metastatic tumor)
- lumbar puncture may show evidence of inflammation, infection or tumor

Treatment

- depending on the specific cause

Orbital Apex Syndrome

- Clinical features are the same as cavernous sinus syndrome, plus ipsilateral optic nerve dysfunction is present (Fig. 6.19).
- Causes and investigations are the same as for cavernous sinus syndrome.

BILATERAL MULTIPLE NERVE PALSIES

Causes include:

- bilateral cavernous sinus lesions (see earlier)—e.g., pituitary adenoma with extension to both cavernous sinuses
- bilateral orbital apex syndrome (rare)
- acute or chronic meningitis
- Guillain–Barré syndrome (GBS) and Miller Fisher variant
- Wernicke encephalopathy

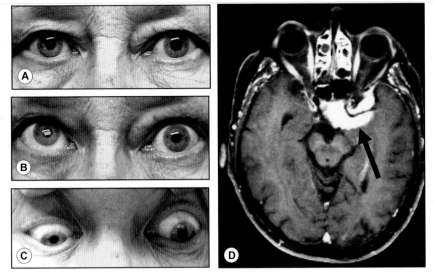

Fig. 6.19 (A–D) Left orbital apex syndrome due to sphenoid wing meningioma. There is a left partial third nerve palsy with pupil involvement (decreased elevation and depression of left eye and left mydriasis), decreased left corneal sensation, and decreased left visual acuity with left RAPD.

Meningitis

Causes

- Acute infections, e.g., acute bacterial meningitis.
- Chronic infections, e.g., fungal, tuberculosis, syphilis.
- Sarcoidosis.
- Cancer, including diffuse meningeal metastasis from solid tumors such as breast cancer ("carcinomatous meningitis").
- Any of the cranial nerves may be affected, including one or more of the third, fourth, or sixth nerves on one or both sides.
- The classic photophobia and neck stiffness of acute meningitis may be absent with the chronic causes.
- Diagnosed on MRI and lumbar puncture.

Guillain–Barré Syndrome and Miller Fisher Variant

Symptoms and Signs

- GBS:
  - Progressive ascending symmetric limb weakness with areflexia.
  - Minimal or no sensory loss.
  - Respiratory paralysis can occur.
  - Probably a postinfectious autoimmune demyelinating polyneuropathy that mainly affects the cranial nerves and peripheral motor nerves.

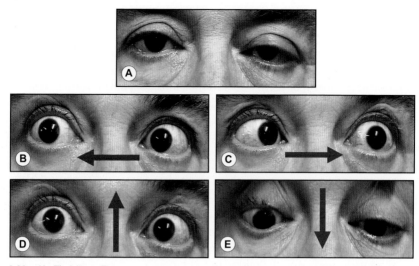

Fig. 6.20 (A–E) Miller Fisher syndrome: ataxia, areflexia, and ophthalmoplegia. This man developed diplopia and problems walking a few days after gastroenteritis. The *arrows* indicate the direction the patient was attempting to look.

- Miller Fisher syndrome (MFS) (Fig. 6.20 and Video 6.15):
  - Triad of ataxia, areflexia, and ophthalmoplegia (but not all are always present).
  - No significant limb weakness.
- Both GBS and MFS can have one or more of the following ophthalmic complications:
  - Any pattern of bilateral partial or complete ophthalmoplegia, often with diplopia.
  - Unilateral or bilateral ptosis.
  - Pupillary abnormalities (including bilateral dilated unreactive pupils).
  - Autoimmune optic neuritis.
  - Papilledema.
- Urgent investigation and treatment are required as an inpatient in an acute neurology ward.

Wernicke Encephalopathy

- Cause: thiamine deficiency (usually as a result of chronic alcohol use disorder); this causes degeneration of the ocular motor nerves and vestibular nuclei in the brainstem.
- Symptoms and signs: triad of ataxia, confusion, and ophthalmoplegia.
  - Any pattern of bilateral partial or complete ophthalmoplegia, including:
  - Bilateral sixth nerve palsy.
  - Horizontal or vertical gaze palsies.
  - INO and/or
  - Upbeat, downbeat or gaze-evoked nystagmus.
- Urgent inpatient investigation and treatment.

Brain Disease

INTERNUCLEAR OPHTHALMOPLEGIA

Causes

- brainstem (midbrain or pons) stroke, tumor, infection, inflammation, MS
- Wernicke encephalopathy (thiamine deficiency)
- pernicious anemia causing B12 deficiency

Mechanism (Fig. 6.21)

- INO occurs when the medial longitudinal fasciculus (MLF) on one side is damaged.
- The sixth nerve nucleus in the pons is the "center for lateral gaze": it contains:
  - Sixth nerve motor neurons that innervate the ipsilateral lateral rectus.
  - Interneurons which immediately cross the midline to ascend in the contralateral MLF, to synapse on medial rectus motor neurons in the contralateral half of the third nerve nucleus in the midbrain.
- A lesion of the MLF on one side thus causes loss of adduction of the ipsilateral eye on lateral gaze to the other side.

Symptoms

- diplopia (if unilateral and mild, this may only be noticed on side gaze)
- oscillopsia (movement of the visual world—"jumping" images) in side gaze
- ± other symptoms of brainstem disease (e.g., vertigo, limb numbness or weakness)

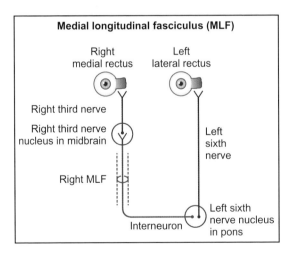

Fig. 6.21 Schematic anatomy of the medial longitudinal fasciculus.

Signs

Unilateral INO (Fig. 6.22)
- Primary position exotropia (except in mild cases).
- Decreased adduction of the ipsilateral eye, e.g., in a right INO, the right eye cannot adduct fully on attempted left gaze.
  - Convergence: in many cases of INO, ipsilateral eye adduction is better with convergence than with smooth pursuit testing (this is because the neural "instructions" for convergence do not travel via the MLF).
- Abducting nystagmus of the contralateral eye, e.g., in a right INO, on attempted left gaze the left eye exhibits a coarse left-beating jerk nystagmus.

Bilateral INO (Video 6.16)
- large exotropia
- decreased adduction of both eyes with bilateral abducting nystagmus
- sometimes termed "WEBINO" (wall-eyed binocular INO)

Differential Diagnosis
- partial third nerve palsy or myasthenia gravis
- note: if a patient has isolated unilateral medial rectus weakness, the diagnosis is more likely to be INO than partial third nerve palsy

Investigations
- If not known to have MS, urgent referral to a neurologist, plus MRI brain with contrast (concentrating on the brainstem) to exclude a brainstem tumor or stroke.

Treatment
- If due to MS: usually resolves with time (there may be residual adduction weakness).
- Others: treat the cause if possible.

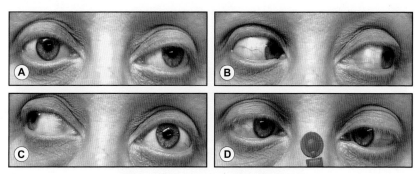

Fig. 6.22 Left internuclear ophthalmoplegia. (**A**) Left exotropia in primary position. (**B**) Full abduction of left eye on left gaze. (**C**) Decreased adduction of the left eye on attempted right gaze (left eye adducting saccades were slow and there was abducting nystagmus of the right eye in right gaze). (**D**) Improved adduction of the left eye on convergence to a near target (present in some but not all cases of internuclear ophthalmoplegia).

SKEW DEVIATION

This is a general term for any vertical or oblique deviation caused by a brainstem lesion that is not a nuclear or fascicular third or fourth nerve palsy.

Causes

- brainstem (midbrain, pons or medulla) stroke, tumor, infection, inflammation, or MS

Symptoms

- Vertical, oblique, and/or torsional diplopia.
- There may also be other brainstem symptoms, e.g., vertigo, oscillopsia, arm or leg numbness or weakness.

Signs (Fig. 6.23, Video 6.17)

- Vertical or oblique deviation in the primary position (hypertropia or hypotropia, ± esotropia or exotropia).
- The deviation may be comitant (same amount of deviation in all positions of gaze) or incomitant (more deviation in one direction of gaze than in another).
- There may be a visible limitation of eye movements, or eye movements may appear "full."
- Sometimes the patient adopts a head tilt.
- Almost any pattern of motility disturbance; can very closely mimic a fourth nerve palsy.
- Intorsion of the hypertropic eye when torsion is measured or the fundus observed.
- Sometimes alternating hypertropia (right eye higher on right gaze, left eye higher on left gaze).

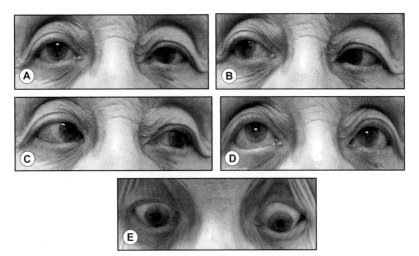

Fig. 6.23   (A–E) Skew deviation after a stroke. Right eye is hypertropic.

Differential Diagnosis

- Fourth nerve palsy:
  - In most skews, the hypertropic eye is incyclotorted (not excyclotorted as in a fourth); you can measure this with double Maddox rods (see p. 42) and look for fundus intorsion.
  - There are almost always other brainstem symptoms and signs with a skew, that are absent in a fourth nerve palsy.
- Partial third nerve palsy: this is suggested by a vertical deviation with ptosis or pupil changes.
- Myasthenia: history of variability or fatigability is suggestive of myasthenia.

Investigations

- urgent neurology assessment
- urgent MRI brain with contrast, concentrating on the brainstem

Treatment

- Treat cause if possible.
- If stable for at least 6 months and no recovery, vertical rectus muscle surgery may sometimes help the patient regain single vision in the primary position.

SUPRANUCLEAR OPHTHALMOPLEGIAS

- The key feature of supranuclear ophthalmoplegias is that some types of eye movements are more severely affected than others; this does not happen with muscle, neuromuscular junction, or nerve disease, in which all types of eye movement are affected equally.
- In most supranuclear motility disease, saccades are affected earliest and most severely, and the VOR is affected latest and least severely, with smooth pursuit being in between.
- For example, in a supranuclear vertical gaze palsy:
  - The patient may not be able to initiate an upward saccade at all (there is no eye movement at all when you ask them to "look up").
  - They can pursue a target moving upward, although upward pursuit is limited in extent.
  - But on VOR testing ("doll's-head," in which the patient's head is "nodded" back and forth—see p. 38), the eyes move upward to their normal full extent.
  - This shows that the lesion must be in the motor "chain of command" above the level of the ocular motor nerve nuclei ("supranuclear"), because a lesion at the nuclear level or below would cause equal paralysis of all types of eye movements.
- Supranuclear ophthalmoplegias include:
  - Dorsal midbrain syndrome.
  - Vertical saccadic palsy due to midbrain disease.
  - Horizontal saccadic palsy due to pontine disease.
  - Progressive supranuclear palsy (PSP).

Dorsal Midbrain Syndrome

- This is a syndrome consisting of one or more of:
  - supranuclear upgaze palsy
  - abnormal convergence
  - eyelid retraction
  - abnormal pupils

Causes

- pineal region tumors (including pinealoma) compressing the dorsal midbrain
- hydrocephalus (causes dilation of the cerebral aqueduct in the midbrain)
- stroke or MS

Mechanism

- damage to the upper dorsal midbrain including the posterior commissure (contains fibers coordinating upward eye movements) and pupil and convergence pathways

Symptoms

- (sometimes) diplopia, due to associated skew deviation or (if only at near) convergence insufficiency
- difficulty with reading and near vision (usually due to convergence insufficiency)
- painful oscillopsia induced by attempted upgaze

Signs (Fig. 6.24 and Video 6.18)

One or more of:
- Supranuclear upgaze palsy
  - Severe limitation of upward eye movements.
  - Poor or absent upward saccades and smooth pursuit.
  - Vertical VOR (tested by "doll's-head") and Bell phenomenon (uprolling of the eye on attempted eye closure) are relatively intact.

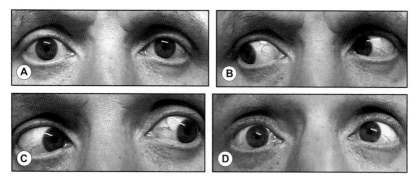

Fig. 6.24 (A) Dorsal midbrain syndrome due to hemorrhage into a pineal tumor. This man can pursue and saccade right and left (B, C); however, on attempting to saccade upward, he experiences painful convergence retraction nystagmus (there are bilateral adducting spasms) and upgaze is severely limited (D).

- Abnormal convergence
  - Convergence retraction nystagmus in some patients: (often painful) jerk convergence movements triggered by attempted upward saccades.
  - Many patients have poor convergence (secondary convergence insufficiency).
  - Others develop convergence spasm.
- Eyelid retraction: bilateral upper eyelid retraction in some patients.
- Abnormal pupils: bilateral large pupils with light-near dissociation (poor reaction to light, better reaction to near) in some patients.

Investigations

- urgent neurology assessment
- MRI brain with contrast with special views of the midbrain and pineal region

HORIZONTAL GAZE PALSY (VIDEOS 6.19 AND 6.20)

The sixth nerve nucleus in the pons is the center for conjugate lateral gaze. It contains both primary motor neurons to the ipsilateral lateral rectus and interneurons to the contralateral medial rectus (see Fig. 6.21). Therefore, a lesion of the left sixth nerve nucleus will cause a deficit of abduction of the left eye and a deficit of adduction of the right eye—a left conjugate gaze palsy.

HORIZONTAL SACCADIC PALSY

Causes

- Pontine lesions affecting the paramedian pontine reticular formation (PPRF).
- Stroke, MS, tumor.
- The patient may or may not have diplopia; if diplopia is present, it is often caused by an associated sixth nerve palsy.

Mechanism

- The PPRF is the saccadic generator for horizontal saccades.
- If it is destroyed by a small lesion, there is selective loss of horizontal saccades, with preservation of other movements.

VERTICAL GAZE PALSY (VIDEO 6.21)

The midbrain contains the centers for conjugate vertical gaze, including the rostral interstitial nucleus of the MLF (riMLF). Midbrain lesions may therefore result in a deficit in the vertical movement of both eyes—upgaze, downgaze, or both.

VERTICAL SACCADIC PALSY

Causes

- Midbrain lesions affecting the riMLF: stroke, MS, tumor.
- Metabolic disease, e.g., Niemann-Pick.
- The patient may or may not have diplopia; if diplopia is present, it is often caused by an associated skew deviation.

Mechanism

- The riMLF is the saccadic generator for vertical saccades.
- If it is destroyed by a small focal lesion, there is selective loss of vertical saccades (downwards worse than upwards) with relative preservation of other eye movements including horizontal saccades.

Progressive Supranuclear Palsy

- An idiopathic degenerative disease of the brainstem of elderly patients which is usually fatal within a decade.
- This begins as a selective impairment of downward vertical saccades, with relatively preserved downwards pursuit and VOR.
- As the disease progresses, upward and horizontal saccades are also lost, followed by smooth pursuit and convergence, whereas VOR is still relatively preserved (Fig. 6.25, Video 6.22).
- Finally, VOR is lost because of damage to the ocular motor nuclei (the palsy becomes nuclear as well as supranuclear), resulting in a bilateral complete external ophthalmoplegia.
- Often, the eyes remain straight in primary position, although primary position diplopia is not uncommon; diplopia at near due to secondary convergence insufficiency is very common.
- MRI changes become visible as the brainstem damage progresses.
- There is no curative treatment but the patient's symptoms of diplopia while reading may be helped by single-vision prism reading spectacles that replace the absent convergence and do not require the eyes to move down, as bifocals do.

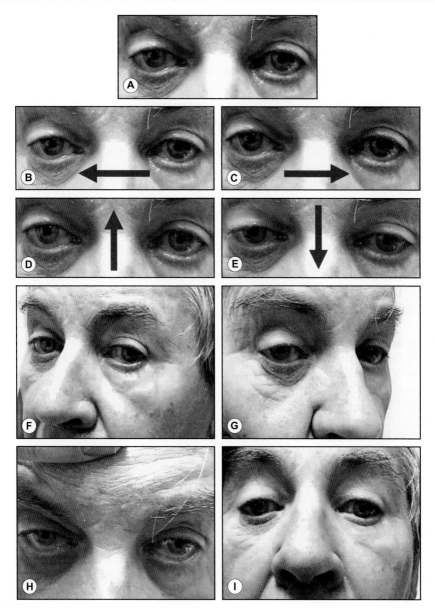

Fig. 6.25 (**A**) Progressive supranuclear palsy. (**B–E**) The *arrows* show the attempted direction of gaze when the patient tried to pursue a slowly moving target; there was very little movement in any direction. Attempted saccades also gave little movement in any direction. "Doll's-head" vestibulo-ocular reflex (VOR) stimulation was then performed (the patient's head was held in the examiner's hands and turned first from side-to-side to stimulate horizontal VOR (**F, G**), then "nodded" up and down to stimulate vertical VOR) (**H, I**). This doll's-head VOR stimulation led to a greatly increased range of eye movement compared with pursuit or saccades (in contrast to chronic progressive external ophthalmoplegia due to myopathy, in which all types of movement including VOR are affected equally).

Other Causes of Diplopia

DECOMPENSATED CHILDHOOD STRABISMUS

If a patient with a history of a childhood strabismus (with or without patching or strabismus surgery) develops double vision, there are two possibilities:

- the patient has acquired diplopia of a completely unrelated cause (e.g., has a meningioma that has caused a sixth nerve palsy on top of a preexisting asymptomatic congenital esotropia) or
- the patient has developed diplopia related to their old strabismus, by either of the mechanisms described below.

Mechanism

- "Loss of motor control": patients who previously had "straight" eyes with no diplopia
  - Particularly in the case of intermittent exotropia and congenital fourth nerve palsy, young patients with "latent" strabismus can often keep their eyes aligned "with effort" (consciously or unconsciously). These patients often only notice diplopia (and notice their eye "turn") when they are tired or have had alcohol.
  - However, with age, illness, or trauma, there can be "loss of control" that can cause either intermittent or persisting diplopia due to intermittent or persisting misalignment of the eyes.
  - This loss of control can happen gradually or suddenly (particularly after illness).
- "Loss of suppression": patients who previously had constantly turned eyes but no diplopia
  - If children develop strabismus of any cause, the developing brain "switches off" the image from the deviated eye, to avoid diplopia (cortical "suppression").
  - These patients often have obviously misaligned eyes but do not notice diplopia.
  - However, at any stage later in life, the mechanism of suppression can be lost and the patient appreciates diplopia for the first time.
  - It isn't clearly understood why this happens but in some cases it appears to be precipitated by illness, a change in spectacle strength, or a change in the angle of the strabismus.

Approach

- First, make sure you are not missing acquired strabismus of a different cause (be suspicious of this if you find limitation of movement, decreased sensation, unequal pupils, slow saccades, or any other "neurologic" signs).
- Then perform careful orthoptic measurements of sensory and motor function and assess what treatment is possible.

Treatment

- This is complex (see a strabismus text) but may include prism spectacles, botulinum toxin injection, or strabismus surgery.

DECOMPENSATED PHORIA

Check that your patient meets ALL the following clinical diagnostic criteria before you make this diagnosis!

This should NOT be used as a term for every case of acquired diplopia for which an obvious cause is not present!

CLINICAL DIAGNOSTIC CRITERIA FOR DECOMPENSATED PHORIA

The patient must have ALL of the following:

HISTORY

- history of HORIZONTAL diplopia that is (at least initially) INTERMITTENT
- no severe headache, pulsatile tinnitus, or neurologic symptoms (if present, suspect primary intracranial disease)
- no arm or leg weakness, hoarse voice, problems swallowing or breathing, or history of an intermittent ptosis
- no eye or orbital pain
- no symptoms of GCA (p. 85) (if over 50)

EXAMINATION

- no limitation of eye movement in any direction
- normal velocity horizontal and vertical saccades
- the deviation measures the same on prism cover test in all directions of gaze
- decreased horizontal prism fusional amplitude
- no increase in the amount of diplopia on sustained side or upgaze
- normal corneal and facial sensation
- normal orbicularis and facial muscle power
- normal pupils: no anisocoria, no RAPD
- no ptosis visible and no ptosis develops on sustained upgaze
- normal visual fields to confrontation

THIS IS A DIFFICULT AND POTENTIALLY RISKY DIAGNOSIS TO MAKE. IF IN ANY DOUBT, ASK FOR A NEURO-OPHTHALMIC OPINION.

Mechanism

- Many people have some tendency to develop diplopia occasionally, when tired or sick, due to a preexisting phoria (latent strabismus).
- Usually patients can control their phorias with their fusional ability (the ability to align both eye images by controlling eye position).
- If fusion breaks down, the latent strabismus becomes a manifest tropia and the patient appreciates diplopia.
- Sometimes there is spontaneous breakdown of a phoria; in other cases, there seems to be a clear precipitant (systemic illness, trauma, change of spectacle prescription, decrease in vision in one or both eyes due to eye disease).

Symptoms

- Initially intermittent horizontal diplopia (often the patient will report intermittent diplopia for many months or years, especially when tired or sick).
- The patient may give a history of intermittently closing one eye to see clearly.

Signs

- If "phoric" (latent strabismus): no movement on cover test but a latent esophoria or exophoria is demonstrated on alternate cover test (pp. 31–33).
- If "tropic" (the latent strabismus has become manifest): comitant esotropia or exotropia—the patient may be able to transiently "straighten" the eyes with effort.

- NO:
  - Limitation of movement in any direction on testing eye movements.
  - Decrease in saccade velocity.
  - Change in the angle of deviation on prism cover test in different directions of gaze.
  - Other neuro-ophthalmic signs (decreased corneal or facial sensation, facial weakness, ptosis, unequal pupils, ocular injection, proptosis).

Approach

- First, make sure you are not missing acquired strabismus of a different cause (e.g., a nerve palsy due to a tumor).
- Then perform careful orthoptic measurements of sensory and motor function and assess what treatment is possible.

Investigations

- To exclude other serious causes of diplopia, if there is any suspicion that other disease is present.
- It is not uncommon for patients with serious disease causing diplopia to be initially dismissed as "decompensated phoria" if an obvious cause is not seen; refer to a neuro-ophthalmologist if there is any uncertainty regarding the diagnosis.

Treatment

- If diplopia is only occasional, often no treatment is required, once patients are reassured regarding the condition. If diplopia is constant, strabismus surgery may be required.

CONVERGENCE INSUFFICIENCY

The hallmark of this condition is horizontal double vision only at near.

Causes

- SECONDARY convergence insufficiency:
  - Brain disease causing supranuclear paresis of convergence (e.g., dorsal midbrain syndrome due to pineal tumor or hydrocephalus; Parkinson disease; PSP).
  - Partial third nerve palsy, myasthenia, or muscle disease causing weakness of one or both medial recti.
- PRIMARY (idiopathic) convergence insufficiency:
  - This mainly affects otherwise well young women; convergence is poor with normal medial rectus function and no other abnormalities on a full neuro-ophthalmic examination.

Symptoms

- (Usually intermittent) horizontal diplopia at near (no diplopia at distance).
- Often there is a feeling of "eyestrain" (asthenopia) after prolonged reading.
- Diplopia and eyestrain resolve when the patient closes the eyes or stares into the distance for a few minutes.
- There may be other neuro-ophthalmic symptoms in patients with secondary convergence insufficiency.

Signs

- Secondary convergence insufficiency
  - Near point of convergence is further from the patient's eyes than usual (how to measure: see p. 38).
  - There is almost always some other detectable abnormality (although this may be subtle), e.g., limitation of adduction of one or both eyes; slow adducting saccades; convergence retraction nystagmus or decreased upgaze in dorsal midbrain syndrome; lid or pupil changes; Parkinsonian tremor.
- Primary convergence insufficiency
  - NO abnormalities on a full neuro-ophthalmic examination other than a near point of convergence which is further from the patient's eyes than usual.
  - Full adduction and fast adducting saccades in both eyes.
  - Decreased convergence amplitude on prism testing of fusional range.

Investigations

- Suspected secondary convergence insufficiency: MRI brain with contrast, concentrating on the brainstem; neuro-ophthalmic opinion if this is normal.
- Primary convergence insufficiency: no investigations needed but refer to a neuro-ophthalmologist if there is any doubt about the diagnosis.

Treatment

- Secondary convergence insufficiency: treat the underlying lesion if necessary; giving the patient reading glasses with base-in prism is often of great benefit.
- Primary (idiopathic) convergence insufficiency
  - Cycloplegic refraction (correcting undetected or undertreated hypermetropia may help).
  - Convergence exercises ("pencil push-ups"): the patient is instructed in various exercises to strengthen convergence; these are performed several times a day for at least a few months.
  - Surgical intervention is usually avoided.

CONVERGENCE SPASM

- This is the opposite of convergence insufficiency: too much convergence causes an intermittent or constant esotropia with horizontal diplopia, worse for distance than for near.
- Usually part of the condition called spasm of the near reflex (i.e., accommodation also increased and pupils are miotic).

Causes

- SECONDARY convergence spasm due to brain disease, e.g., some cases of dorsal midbrain syndrome.
- PRIMARY (idiopathic) convergence spasm
  - Mainly affects otherwise well young women; intermittent spasms of excess convergence are present.
  - Some patients have uncorrected hypermetropia.
  - In some patients, related to psychologic problems.

Symptoms

- Intermittent diplopia (for both distance and near or just for distance).
- Eye ache or "eyestrain."
- In some, blurred vision at distance (due to spasm of accommodation causing acquired myopia).
- In secondary convergence spasm, there may be symptoms of underlying brainstem disease.

Signs

- Esotropia (left, right or alternating): this usually cannot be sustained for a long period and resolves on prolonged cover of one eye.
- With both eyes open, abduction may seem to be limited (simulating a sixth nerve palsy), but if each eye is covered or patched in turn, full abduction of the uncovered eye can usually be demonstrated.
- Pupils: miosis (due to overaction of the pupillary near response; if miosis absent, or if pupils are large or unreactive, suspect secondary convergence spasm).
- Acquired myopia on undilated retinoscopy with both eyes open (due to spasm of accommodation increasing the eye's refractive power).
- In secondary convergence spasm, there are usually other signs of dorsal midbrain syndrome or other midbrain disease (e.g., decreased upgaze or convergence retraction nystagmus on attempted upward saccades).

Investigations

- MRI brain with contrast concentrating on the brainstem if there are symptoms or signs suspicious for secondary convergence spasm.
- Neuro-ophthalmic referral if there is any doubt regarding the cause.

Treatment

- Secondary convergence spasm: treat the underlying disease; if spasm is provoked by trying to focus at near, give the patient reading glasses with base-in prism.
- Primary convergence spasm: try to "break the cycle" of spasm
  - Hypermetropic spectacles or bifocals if uncorrected hypermetropia is present.
  - Cycloplegic drops.
  - Occlude inner half of spectacle lenses.
  - Psychologic counseling helps in some cases.

DIVERGENCE PARALYSIS/INSUFFICIENCY

Beware this pattern of eye movements. In many cases it is due to a slowly progressive mild unilateral or bilateral sixth nerve palsy.

Causes

- unilateral or bilateral partial sixth nerve palsy due to tumor (e.g., pontine glioma, clival meningioma)
- myasthenia (causing bilateral lateral rectus weakness)

Symptoms

- single vision for near but horizontal diplopia for distance

Signs

- esotropia at distance but not at near
- no increase in esotropia on right or left gaze
- no limitation of abduction on right or left gaze

Investigations

- Symptoms or signs highly suggestive of myasthenia: investigate for this.
- All other patients require an MRI brain scan with contrast to look for a pontine or skull base tumor causing unilateral or bilateral partial sixth nerve palsy.

Treatment

- Treat the underlying cause.
- Prisms or strabismus surgery may help in some cases if there are residual problems.

SAGGING EYE SYNDROME

Cause

- Rectus muscles are connected by connective tissue ligaments or bands, and the band that connects the lateral rectus and superior rectus muscles normally suspends the lateral rectus vertically within the orbit against inferior tension exerted by the inferior oblique muscle.
- With aging, this band can progressively elongate and rupture, resulting in strabismus that often is acute in onset and painless.

Signs

- mild to moderate esotropia with the characteristics of a divergence insufficiency from the weakened action of the lateral rectus
- hypotropia from the weakened action of the superior rectus
- a combination of an esotropia and hypotropia

Significance

- may occur acutely or subacutely
- may mimic a partial third or sixth nerve palsy

Examination

- full or nearly full extraocular movements despite strabismus
- normal-velocity saccades
- no neurological symptoms or signs
- high or absent upper lid crease
- deep superior sulcus or even ptosis due to the involutional changes involving the eyelid and levator tendon

Imaging

- Orbital CT or MRI shows marked elongation and significant displacement of all four rectus muscles away from the orbital center.
- Lateral rectus is displaced inferiorly.
- Superior rectus is displaced medially.

Treatment

- extraocular muscle surgery

HEAVY EYE SYNDROME

- Occurs in patients with high axial myopia (i.e., >8 D).
- A strabismus that mimics that of thyroid eye disease; however, patients with this condition have no clinical or laboratory evidence of thyroid eye disease.

Signs

- comitant esotropia typically associated with limited ductions (unlike sagging eye syndrome)
- no ptosis

Etiology

- stretching of the connective tissue band between the superior and lateral rectus muscles related to compression of the band by the myopic (elongated) eye
- strabismus similar to that which occurs in the sagging eye syndrome (see above) but presents earlier in life, usually in the 30s and 40s.

Imaging

- On coronal MRI sequences, the stretched connective tissue band may be seen with the lateral rectus muscle tightly apposed to the globe and inferiorly displaced (in contrast to findings of sagging eye syndrome, in which the lateral rectus is displaced both inferiorly and away from the globe).

Significance

- Because of the limited ductions, patients with the heavy eye syndrome are likely to be thought to have an ocular motor nerve paresis.

Treatment

- Heavy eye syndrome usually is treated with surgery.

"Seeing Things"

Introduction

Patients may "see things" because of disease of the:

- eye
- optic nerve
- brain

Occasionally, patients complain of visual symptoms other than blurred vision, field loss, transient visual loss or double vision. These unusual visual symptoms include:

- Visual illusions: The patient has abnormal visual perception of a viewed object (an object that is really there "looks funny").
- Visual hallucinations: The patient has a visual sensation that does not correspond to a real object (they see something that isn't really there). Visual hallucinations may be simple (e.g., flashes of light from a posterior vitreous detachment) or complex (e.g., seeing the image of a person who is not really present).

As eye care professionals, we need to realize that serious brain disease can present with very unusual-sounding visual complaints. If a patient's visual phenomena are not consistent with visible intraocular disease and are not the visual prodrome of migraine (p. 188), we would recommend referral to a neuro-ophthalmologist or neurologist. If this is not possible, perform brain magnetic resonance imaging (MRI) as an initial investigation.

EYE DISEASE

- Eye disease can cause visual hallucinations or visual illusions. A very common simple visual hallucination is the sensation of flashes of white light from posterior vitreous detachment or retinal tear, and patients with bilateral (and, occasionally, unilateral) poor vision from any ocular cause often experience simple or complex visual hallucinations (Charles Bonnet syndrome). A rare retinal cause of simple visual hallucinations is cancer-associated retinopathy, resulting in intrusive colored flashes. Visual illusions caused by ocular disease include haloes around lights from acute glaucoma or cataracts and metamorphopsia from macular disease.

OPTIC NERVE DISEASE

- Compression of an optic nerve by an orbital or brain tumor can cause the simple hallucination of flashes or sparkles of white or colored light. Patients with optic neuritis or anterior ischemic optic neuropathy (AION) may have similar complaints.

BRAIN DISEASE

- Brain disease is a common cause of both visual hallucinations and visual illusions. By far, the most common visual phenomena of brain disease are the simple visual hallucination of migraine. Seizures and posterior cortical disease including brain tumors, metabolic diseases, and dementing illnesses can cause complex, long-lasting hallucinations (e.g., seeing flowers, animals, monsters, or people who aren't really there). On the other hand, some patients with serious central nervous system (CNS) disorders that affect the higher visual areas can present first to ophthalmologists with strange-sounding visual illusions (e.g., a viewed object stays in vision even when the patient looks away (palinopsia); moving objects look stationary or leave a blurred or multiple-image trail (palinopsia); objects look distorted or warped (cerebral metamorphopsia); double or multiple images are seen with each eye (polyopia). Patients with focal brain lesions causing hallucinations or visual illusions often have hemianopic visual field defects detectable on perimetry, and the illusions or hallucinations are in the hemifield with the defect.
- Although patients with psychiatric illnesses may have visual hallucinations, such patients believe that what they are seeing is REAL, whereas patients with hallucinations from eye or brain disease usually know that what they are seeing is NOT REAL!

Examination Checklist

"SEEING THINGS"

Have you asked about, and looked for, all the following key features?

History

- ☐ What exactly is the patient seeing?
  - ☐ Detailed description (ideally from patient but may have to ask accompanying family member/friend if patient has ever described what he/she is seeing).
  - ☐ One or both eyes?
  - ☐ Where in the visual field (all over, central, to the side)?
  - ☐ When did it start?
  - ☐ Speed of onset?
  - ☐ Development over time?
  - ☐ Has it stopped now?
  - ☐ Is it getting better, staying the same, or still worsening?
  - ☐ Transient visual loss?

☐ Other ophthalmic symptoms: is the vision otherwise normal or is there also blurred vision, field loss or double vision?

☐ Neurologic symptoms, e.g., headaches, numbness, weakness, memory loss, personality change?

☐ Previous medical and surgical history: cancer, dementia, potentially toxic medications?

☐ Social history: smoker, alcohol, illicit drugs?

☐ If patient over 50: symptoms of giant cell arteritis (GCA)?

☐ System review questions: any clues to the cause anywhere in the body?

Examination

☐ Visual acuity.

☐ Color vision testing.

☐ Visual field defect to confrontation?

☐ Eye movements.

☐ Pupils.

   ☐ Relative afferent pupillary defect (RAPD)?

   ☐ Anisocoria?

☐ Eyelids: ptosis?

☐ Orbits?

☐ Decreased corneal or facial sensation to light touch?

☐ Orbicularis and facial strength?

☐ If patient over 50: palpate temporal arteries.

☐ Measure blood pressure: in all cases, especially if disc swelling is present.

☐ Full neurologic examination: in all cases of unexplained visual phenomena.

Plus: Perform Perimetry

☐ IN ALL CASES

Visual Illusions (Table 7.1 and Fig. 7.1)

METAMORPHOPSIA (FIG. 7.2)

Definition

- distortion of the shape or size of visible objects

Types

- Metamorphopsia: objects are seen warped or distorted.
- Micropsia: objects are seen smaller than they really are.
- Macropsia: objects are seen larger than they really are.

Causes

- retinal, e.g., choroidal neovascular membrane
- cerebral
  - parietal tumor or stroke
  - complex partial seizures (a common cause of macropsia or micropsia)
  - migraine

TABLE 7.1 ■ **Visual Illusions**

Symptom	Name	Possible Cause
Distortion of visible objects that disappears on covering one eye	Retinal metamorphopsia	Choroidal neovascular membrane; central serous retinopathy; other macular diseases
Distortion of visible objects that persists on covering either eye	Cerebral metamorphopsia	Parietal tumor or stroke; epilepsy; migraine
Double vision that does not change on covering either eye	Cerebral diplopia	Parieto-occipital tumor or stroke; migraine
Multiple images that do not change on covering either eye	Cerebral polyopia	Parieto-occipital tumor or stroke; migraine
Seeing a persisting afterimage of an object (or a previously viewed object reappears minutes later)	Palinopsia (visual perseveration)	Parieto-occipital tumor or stroke; illegal drug use
Moving objects leave behind multiple images or a "comet trail"	Cerebral polyopia for moving objects	Parieto-occipital tumor or stroke; migraine
Moving objects look stationary	Akinetopsia	Bilateral occipito-temporal lesions

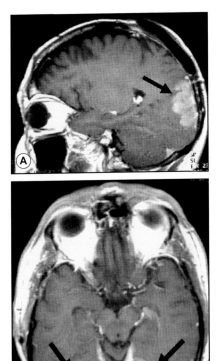

Fig. 7.1 (A, B) This patient, who had suffered multiple recurrences of an occipital meningioma, complained of multiple complex visual illusions, including cerebral polyopia for moving objects, akinetopsia, and palinopsia.

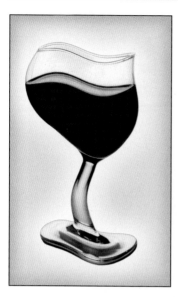

Fig. 7.2 Metamorphopsia: objects are seen as distorted.

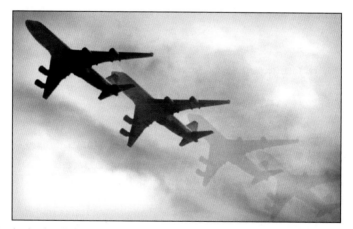

Fig. 7.3 Cerebral polyopia for moving objects. In this case, a moving airplane leaves a trail of multiple still images.

DIPLOPIA OR POLYOPIA (FIG. 7.3)

Definition

- Two or multiple images are seen of a single object.

Causes

- Monocular diplopia or polyopia
  - corneal scar
  - high astigmatism

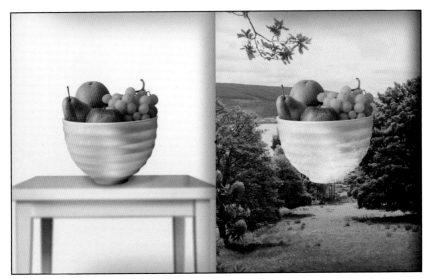

Fig. 7.4 Palinopsia (visual perseveration). In this case, a fruit bowl seen earlier reappears when the patient is viewing a landscape.

- cataract
- decentered or tilted intraocular lens
- iridectomy
- misaligned spectacles
- Binocular diplopia: misalignment of the eyes.
- Cerebral diplopia or polyopia
  - Each eye sees the same two (or multiple) images.
  - No change in image appearance viewing with right eye, left eye, or both eyes.
  - Images persist despite viewing through a pinhole.
  - Due to parieto-occipital tumor or stroke; or migraine.
- Cerebral polyopia for moving objects: a moving object leaves multiple still images or a blurred trail.

PALINOPSIA (VISUAL PERSEVERATION) (FIG. 7.4)

Definition

- Once viewed, an object persists in view despite fixation being shifted away or reappears in view seconds or minutes later despite no longer being present or looked at.

Causes

- parieto-occipital tumor, stroke, traumatic brain injury

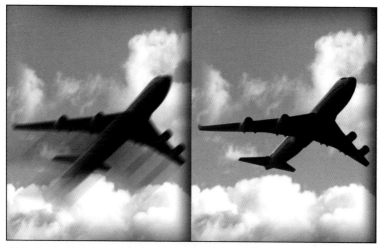

Fig. 7.5   Akinetopsia: the sensation of lack of movement. In this case, a rapidly moving airplane is seen as standing still.

AKINETOPSIA (FIG. 7.5)

Definition

- Smoothly moving objects look stationary or "jump" from place to place.

Causes

- bilateral occipitotemporal lesions

Visual Hallucinations (Table 7.2)

SIMPLE VISUAL HALLUCINATIONS (FIG. 7.6)

Definition

- Simple positive visual phenomena are seen, with no corresponding real object.

Examples

- flashes or sparkles of white or colored light
- zig-zags
- simple patterns
- "visual snow": the sensation of "snowy" or "pixelated" vision, throughout the whole visual field of both eyes

TABLE 7.2 ■ Visual Hallucinations

Symptom	Name	Possible Cause
One or more of flashing lights, stationary lights, sparkles, zig-zag lines, other patterns	Simple visual hallucinations	Retinal disease; optic nerve disease; migraine; occipital tumor; occipital epilepsy; moderate or severe visual loss (Charles Bonnet syndrome)
Seeing objects or people that aren't there.	Complex visual hallucinations	Dementia; metabolic disease; illegal drug use; occipital tumor; occipital epilepsy; moderate or severe visual loss (Charles Bonnet syndrome)

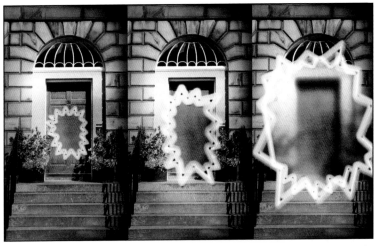

Fig. 7.6   A common example of a simple visual hallucination: the visual prodrome of migraine. The patient sees a slowly expanding area of blurred vision bounded by flashing or zig-zag lines (scintillating scotoma).

Causes

- posterior vitreous detachment or retinal detachment (common)
- compression of the optic nerve/s or chiasm by tumor (rare)
- visual aura of migraine (very common)
- occipital lobe tumor, epilepsy, stroke, or arteriovenous malformation (rare)
- blind both eyes (Charles Bonnet syndrome, common)
- idiopathic (e.g., "visual snow")

COMPLEX VISUAL HALLUCINATIONS (FIG. 7.7)

Definition

- Complex positive visual phenomena are seen, with no corresponding real object.

Examples

- seeing animals, objects, or people that are not really present

Causes

- dementia (common)
- illegal or medicinal drug use (common)
- occipital tumor
- complex partial seizures/occipital epilepsy
- blind both eyes
    - Charles Bonnet syndrome, common.
    - It is important to reassure the patient that they are not "going mad"!

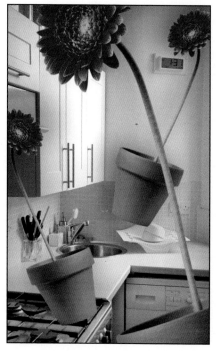

Fig. 7.7 An example of a complex visual hallucination.

Visual Snow Syndrome

This condition is considered by some to be an illusion created by disordered visual processing; however, others see it as normal noise in the visual system that most persons dampen out. On the other hand, the palinopsia that some patients with visual snow experience **is** definitely an illusion.

DEFINITION

- diffuse, small, dynamic dots throughout the visual field often described like "static" or "looking through a snowstorm"
- a constant symptom that does not impair visual acuity or color vision
- a chronic process that patients may not realize is abnormal until pointed out

CAUSES

- currently unknown but thought to be due to hypersensitivity of the visual pathway
- strong comorbidity of migraine, leading to theories that the condition may have related pathophysiology

DIAGNOSIS

- clinical
- normal exam and testing, including neuroimaging and electrophysiological tests (e.g., visual evoked potential [VEP] and electroretinography [ERG])

TREATMENT

- inconsistent benefit from medications such as lamotrigine, carbamazepine, naproxen, sertraline
- emphasize to patient normal exam and testing, reassure that it is a benign condition and that the patient is "not crazy" and will "not go blind" from its effects
- lifestyle modification (e.g., dull paper, tinted glasses, lowering ambient brightness)
- ultimately a risk/benefit discussion regarding use of medication

CHAPTER 8

Abnormal Movement or Orientation of the Visual World

Introduction

Patients may notice abnormal movement of the visual world because of disease of the:

- inner ear
- brain

Occasionally, your patients may complain that they feel like their vision is moving or shaking: this illusory movement of a truly stable environment is called oscillopsia. These sensations can be very disturbing and disabling for the patient. If the patient is examined while they are having these symptoms, the patient is usually seen to have nystagmus (repetitive abnormal eye movements).

As eye care professionals, we need to realize that serious disease can present with abnormal movement of the visual world and nystagmus. In general, nystagmus associated with oscillopsia is due to new-onset inner ear or brain pathology and requires urgent investigation. By contrast, patients who have nystagmus but do not notice the visual world moving have almost certainly had the nystagmus since early childhood (congenital sensory nystagmus due to blindness or congenital idiopathic nystagmus) (see Chapter 9).

We recommend that all patients with unexplained oscillopsia be evaluated by a neuro-ophthalmologist. If this is not possible, magnetic resonance imaging (MRI) brain with contrast is the necessary first investigation.

INNER EAR DISEASE

- Probably the most common cause of nystagmus is vertigo due to inner ear diseases (e.g., an ear infection or Ménière disease). These conditions usually present to neurologists or ear specialists rather than to ophthalmologists. In contrast to brain causes of oscillopsia, the oscillopsia and nystagmus of inner ear disease are almost always transient and resolve within a week; there are also often other symptoms such as deafness or ear pain that help localize the disease.

BRAIN DISEASE

- Most patients with nystagmus due to brain disease present to neurologists with multiple neurologic symptoms; an ophthalmologist is often only consulted once the cause has already been diagnosed on MRI and other tests. Occasionally, however, patients with acquired nystagmus present first to ophthalmologists complaining of "moving" or "jumping" vision.
- Brain disease can also cause the illusion of abnormal movement or orientation of the visual world with absolutely normal eye movements. Akinetopsia occurs when brain disease results in the loss of movement perception. Visual allesthesia due to brain disease results in the visual world being seen "tilted."

TYPES OF EYE MOVEMENT DISORDERS CAUSING ABNORMAL MOVEMENT OF THE VISUAL WORLD

This is a vast and complex topic, but most cases can be classified in a basic way as one of (or a combination of) the following:

- Primary position nystagmus: the eyes are moving while the patient is looking straight ahead; due to inner ear, cerebellar, or brainstem disease, medications, or drugs.
  - jerk nystagmus (sidebeat, upbeat, downbeat) (Videos 8.1, 8.2, and 8.3)
  - pendular nystagmus (Video 8.4)
  - torsional (rotary) nystagmus (Video 8.5)
  - see-saw nystagmus (Video 8.6)
  - periodic alternating nystagmus (Video 8.7)
- Gaze-evoked nystagmus: the eyes are stationary with the patient looking straight ahead but start to move when the patient looks in other directions; due to cerebellar or brainstem disease, medications, or drugs (Video 8.8).
- Superior oblique myokymia: the superior oblique muscle intermittently fires, causing intermittent oscillopsia and/or vertical diplopia; idiopathic or due to vascular compression of the fourth nerve root (Video 8.9).
- Saccadic intrusions: an unwanted and involuntary series of saccades disrupts fixation; due to a paraneoplastic syndrome or brain disease (Videos 8.10–8.14).
- Loss of the vestibulo-ocular reflex (VOR): the patient experiences "jumping" of the visual world when moving or walking due to loss of the usual VOR compensatory movements; due to cerebellar or brainstem disease.

Examination Checklist

ABNORMAL MOVEMENT OF THE VISUAL WORLD

Have you asked about, and looked for, all the following key features?

History

- ☐ The abnormal movement
  - ☐ What does the patient notice? Does the world seem to move up and down, side-to-side, or rotate around?

- ☐ Does it seem to affect one or both eyes?
- ☐ When did it start?
- ☐ Precipitating factors?
- ☐ Does it happen at rest or only with head or body movement?
- ☐ Does it occur only with the body or head in a particular position (e.g., lying on the right side)?
- ☐ Constant or intermittent? If intermittent, how long do episodes last?
- ☐ Getting better or worse or staying the same?
- ☐ Any neurologic symptoms?
  - ☐ Deafness or tinnitus? (suspect vestibular schwannoma)
  - ☐ Problems with balance?
  - ☐ Headache?
  - ☐ Current or previous numbness, weakness, problems walking or talking?
- ☐ Any other ophthalmic symptoms: blurred vision, double vision, or field loss?
- ☐ Previous medical and surgical history: cancer, atherosclerotic risk factors, medications (e.g., sedatives, lithium)?
- ☐ Social history: smoker, alcohol, illicit drugs?
- ☐ If patient over 50: symptoms of giant cell arteritis (GCA)?
- ☐ System review questions: any clues to the cause anywhere in the body?

Examination

- ☐ Visual acuity.
- ☐ Color vision testing.
- ☐ Visual field testing to confrontation.
- ☐ Eye movement testing.
  - ☐ Are any abnormal ocular movements (e.g., nystagmus) visible in primary position or in other directions of gaze?
  - ☐ Are the eyes aligned in primary position?
  - ☐ Smooth pursuit testing of range of eye movement.
  - ☐ Saccades: horizontal, then vertical.
  - ☐ Convergence.
  - ☐ VOR ("doll's-head").
- ☐ Pupils
  - ☐ Relative afferent pupillary defect (RAPD)?
  - ☐ Anisocoria?
- ☐ Eyelids: ptosis?
- ☐ Orbits.
- ☐ Decreased corneal or facial sensation to light touch?
- ☐ Orbicularis or facial weakness?
- ☐ If patient over 50: palpate temporal arteries.
- ☐ Full neurologic examination: in all cases of unexplained oscillopsia.

Plus: Perform Perimetry if

- ☐ field defect to confrontation, or
- ☐ decreased visual acuity, color vision, or RAPD

Oscillopsia

DEFINITION

- An illusory to-and-fro movement of the environment.
- May be horizontal, vertical, torsional, or a combination of these directions.
- Usually caused by an acquired instability of fixation from vestibular or neurologic disorders.
- When oscillopsia is produced or accentuated by head movement, it is usually of vestibular origin.

CAUSES

- acquired nystagmus
- saccadic intrusions
- superior oblique myokymia
- abnormal VOR

ACQUIRED NYSTAGMUS

Definition

- to-and-fro movement of the eyes

Types

- May be constant or intermittent: if intermittent, may occur only in certain directions of gaze or at near as opposed to distance.
- May be pendular, jerk, or mixed type.
- Pendular (Video 8.15).
  - Movements in each direction are the same amplitude and frequency.
  - Patients describe to-and-fro movement of the world.
- Jerk (Videos 8.2 and 8.3).
  - The frequency of movement in one direction (or phase) is faster than the frequency of movement in the other (fast phase versus slow phase).
  - Patients usually describe movement of the world in the direction of the fast phase.
  - Although jerk nystagmus is described by the direction of the fast phase (e.g., downbeat nystagmus has a downward fast phase and an upward slow phase), it is the SLOW PHASE of the nystagmus that is the pathologic movement; the fast phase is a normal corrective movement.

Common Types of Acquired Nystagmus

Central Vestibular Nystagmus

- downbeat (Video 8.3)
  - drug induced (e.g., alcohol, anticonvulsants, lithium)
  - Chiari malformation (Fig. 8.1)
  - multiple sclerosis (MS)
  - metabolic disorders

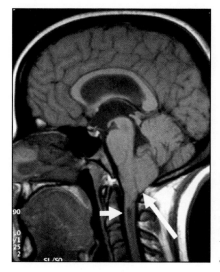

Fig. 8.1 Magnetic resonance image (MRI) of a patient with headaches and oscillopsia due to downbeat nystagmus. Sagittal MRI shows a Chiari malformation: the cerebellar tonsil *(long arrow)* has herniated downward through the foramen magnum. There is an associated cervical spinal syrinx *(short arrow)*.

- hydrocephalus
- encephalitis
- cerebellar degenerations
- upbeat (Video 8.2)
  - lesions of the anterior cerebellar vermis
  - medullary lesions
  - meningitis
  - Wernicke encephalopathy
  - tobacco

Convergence Retraction Nystagmus (Video 8.16)
- a dysconjugate, jerk nystagmus in which the fast phases are inward and the slow phases are outward
- associated with retraction of the globes
- induced by attempted convergence or attempted upward saccades
- indicates damage to dorsal midbrain (e.g., ischemia, compression, hydrocephalus) (Fig. 8.2)
- often part of "Parinaud syndrome" (dorsal midbrain syndrome), that includes:
  - paresis of upward gaze (worse for saccades than pursuit)
  - lid retraction
  - light-near pupillary dissociation (Video 8.17A and B)

See-Saw Nystagmus (Video 8.6)
- dissociated nystagmus in which one eye rises and intorts while the other eye falls and extorts
- indicates damage to midbrain reticular nuclei
- often seen with large suprasellar tumors (e.g., pituitary adenomas, craniopharyngiomas) but not caused by visual loss or visual field defects

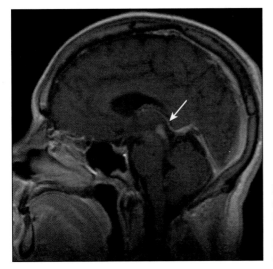

Fig. 8.2 Magnetic resonance image of a patient with convergence retraction nystagmus, as well as other elements of Parinaud syndrome due to sarcoidosis involving the dorsal mesencephalon *(arrow)*.

Periodic Alternating Nystagmus (Video 8.7)
- spontaneous, horizontal, jerk nystagmus that periodically changes direction, usually every 2 minutes
- often caused by lesions at the craniocervical junction (e.g., Chiari malformation)
- also seen with lithium intoxication, MS, Creutzfeldt-Jakob disease

Acquired Pendular Nystagmus (Video 8.15)
- may have horizontal and/or vertical components
- sinusoidal waveform at a frequency of 2–8 cycles/second
- may be dissociated and dysconjugate
- seen in patients with MS, palatal myoclonus, blindness

Rebound Nystagmus (Videos 8.18 and 8.19)
- conjugate, horizontal, jerk nystagmus
- induced by saccade from right or left gaze back to center
- fast phases in direction of saccade (slow phases in direction of prior eccentric gaze)
- a transient phenomenon in which nystagmus rapidly dampens within a few seconds after onset
- caused by chronic cerebellar or, less often, chronic brainstem disease such as MS or cerebellar atrophy

Voluntary Nystagmus (Video 8.20)
- can be produced by about 8% of the population
- rapid, horizontal, conjugate oscillations
- usually unsustained and associated with convergence

SACCADIC INTRUSIONS
- inappropriate saccadic eye movements that intrude on steady fixation
- tend to be rapid and brief

Types and Significance

Square-Wave Jerks (Video 8.10)

- small, conjugate saccades that take the eyes away from fixation position and then return them after about 200 milliseconds
- may be seen in elderly, otherwise healthy persons
- more common in patients with Parkinson disease, cerebellar degenerations, progressive supranuclear palsy, dementia
- asymptomatic

Macrosquare-Wave Jerks (Video 8.11)

- large eye movements that take the eyes off target and then return them after a latency of about 80 milliseconds
- seen in disorders that disrupt cerebellar outflow (e.g., MS)

Macrosaccadic Oscillations (Video 8.12)

- horizontal saccades that occur in bursts
- initially build up and then decrease in amplitude
- occur in patients with midline cerebellar disease

Opsoclonus (Video 8.13)

- multivectoral saccadic oscillations without an intersaccadic interval
- also called "saccadomania"
- may be intermittent or constant
- most often seen in encephalitis or as a paraneoplastic phenomenon

Ocular Flutter (Video 8.14)

- same as opsoclonus except movement only in one plane
- occurs in same settings as opsoclonus

SUPERIOR OBLIQUE MYOKYMIA (VIDEO 8.9)

- Typically brief episodes of vertical or torsional oscillopsia or both.
- Occurs only in one eye; other eye is stable.
- Some episodes described as "shimmering" of environment.
- Attacks usually last less than 10 seconds but may occur many times per day.
- Attacks may be brought on by looking downward, by tilting the head toward the side of the affected eye, and by blinking.

ABNORMAL VESTIBULO-OCULAR REFLEX

- Patients see objects as jiggling or blurred.
- May be constant or episodic.
- When episodic, may be induced by sound (e.g., Tullio phenomenon from dehiscence of bone of superior semicircular canal).
- Damage may be anywhere in the vestibular pathway, e.g., semicircular canals, otoliths, vestibular nerve, vestibular nuclei, or connections with ocular motor nuclei.

TREATMENT OF OSCILLOPSIA

- acquired nystagmus or saccadic intrusions (Video 8.21)
  - baclofen
  - memantine
  - valproate
  - gabapentin
- superior oblique myokymia
  - medical therapy: carbamazepine, propranolol, gabapentin
  - surgical therapy: ipsilateral superior oblique tenectomy combined with ipsilateral inferior oblique myectomy
- superior semicircular canal dehiscence
  - repair of dehiscence
  - local injection of gentamicin

Akinetopsia

DEFINITION

- loss of movement perception

TYPES

- first-order: abnormal displacement of object boundaries that differ in luminance from the background
- second-order: abnormal movement of objects distinguished by texture and stereo disparity, rather than luminance
- attention generated

ETIOLOGY

- Dysfunction of the dorsolateral visual association cortex.
- Usually requires bilateral cerebral lesions; however, more subtle and generally asymptomatic disturbances of motion perception occur with unilateral cerebral lesions.
- Usually lateral aspects of Brodmann areas 18, 19, and 39 (lateral occipital, middle temporal, and angular gyri).

TESTING

- animated displays of moving dots (random-dot cinematograms) or moving gratings to determine motion direction, motion speed, the presence of a motion boundary, and forms defined by motion
- generally experimental

MANIFESTATIONS

- No sensation of motion in depth or of rapid motion.
- Objects that are moving rapidly appear to jump rather than move smoothly.

- Ability to discriminate differences in speed is severely impaired.
- Discrimination of direction is abnormal.
- Minimum and maximum displacements needed to distinguish motion direction are abnormal.
- Use of motion cues for various tasks is impaired.
- May be able to distinguish moving from stationary stimuli.

ASSOCIATED DEFICITS

- may have homonymous field defects
- impaired spatial vision
- impaired perception of form

CAUSES

- tumors
- hemorrhage
- infarction
- degenerations
- metabolic disturbances

TREATMENT

- aimed at etiology

Visual Allesthesia

DEFINITION

- abnormal orientation of the visual world

MANIFESTATIONS

- Environment may appear tilted or rotated (Fig. 8.3).
- Tilt/rotation may be of any amount (e.g., 90 degrees, 180 degrees).
- Tilt is constant.
- Tilt/rotation usually oculocentric (e.g., environment is tilted at same angle regardless of direction of gaze).

CAUSES

- usually ischemia/infarction of lateral medulla (see Fig. 8.3, center, left, and right, and Fig. 8.4)
  - occlusion of ipsilateral vertebral artery
  - occlusion of ipsilateral posterior inferior cerebellar artery
- almost never an isolated phenomenon; usually part of Wallenberg syndrome but may occur from parietal-occipital or occipital lobe disease (see Fig. 8.3, lower left and right)
- may last days to weeks

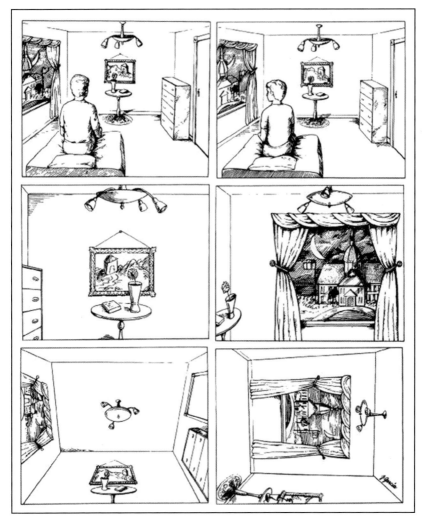

Fig. 8.3 Visual allesthesia in a 70-year-old man who suffered right parieto-occipital damage after placement of a shunt for normal-pressure hydrocephalus. Illustrations on the *left* show the view and orientation when the patient was looking forward. Illustrations on the *right* show the view and orientation when the patient was looking to the left. *Upper left* and *upper right* figures show a third-person view of the patient's room, indicating the head position and the orientation of the environment that would be seen by a normal person looking forward *(left)* and to the left *(right)*. *Center left* and *center right* figures illustrate the appearance of the environment that would be seen by a patient with classic visual allesthesia (e.g., with Wallenberg syndrome) when looking forward *(center left)* and to the left *(center right)*. Note that there is transposition of the visual field. *Lower left* and *lower right* figures illustrate the environmental rotation experienced by the patient. In contrast to the rotation seen by the patient with classic visual allesthesia *(center figures)*, the rotation is independent of head position. (With permission from Girkin, C.A., Perry, J.D., and Miller, N.R. Visual environmental rotation: A novel disorder of visiospatial integration. *J Neuro-Ophthalmol* 19:13–16, 1999.)

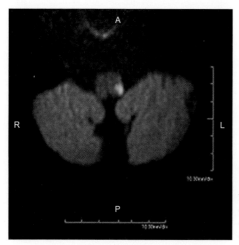

Fig. 8.4 Diffusion-weighted magnetic resonance image of a left lateral medullary infarction due to occlusion of the left posterior inferior cerebellar artery in a patient with Wallenberg syndrome. The *bright area* is indicative of restricted diffusion.

ASSOCIATED MANIFESTATIONS OF WALLENBERG (LATERAL MEDULLARY) SYNDROME

- ipsilateral impairment of pain and temperature sensation over face
- ipsilateral Horner syndrome
- ipsilateral limb ataxia
- contralateral impairment of pain and temperature sensation over trunk and limbs
- dysphagia
- dysarthria

DIAGNOSIS

- by clinical assessment combined with neuroimaging

TREATMENT

- supportive

CHAPTER 9

Abnormal Eye Movements Without Visual Symptoms

Introduction

Abnormal eye movements without visual symptoms may be caused by disease of the:

- eye/s
- extraocular muscles
- brain

Occasionally, a patient will be referred to you because although they are visually asymptomatic (or has had long-standing poor vision in one or both eyes), the eyes have been observed to move in an abnormal fashion. The abnormal eye movements are often observed during an examination by a doctor for another problem (e.g., for headaches) or during a routine eye examination. These incidentally noticed abnormal movements include:

- misaligned eyes without diplopia, e.g., long-standing strabismus since childhood
- abnormal voluntary eye movements without diplopia, e.g., diffuse external ophthalmoplegia or gaze palsy
- repetitive involuntary eye movements without oscillopsia, e.g., congenital idiopathic nystagmus

As eye care professionals, we need to know that although most asymptomatic eye movement disorders are benign, they can rarely be the first sign of serious disease. For example, vertical saccadic palsy may be an early sign of progressive supranuclear palsy (PSP) and horizontal gaze palsy may be the presenting sign of a brainstem tumor. In most cases of brain disease, however, other neurologic symptoms and/or signs are present.

If the patient has a known history of a very long-standing problem that has previously been appropriately investigated (e.g., congenital idiopathic nystagmus), then nothing further needs to be done. However, if there is any doubt regarding the nature of the eye movement disorder, the patient should be evaluated by a neuro-ophthalmologist.

Examination Checklist

ABNORMAL EYE MOVEMENTS WITHOUT VISUAL SYMPTOMS

Have you asked about, and looked for, all the following key features?

History

☐ How was the abnormal movement noticed?
    ☐ On a routine check or was the patient having visual or neurologic symptoms?
    ☐ When was the abnormal movement first noticed?
    ☐ Any previous investigation or treatment?
☐ Previous ophthalmic history: childhood strabismus, poor vision, patching?
☐ Any neurologic symptoms: headache, problems with memory, walking, talking?
☐ Previous medical and surgical history.
    ☐ medications, present or past
    ☐ social history: alcohol, illicit drugs
☐ System review questions: any clues to the cause anywhere in the body?

Examination

☐ Visual acuity.
☐ Visual field testing to confrontation.
☐ Eye movement testing
    ☐ Are the eyes aligned in primary position?
    ☐ Nature of the abnormal movement in primary position.
    ☐ Does the abnormal movement change in other positions of gaze?
    ☐ Smooth pursuit testing of range of eye movement.
    ☐ Saccades: horizontal, then vertical.
    ☐ Convergence.
    ☐ Vestibulo-ocular reflex (VOR, "doll's-head").
☐ Pupils
    ☐ Relative afferent pupillary defect (RAPD)?
    ☐ Anisocoria?
☐ Eyelids: ptosis?
☐ Orbits.
☐ Decreased corneal or facial sensation to light touch?
☐ Orbicularis or facial weakness?
☐ Full neurologic examination: if the patient has neurologic symptoms.

Plus: Perform Perimetry if

☐ field defect to confrontation, or
☐ decreased visual acuity, color acuity, or RAPD

Misaligned Eyes Without Diplopia

POOR VISION OR CHILDHOOD-ONSET STRABISMUS

■ A misaligned eye may be the cause of poor vision (strabismic amblyopia) or poor vision may be the cause of a misaligned eye ("sensory" esotropia or exotropia).

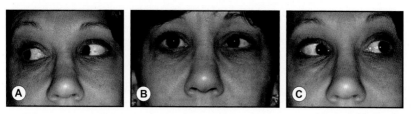

Fig. 9.1 This woman has had a long-standing, asymptomatic, left esotropia since childhood. Note that the eye movements are full and the angle of deviation is the same in all positions of gaze. (**A**) Right gaze. (**B**) Primary position. (**C**) Left gaze.

- Strabismic amblyopia: an eye that is constantly misaligned (usually turned in) in early life will often result in poor vision in the turned eye ("lazy eye").
- "Sensory" deviations: blind eyes tend to turn:
  - In in children ("sensory" esotropia).
  - Out in adults ("sensory" exotropia).
- In all these deviations, there should be no visible restriction of movement of either eye and the deviation should measure the same in all directions of gaze (i.e., the strabismus is "comitant") (Fig. 9.1).
  - The exception to this is Duane syndrome (the patient is often a child or young adult referred with incidentally noticed "sixth nerve palsy" with no diplopia).
- Treatment
  - Surgical treatment is indicated in an adult or older child if the patient is distressed by the appearance of the eyes.
  - However, beware of postoperative diplopia (that can occur even if the vision is poor in one or both eyes); a neuro-ophthalmologist or strabismologist should perform careful preoperative diplopia testing before any surgery is contemplated.

Abnormal Voluntary Eye Movements Without Diplopia

NORMAL AGE-RELATED LOSS OF UPGAZE

- Many normal subjects lose the ability for extreme upgaze with age; the limitation is always the same in both eyes.
- If an asymptomatic elderly patient is incidentally noted to have mild to moderate restriction of upgaze only, with no visual or neurologic symptoms, and otherwise entirely normal eye movements (including fast upward and downward saccades), a sinister cause is very unlikely.

GAZE PALSY

In this condition, the patient cannot look in a particular direction. For example, in a rightward horizontal gaze palsy, neither eye can look to the right (the right eye cannot abduct, the left eye cannot adduct).

HORIZONTAL GAZE PALSY

Example: left horizontal gaze palsy (Video 9.1)

Signs

- Both eyes can look up, down, and to the right, but neither eye can look to the left.
- If acute, the eyes are often tonically deviated to the right.
- In many cases, there is also an esotropia in primary position from concomitant damage to the ipsilateral sixth nerve fascicle, resulting in diplopia.

Cause

- Left abducens (sixth nerve) nucleus lesion in the pons.
- A left abducens nucleus lesion will cause a leftward horizontal gaze palsy because it destroys:
  - The cell bodies of left sixth nerve neurons (so the left lateral rectus won't work).
  - Interneurons that drive right medial rectus subnucleus neurons (so the right medial rectus won't work).

VERTICAL GAZE PALSY

Example: complete vertical gaze palsy

Signs

- Both eyes can look right and left but not up or down.
- VOR ("doll's-head") movement vertically may be present in the absence of voluntary vertical saccades.
- There may or may not be a deviation in primary position causing diplopia as well.

Cause

Bilateral rostral interstitial nucleus of the medial longitudinal fasciculus (riMLF) lesions in the dorsal midbrain (this region generates vertical saccades).

GENERALIZED OPHTHALMOPLEGIA

- Both eyes have poor or absent movements in all directions.
- Often, the eyes remain aligned in primary position, so the patient does not notice diplopia; however, some patients do have diplopia.

Causes

- extraocular muscle disease, for example:
  - a mitochondrial myopathy causing chronic progressive external ophthalmoplegia (CPEO)
  - oculopharyngeal dystrophy
- neuromuscular junction disease, e.g., severe myasthenia or botulism
- disease of the third, fourth, and sixth nerves on both sides, e.g., the Miller Fisher variant of Guillain-Barré syndrome (GBA) (an acute demyelinating polyneuropathy), carcinomatous meningitis, or pituitary apoplexy
- brain disease, e.g., PSP

Importance of Vestibulo-ocular Reflex (VOR, "Doll's-Head") Testing

- In supranuclear brain disease (e.g., PSP or dorsal midbrain syndrome), VOR produces more ocular movement than voluntary saccades or pursuit.
- By contrast, in diffuse ophthalmoplegia of all other causes (e.g., CPEO due to mitochondrial myopathy), all types of eye movement are affected equally (VOR is no better than pursuit or saccades, because the problem is in the extraocular muscles themselves).

CHRONIC PROGRESSIVE EXTERNAL OPHTHALMOPLEGIA (CPEO)

(See p. 207.)

Demographic

- adults of all ages

Cause

- A sporadic or inherited defect in chromosomal or mitochondrial DNA causes a slow degeneration and atrophy of the extraocular muscles.

Signs (Fig. 9.2)

- All eye movements are affected equally ("doll's-head" [VOR] testing does not improve the range of eye movements beyond that seen with pursuit or saccades).

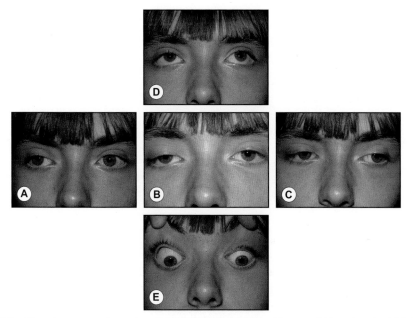

Fig. 9.2 Chronic progressive external ophthalmoplegia. This 15-year-old boy has had bilateral ptosis for several years. He has no diplopia; however, his eye movements are limited in all directions. (**A**) Attempted right gaze. (**B**) Primary position. (**C**) Attempted left gaze. (**D**) Attempted upgaze. (**E**) Attempted downgaze.

- There is a slow loss of extraocular movements over years, which may be unnoticed by the patient until detected on routine examination.
- There may also be one or more of the following:
    - bilateral (or, rarely, unilateral) ptosis
    - bilateral weakness of eye closure
    - pigmentary retinopathy
    - cardiac conduction defects
    - limb muscle myopathy.
- Pupils are always normal.

Investigations

- gene testing on blood (positive in some cases) or muscle biopsy (positive in most cases)

Treatment

- No curative treatment is possible.
- Cardiac investigations.
- Prisms for reading if there is diplopia at near from convergence insufficiency.
- Consider extraocular muscle surgery if strabismus present.
- Ptosis surgery if severe ptosis is present (high risk of corneal exposure if there is also orbicularis weakness; must not raise lids too high).

PROGRESSIVE SUPRANUCLEAR PALSY (PSP)

(See p. 248.)

Demographic

- usually elderly patients

Cause

- a generalized brainstem degenerative disease that destroys supranuclear connections to the ocular motor nerve nuclei

Symptoms

- difficulty reading (because the eyes don't look down)
- difficulty eating (can't see the food on their plate because the eyes don't look down, leading to the "dirty tie" syndrome—they spill their food)

Signs

- Vertical saccades are usually the earliest eye movement affected, with downgaze usually affected first.
- Eventually diffuse ophthalmoplegia.
- Doll's-head (VOR) testing results in better eye movement than that seen with pursuit or saccades (unless the disease is very advanced).
- There may also be one or more of the following:
    - Dementia.
    - Neck rigidity.
    - Problems speaking, swallowing, and walking.

Treatment

- No curative treatment is possible.
- Single lens reading glasses instead of bifocals.
- Prisms for reading if there is diplopia at near from convergence insufficiency.

Repetitive Involuntary Eye Movements Without Oscillopsia

- Adult patients who had onset of nystagmus in early childhood usually do not notice movement of the visual world (in contrast to adults with acquired nystagmus who almost always have severe oscillopsia).
- Adults with childhood-onset nystagmus are sometimes referred to ophthalmologists when an optometrist or doctor notices their constant eye movements on a routine check-up.

TYPICAL CONGENITAL NYSTAGMUS

Causes

- Congenital idiopathic nystagmus (congenital "motor" nystagmus)
  - Often inherited in an autosomal-dominant manner.
  - The eyes and the child are otherwise entirely normal apart from the constant nystagmus.
  - Nystagmus usually is of a jerk type (has a fast phase and slow phase) (Video 9.2).
  - Visual acuity is degraded by the constant eye movement but is usually still reasonable (often in the 20/40–20/100 range).
- Nystagmus associated with early-onset blindness (congenital "sensory" nystagmus)
  - Nystagmus is often pendular (Video 9.3).
  - Visual acuity is very poor due to the congenital or early-onset ocular or visual pathway disease.
- Nystagmus associated with head nodding and torticollis (spasmus nutans) (Video 9.4)
  - May be present at birth or appear within a few years of life.
  - Monocular or binocular but asymmetric.
  - Small amplitude, high frequency.
  - May be jerk, pendular, or mixture.
  - Not all features of the triad always present (e.g., head nodding or torticollis may be absent or minimal).
  - Usually resolves spontaneously in first decade of life.
  - Vision usually good.
  - Usually benign but may be associated with optic pathway glioma.

Signs

- Horizontal, uniplanar, conjugate, jerk, pendular, or jerk-pendular nystagmus (the eyes move horizontally no matter what the direction of gaze).
- In the "motor" type, there usually is a "null point" in which the amplitude of nystagmus is minimized and the nystagmus almost always dampens during attempted near viewing.

- In spasmus nutans, nystagmus horizontal, monocular or bilateral asymmetric, high frequency, small amplitude, often with head nodding and/or torticollis.

Investigations

- Every child with nystagmus requires careful investigation (preferably by a pediatric ophthalmologist).
- An adult with known congenital nystagmus that was previously appropriately investigated requires no further work-up.

Treatment

- Usually, the only "treatment" required is to reassure the referring practitioner.
- Various surgical procedures on the extraocular muscles may diminish (although not stop) congenital motor nystagmus.
- Contact lenses may reduce congenital motor nystagmus.
- Congenital motor nystagmus sometimes decreases with age.
- The benign form of spasmus nutans spontaneously resolves.

LATENT NYSTAGMUS

- No nystagmus is noticed with both eyes open, but on covering one eye, jerk nystagmus develops with its fast phase toward the uncovered eye.
- This is usually no problem for the patient but may be discovered when one eye is covered during routine testing.
- If the patient loses vision in his or her fixating eye, latent nystagmus may become constant ("manifest" latent nystagmus).

ACQUIRED NYSTAGMUS WITH POOR VISION

- Both eyes becoming blind at any age can result in pendular or roving nystagmus.
- A blind patient developing nystagmus of another (e.g., neurologic) cause will not notice oscillopsia.

SQUARE-WAVE JERKS

- These are (usually horizontal) back-to-back saccades that "step" both eyes together away from fixation then immediately return them to primary position (Video 9.5).
- They are usually small and often require careful observation to detect.
- Normal subjects show a few small square-wave jerks every minute and these increase with age.
- Neurodegenerative disorders such as Parkinson disease result in an increase in the number and amplitude of square-wave jerks.
- Square-wave jerks are asymptomatic and cause no problems for the patient; they are of diagnostic interest only.

CHAPTER **10**

Unequal Pupils

Introduction

Unequal pupils (anisocoria) may be caused by disease of the:

- eye
- orbit
- brain
- neck
- upper chest

Patients occasionally present because a difference in the sizes of their pupils has been noticed by their family, an examining practitioner, or the patient themselves. Alternatively, you might notice anisocoria while examining the patient for another complaint.

As eye care professionals, we all need to have a practical plan for assessing patients with unequal pupils. On history and examination, we need to decide if the patient can be clinically diagnosed and reassured (e.g., Holmes-Adie tonic pupil) or requires referral or investigation (e.g., Horner syndrome).

Anisocoria can be physiologic or pathologic. Physiologic anisocoria is common: one in five normal subjects has a slight but noticeable difference in the size of their pupils. Physiologic anisocoria can be recognized because the patient is asymptomatic, both pupils constrict briskly to light and dilate briskly to dark, there is no ptosis, and ocular movements are normal.

Pathologic anisocoria is due to disease in one of three places:

- in the iris itself
- in the neural pathway that causes pupil constriction (the parasympathetic chain)
- in the neural pathway that causes pupil dilation (the sympathetic chain)

IRIS DISEASE

- Overall, the most common cause of pathologic anisocoria seen by eye care providers is change in the iris itself, most often due to previous cataract or corneal surgery. Previous blunt trauma can also cause persisting traumatic mydriasis. Infrequently, the patient may have (purposefully or accidentally) instilled a dilating or constricting substance into the eye.

PARASYMPATHETIC CHAIN DISEASE (BRAIN, THIRD NERVE, CILIARY GANGLION)

- Third nerve disorders can very rarely present with just a dilated pupil but almost always ptosis, motility disturbance, or both signifies that a partial third nerve palsy is present. More commonly, ciliary ganglion disease of unknown cause results in the Holmes-Adie tonic pupil syndrome, which can be recognized by light-near dissociation, spiraling of the iris on slit-lamp examination, and the absence of other neurologic symptoms or signs other than (sometimes) areflexia.

SYMPATHETIC CHAIN DISEASE (BRAIN, NECK, UPPER CHEST)

- Horner syndrome is caused by a lesion anywhere in the sympathetic chain that descends from the hypothalamus in the center of the brain down through the brainstem and cervical spinal cord, runs across the top of the lung, then ascends with the internal carotid artery (ICA) upward through the neck and then forward through the cavernous sinus to reach the orbit. Common causes for Horner syndrome include a tumor compressing any part of the chain in the head, neck, or upper chest; an ICA dissecting aneurysm in the neck; a presumed ischemic insult due to atherosclerosis; or a congenital defect in the sympathetic chain.

Examination Checklist

UNEQUAL PUPILS

Have you asked about, and looked for, all the following key features?

History

- ☐ How was the anisocoria first noticed: on a routine check or was the patient having visual or neurologic symptoms?
- ☐ Any ophthalmic symptoms?
  - ☐ Blurred vision or field loss? (possible orbital apex tumor)
  - ☐ Transient visual loss? (ICA dissection)
  - ☐ Diplopia? (possible partial third nerve palsy from aneurysm or tumor)
- ☐ Previous ophthalmic history: eye trauma or surgery? (possible traumatic mydriasis)
- ☐ Any neurologic symptoms: headache, numbness, or weakness?

- ☐ Previous medical and surgical history
  - ☐ Cancer?
  - ☐ Use of topical agents or inhalants (e.g., antiasthmatic nasal sprays)
  - ☐ Previous neck trauma, e.g., car accident "whiplash" injury, chiropractic manipulation, or roller-coaster ride? (possible Horner syndrome from ICA dissection).
- ☐ If patient over 50: symptoms of giant cell arteritis?
- ☐ System review questions
  - ☐ Hemifacial, neck, or arm pain? (possible Horner syndrome from ICA dissection)
  - ☐ Any clues to the cause anywhere in the body?

Examination

- ☐ Visual acuity.
- ☐ Color vision testing.
- ☐ Visual field testing to confrontation.
- ☐ Eye movement testing.
- ☐ Pupils
  - ☐ Estimate pupil sizes.
  - ☐ Do both pupils constrict rapidly and fully to light? If not, do they constrict to near?
  - ☐ Do both pupils dilate rapidly and fully in the dark?
  - ☐ Relative afferent pupillary defect (RAPD)?
- ☐ Eyelids: ptosis? (possible partial third nerve palsy or Horner syndrome).
- ☐ Orbits.
- ☐ Decreased corneal or facial sensation to light touch?
- ☐ If possible Horner syndrome:
  - ☐ Examine the neck (lumps or lymphadenopathy?).
  - ☐ Examine the hands (clawing or finger abduction or adduction weakness?).
  - ☐ "Spoon test" for facial sweating (p. 296).
- ☐ If patient over 50: palpate temporal arteries.
- ☐ Full neurologic examination: if the patient has neurologic symptoms.

Plus: Perform Perimetry if

- ☐ field defect to confrontation, or
- ☐ decreased visual acuity, color acuity, or RAPD

Management Flowchart

UNEQUAL PUPILS

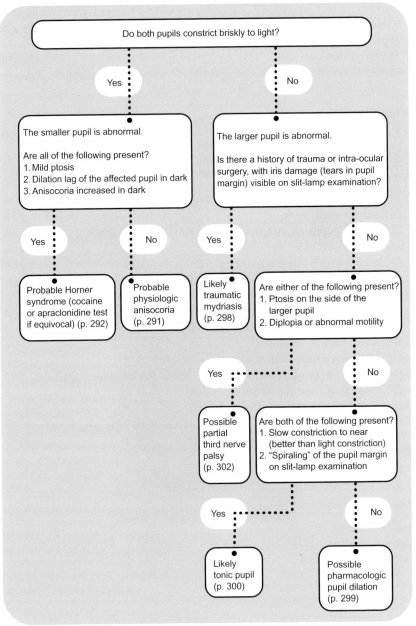

Approach to Anisocoria

DEFINITION

- a difference in the size of the pupils

ETIOLOGY

- may be caused by dysfunction of sympathetic or parasympathetic pathway

RULE

- never caused by an afferent pathway lesion unless that lesion *also* affects efferent sympathetic or parasympathetic pathway

QUESTION

- What is the most important question to answer in a patient with anisocoria?

ANSWER

- Are both pupils normally reactive to light or is one (or both) poorly reactive?

EXPLANATION

- If both pupils are reactive, the lesion is probably in the sympathetic pathway because pupillary constriction (parasympathetic pathway) is intact, whereas if one pupil is poorly or nonreactive (and there is no RAPD!), the lesion is probably in the parasympathetic pathway (brainstem, third nerve, ciliary ganglion, short ciliary nerves, iris sphincter).

Anisocoria With Normally Reactive Pupils

DIFFERENTIAL DIAGNOSES

- common
  - physiologic anisocoria
  - Horner syndrome
- uncommon: intermittent pupillary mydriasis of the young (some cases)

PHYSIOLOGIC ANISOCORIA (FIG. 10.1)

- Present in 15%–20% of normal people.
- Present at birth.
- May be very obvious or very subtle.
- May change both size and side by hour.
- No visual effects.

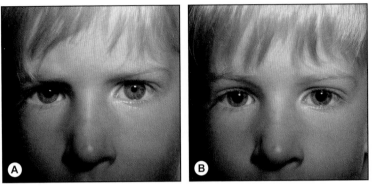

Fig. 10.1   Physiologic anisocoria in a child. (**A**) Before pharmacologic testing with topical 4% cocaine. There is obvious anisocoria with the left pupil smaller than the right. Both pupils reacted normally to light. (**B**) Forty-five minutes after topical instillation of 4% cocaine on both sides, both pupils are widely dilated.

- If the patient is asymptomatic and there is normal motility and no ptosis, no pharmacologic testing or other investigations are required.
- Occasionally, however, if by coincidence there is a mild ptosis of another cause, there can be concern that the patient could have Horner syndrome.
- Pharmacologic testing to differentiate physiologic anisocoria from Horner syndrome:
    - The transmitter substance at the neuromuscular junction of the sympathetic pathway is norepinephrine.
    - 10% cocaine blocks the reuptake of norepinephrine.
    - Patients with physiologic anisocoria have normal release of norepinephrine at the junction of the sympathetic neuron and the iris dilator.
    - A patient with physiologic anisocoria will show dilation of both pupils 45 minutes after two drops of 10% cocaine are instilled in both eyes (compared with Horner syndrome in which there is no dilation) (see Fig. 10.1).

HORNER SYNDROME (FIG. 10.2 AND VIDEO 10.1)

- Results from damage to the oculosympathetic system.
- Damage may affect first-, second-, or third-order neuron in pathway.

Signs

- anisocoria with smaller pupil on side of lesion
- pupils normally reactive to light (actually, Horner pupil is hyperreactive to light)
- ipsilateral upper eyelid ptosis (from involvement of Muller's muscle)
- upside-down ptosis of ipsilateral lower lid (lower lid slightly higher)
- apparent enophthalmos (from ptosis of upper and lower lids)

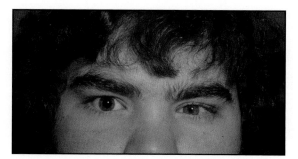

Fig. 10.2 Left Horner syndrome in a young man after a roller-coaster ride. Note anisocoria with the left pupil smaller than the right. Both pupils were normally reactive to light. Note associated left upper and lower lid ptosis. The patient was subsequently found to have a left internal carotid artery dissection.

TABLE 10.1 ■ Summary of Pharmacologic Testing for Horner Syndrome

Site	For Diagnosis		For Localization	
	Cocaine	Apraclonidine	Hydroxyamphetamine	1% Phenylephrine
Normal	Dilates	No change	Dilates	No change
Central or preganglionic	No/minor change	Dilates	Dilates	No change
Postganglionic	No change	Dilates	No change	Dilates

Pharmacologic Testing to Confirm the Diagnosis of Horner Syndrome (Table 10.1)

- Regardless of the location of the lesion along the sympathetic pathway, patients with Horner syndrome have a reduced rate of norepinephrine release at the iris dilator neuromuscular junction.
- 10% cocaine will not dilate a Horner pupil (or will dilate it minimally) (Fig. 10.3).
- Place two drops of 10% cocaine in each eye.
- Place cocaine in the eye with the smaller pupil first.
  - Why? Because topical cocaine is a major ocular irritant. If cocaine drops are put in the eye with the larger pupil first, the patient may squeeze the lids tightly while you are trying to put drops in the other eye. Then, if the smaller pupil fails to dilate, it could be because it is a Horner pupil *or* because the drops didn't get into the eye because of squeezing of the eyelids. If the cocaine drops are placed first in the eye with the smaller pupil, the latter argument cannot be made.
- Wait 45 minutes.
- Examine the pupils in dim light or a dark room.
  - Why? Because cocaine affects only the sympathetic system, not the parasympathetic system. If the pupils are examined in bright light, they may constrict and the effects of the cocaine may not be appreciated.

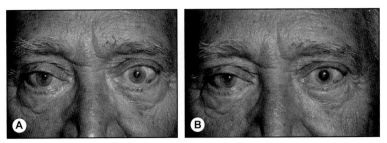

Fig. 10.3   Results of pharmacologic testing with 4% cocaine in a man with a right Horner syndrome. (**A**) Before instillation of cocaine, the patient has anisocoria with the right pupil smaller than the left. Both pupils were normally reactive to light. (**B**) Forty-five minutes after topical instillation of 4% cocaine on both sides, the right pupil remains small, whereas the left pupil is widely dilated.

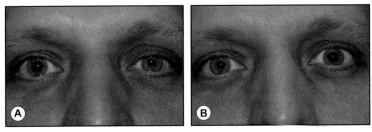

Fig. 10.4   Results of pharmacologic testing with 0.5% apraclonidine in a patient with a left Horner syndrome. (**A**) Before instillation of apraclonidine, there is anisocoria with the left pupil smaller than the right. Both pupils reacted normally to light. (**B**) Forty-five minutes after topical instillation of 0.5% apraclonidine, there is reversal of the anisocoria, with the left pupil larger than the right.

- Why bother with a cocaine test if the patient has anisocoria and ipsilateral ptosis?
  - Because 15%–20% of normal people have physiologic anisocoria and if such a patient has unilateral ptosis from another condition (e.g., age-related levator dehiscence), there is a 50% chance that the ptosis and the miotic pupil will be on the same side.
- Is there an alternative to the cocaine test?
  - Cocaine drops may be hard or impossible to obtain.
  - One can use apraclonidine instead.
  - Apraclonidine is an alpha-adrenergic receptor agonist.
  - It reduces aqueous production and lowers intraocular pressure (IOP).
  - A 1% solution will dilate a Horner pupil (1.0–4.5 mm), with no change in the normal pupil (often reversing anisocoria!) (Fig. 10.4).
  - A 0.5% solution will work just as well.
  - Apraclonidine can cause lethargy and bradycardia in infants, so should not be used in children, especially infants.

Causes

- The sympathetic pathway is a long one. The causes of Horner syndrome are very different depending on the location of the process:
  - central (first order)—head or neck
    - brainstem stroke
    - brainstem tumor
    - spinal cord tumor
    - cervical spondylosis
  - preganglionic (second order)—neck or chest
    - apical lung tumor
    - ICA dissection
    - iatrogenic (from neck or chest surgery)
  - postganglionic (third order)—head or neck
    - ICA dissection (Fig. 10.5)
    - cavernous sinus tumor or inflammation
    - autonomic trigeminal cephalalgias (e.g., cluster headache, paroxysmal hemicrania, short-lasting unilateral neuralgiform headache with conjunctival injection and tearing [SUNCT syndrome])
    - iatrogenic (neck surgery)

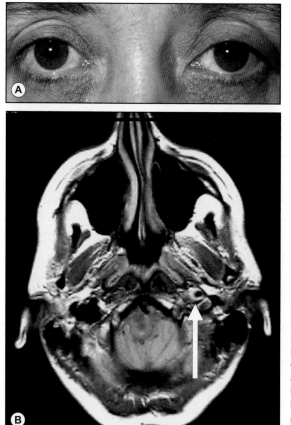

Fig. 10.5 Left Horner syndrome. (**A**) This 28-year-old woman was noticed by her husband to have left ptosis and anisocoria 2 days after experiencing "whiplash" in a car accident. (**B**) Magnetic resonance imaging of the neck revealed a left internal carotid artery dissection *(arrow)*. Anticoagulation was given to prevent a stroke.

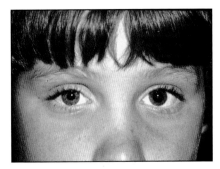

Fig. 10.6 Iris heterochromia in a child with a congenital right Horner syndrome. In addition to right ptosis and anisocoria with the right pupil smaller than the left (both pupils reacted normally), the right iris is lighter than the left.

Clinical Clues to the Location of the Lesion

- Some patients with presumed Horner syndrome have other signs or symptoms that aid in diagnosis.
  - Heterochromia of irides suggests congenital or very long-standing lesion (Fig. 10.6).
  - Facial and/or neck pain suggests carotid dissection causing a postganglionic Horner syndrome.
  - Ipsilateral sixth nerve paresis suggests a cavernous sinus lesion but may also result from a brainstem lesion.
  - Loss of sweating on the side of the Horner pupil suggests a central or preganglionic lesion; the spoon test checks for this.
    - Attempt to slide a smooth metal object like the underside of a spoon across the forehead.
    - Patients with a central or preganglionic Horner syndrome will have dry skin on the side of the lesion, whereas patients with a postganglionic syndrome will have normally hydrated skin bilaterally.
    - The object thus will not slide easily along the side of the forehead in a patient with an ipsilateral central or preganglionic Horner syndrome compared with the opposite side but will slide equally on both sides of the forehead in a patient with a postganglionic Horner syndrome.
  - Multiple ipsilateral ocular motor nerve paresis suggests a postganglionic lesion.
  - Double vision suggests cavernous sinus disease.
  - Hand weakness or clawing suggests a cervical cord lesion.

Pharmacologic Testing to Determine the Location of the Lesion

- Paredrine (1% hydroxyamphetamine) stimulates release of norepinephrine from the presynaptic portion of the neuromuscular junction; it
  - Dilates a normal pupil.
  - Dilates central and preganglionic Horner pupils.
  - Will not dilate a postganglionic Horner pupil (*but* may be false-negative if used within 7–10 days of the onset of an acute postganglionic Horner syndrome, as it can take this long for stores of norepinephrine to be depleted!).

- Phenylephrine (1%) will dilate a postganglionic Horner syndrome (due to denervation sensitivity) but not a preganglionic Horner syndrome.
- Responses are consistent with both agents.

Investigations

- central or preganglionic
    - cervical spine films in flexion and extension
    - chest computed tomographic (CT) scan
    - brain magnetic resonance imaging (MRI), with detailed views of brainstem; plus MRI and magnetic resonance angiogram (MRA) or CT and CT angiogram (CTA) of the neck
- postganglionic
    - MRI brain (with detailed views of skull base and cavernous sinus); MRI/MRA or CT/CTA of neck

INTERMITTENT UNILATERAL PUPILLARY MYDRIASIS (SYMPATHETIC FORM) (FIG. 10.7)

- One pupil transiently becomes large and/or distorted, but remains briskly reactive to light.
- May occur as part of a migraine attack or as an isolated phenomenon, usually in young adults.
- About 50% of patients who have attacks unassociated with migraines have a history of migraines.
- Often asymptomatic but may be associated with blurred vision, photophobia, or both.
- Normal reaction to light and normal accommodation.
- The pupil in these cases may be peaked (i.e., tadpole pupil).
- Lasts 15 minutes to several hours.

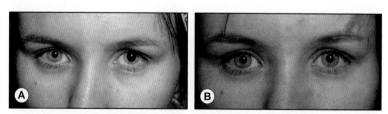

Fig. 10.7 Intermittent unilateral mydriasis (sympathetic form). The patient was a nurse who was noted by the surgeon to have anisocoria. She had no visual symptoms. (**A**) There is anisocoria with the left pupil larger than the right. Both pupils reacted normally to light and the patient had normal accommodation. (**B**) Two hours later, the woman's pupils are isocoric.

Anisocoria With One Pupil That Is Poorly Reactive or Nonreactive to Light

DIFFERENTIAL DIAGNOSES

- iris sphincter damage (traumatic mydriasis)
- pharmacologic blockade
- tonic pupil
- third nerve palsy
- intermittent unilateral pupillary mydriasis (parasympathetic form)

EVALUATION

- Perform a slit-lamp examination to look for iris sphincter damage.
- Check for other evidence of third nerve paresis (e.g., ptosis, exodeviation, hyper- or hypotropia or phoria).
- The diagnosis is usually clinically apparent. However, in a minority of cases, pharmacologic testing is required:
  - Use 1% pilocarpine for a widely dilated, nonreactive pupil (possible pharmacologic dilation).
  - Use 1% tropicamide for a markedly constricted, nonreactive pupil (possible pharmacologic constriction).
  - Use 0.1% pilocarpine for a moderately dilated pupil with sector paralysis, vermiform movements, or light-near dissociation with tonic redilation (possible tonic pupil).

IRIS SPHINCTER DAMAGE (TRAUMATIC MYDRIASIS) (FIG. 10.8)

- pupil usually irregularly dilated
- some reaction usually present
- easily detected using slit-lamp biomicroscopy

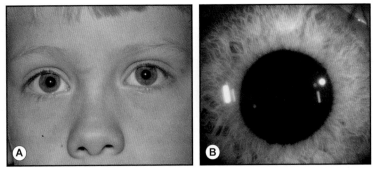

Fig. 10.8   Anisocoria from iris damage. This child had experienced blunt trauma to the right orbit several months earlier, resulting in blurred vision and a red eye. (**A**) There is anisocoria with the right pupil larger than the left. The right pupil reacted sluggishly. Note slight irregularity of the iris. (**B**) Magnified view of the right iris reveals iris sphincter tears.

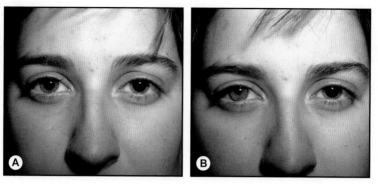

Fig. 10.9 Anisocoria from pharmacologic blockade. The patient was a 19-year-old college student who was to take final examinations later in the week. She complained of blurred vision in her left eye. (**A**) The left pupil is widely dilated. It did not react to light stimulation. The right pupil reacted normally to light. (**B**) Thirty minutes after topical instillation of 1% pilocarpine on both sides, the right pupil is constricted but the left pupil is unchanged in size.

PHARMACOLOGIC BLOCKADE (FIG. 10.9)

- Never due to systemic absorption.
- May be purposeful or by mistake.
- Causes largest fixed, dilated pupils and smallest fixed, miotic pupils.
- Cannot be overcome by topical agents.
- Most cases of pharmacologic pupillary blockade are caused by parasympatholytic agents, but in some cases, the offending agent is a topical parasympathomimetic agent.

Topical Parasympatholytic Agents (Causing Dilated Pupil/s)

- Topical parasympatholytic agents include:
  - Atropine.
  - Scopolamine (patch for seasickness/postoperative nausea).
  - Anticholinergic nasal sprays (inhalants).
  - Ipratropium bromide (e.g., in Atrovent).
  - Plants, e.g., datura (cornpicker's pupil).
  - Flea collar material.
- Testing for parsympatholytic pharmacologic blockade:
  - Place two drops of 1% pilocarpine in each lower cul-de-sac.
  - Wait 45 minutes and observe.
  - Anything less than full constriction is a positive test for pharmacologic blockade (Fig. 10.9).

Topical Parasympathomimetic Agents (Causing Constricted Pupil/s)

- Organophosphate pesticide (causes nonreactive miotic pupil).
- Testing for parasympathomimetic pharmacologic blockade:
  - Place two drops of 1% tropicamide in each lower cul-de-sac.
  - Wait 45 minutes and observe.
  - Anything less than full dilation is a positive test for pharmacologic blockade.

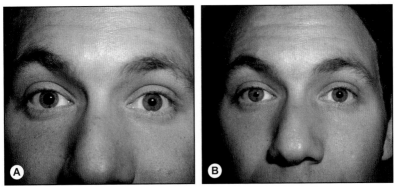

Fig. 10.10   Tonic pupil. (**A**) The right pupil is much larger than the left and does not react to light. (**B**) Forty-five minutes after a solution of 0.1% pilocarpine is instilled in each lower cul-de-sac, the right pupil is markedly constricted, whereas the left pupil is unchanged.

TONIC PUPIL (FIG. 10.10 AND VIDEO 10.2)

- caused by damage to the ciliary ganglion and/or short ciliary nerves
- may be mistaken for pharmacologic blockade but usually not as dilated as pharmacologically dilated pupil

Signs

- dilated pupil
- sluggish or no reaction to light
- sluggish or no reaction to near (but when present, reaction to near better than to light)
- slow redilation after constriction (very important)
- sector iris paralysis
- vermiform movements of iris
- constricts to 0.1% pilocarpine

Etiology

- Features based on:
  - Number of fibers for pupillary constriction versus accommodation in the ciliary ganglion.
  - Aberrant regeneration in the peripheral nervous system.
  - Denervation supersensitivity.
- Number of fibers for pupillary constriction versus accommodation in the ciliary ganglion
  - About 95% of fibers in the ciliary ganglion are for accommodation.
  - Accommodation is more likely to be spared in ciliary ganglion damage.
  - Regeneration is more likely to occur from fibers destined for ciliary body for accommodation.

- Aberrant regeneration
  - After injury to a peripheral nerve, both injured and uninjured fibers regenerate.
  - Fibers originally intended for the ciliary body may regenerate to the iris sphincter; the pupil will constrict during near viewing but not to light.
- Denervation supersensitivity
  - An organ deprived of its postganglionic nerve supply becomes supersensitive to the transmitter substance.
  - The iris sphincter becomes supersensitive to acetylcholine and similar substances (e.g., pilocarpine).
  - Once constriction of the pupil is achieved, supersensitivity of the iris sphincter prevents normal, rapid redilation.

Causes

- classification of tonic pupil syndromes
  - local
  - with systemic or neurologic dysfunction
  - Adie (Holmes-Adie) syndrome
- local tonic pupils
  - tumor
  - trauma
  - inflammation (especially herpes zoster)
  - iatrogenic (lateral orbital exploration)
  - amyloid
- systemic/neuropathic tonic pupils
  - more often bilateral than other syndromes
  - diabetes mellitus
  - myotonic dystrophy
  - dysautonomic syndromes
    - Riley-Day
    - Shy-Drager
    - acute pandysautonomia
    - HIV autonomic neuropathy
  - paraneoplastic
- Adie (Holmes-Adie) syndrome
  - usually unilateral (4% become bilateral each year)
  - women more often affected than men (5:1)
  - usually occurs in early adulthood or middle age (20–50 years)
  - accommodation reduced or absent
  - absent deep tendon reflexes in 50%–75%
  - natural history is for pupil to become smaller and accommodation to improve
  - etiology unknown: possibly viral or autoimmune

Pharmacologic Testing for Tonic Pupil (Fig. 10.10)

- In most cases of tonic pupil, the diagnosis is obvious clinically and no pharmacologic testing is required. However, if the diagnosis is unclear, dilute pilocarpine testing can be performed:
  - Place two drops of 0.1% pilocarpine in the lower cul-de-sac of each eye.
  - Wait 45 minutes and assess.
  - Tonic pupil will constrict (markedly).
  - Normal pupil will not constrict.
  - Some third nerve palsy pupils will also constrict to this strength of pilocarpine.
    - Why? It is thought that some efferent pupillomotor fibers either bypass the ciliary ganglion or pass through it without synapsing.

THIRD NERVE PALSY (FIG. 10.11)

(See p. 219.)

Isolated anisocoria from third nerve palsy:
- The pupil is never widely dilated and nonreactive.
- In a patient with a mildly dilated, less-reactive pupil
  - Ask about episodic eyelid droop or diplopia.
  - Check the position of lids.
  - Test for exodeviation on gaze toward the opposite side.
  - Test for ipsilateral hypotropia in upgaze and hypertropia in downgaze.

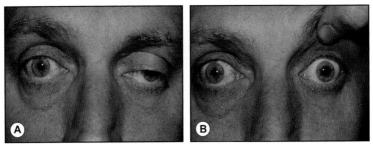

Fig. 10.11 Anisocoria in the setting of a left third nerve palsy. (**A**) The patient has a moderate left ptosis and a left exotropia. (**B**) When the left upper lid is raised, the left pupil can be seen to be dilated. It was minimally reactive to light. The patient subsequently was found to harbor an intracranial aneurysm.

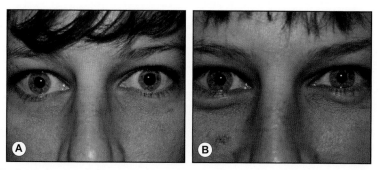

Fig. 10.12   Intermittent unilateral pupillary mydriasis (parasympathetic form). The patient was a physician with a long history of severe migraine headaches. During one of the headaches, she noted blurred vision in her left eye and noted that her left pupil was larger than her right. (**A**) There is anisocoria with the left pupil larger than the right. The left pupil reacted very sluggishly to light; the right pupil reacted normally. The patient underwent a magnetic resonance imaging and magnetic resonance angiography that revealed no intracranial pathology. (**B**) Three hours later, the patient's pupils are isocoric and normally reactive.

INTERMITTENT UNILATERAL PUPILLARY MYDRIASIS (PARASYMPATHETIC FORM) (FIG. 10.12)

- One pupil transiently becomes large and poorly reactive to light.
- May be associated with migraine or occur as an isolated event, usually in young adults.
- Even when not associated with migraine, 50% of patients have a history of migraines.
- Poor reaction of the dilated pupil and reduced (or absent) accommodation.
- No ocular motor dysfunction or ptosis.
- Lasts 15 minutes to several hours.
- MRI may show enhancement of the third nerve.

Ptosis

Introduction

Ptosis may be due to disease of the:

- eyelid
- levator muscle
- neuromuscular junction
- third nerve
- brain
- neck
- upper chest

Patients often present complaining that one or both upper eyelids are "drooping" or a ptosis may be incidentally noticed on examination by the patient's doctor or optometrist.

As eye care professionals, we need to remember that serious disease can first present with ptosis and to have a practical plan for assessing patients with ptosis to avoid missing these potentially life-threatening causes.

The most common cause of either unilateral or bilateral ptosis is age-related dehiscence or disinsertion of the levator aponeurosis. Not infrequently, ptosis is the initial presentation of myasthenia gravis. Other less common but important causes include partial third nerve palsy due to aneurysm or tumor or Horner syndrome from internal carotid artery (ICA) dissection or a tumor in the head, neck, or upper chest.

The cause of ptosis can normally be diagnosed clinically (see management flowchart, p. 308). However, in some cases, further investigations are required, e.g., tests for myasthenia, neuro-imaging, or muscle biopsy for genetic testing.

Examination Checklist

PTOSIS

Have you asked about, and looked for, all the following key features?

History

- ☐ The ptosis
  - ☐ When did it start?
  - ☐ Speed of onset?
  - ☐ Development over time?
  - ☐ Variation through the day or from day to day? (possible myasthenia)
  - ☐ Getting better or worse or staying the same?
- ☐ Other ophthalmic symptoms
  - ☐ Transient visual loss? (possible ICA dissection causing Horner syndrome)
  - ☐ Double vision? (possible myasthenia, or tumor/aneurysm causing partial third or Horner)
  - ☐ Pain?
  - ☐ Blurred vision?
  - ☐ Field loss?
- ☐ Previous medical and surgical history
  - ☐ Recent head or neck trauma? (possible ICA dissection causing Horner syndrome)
  - ☐ Recent neck or chest surgery?
  - ☐ Cancer? (possible head, neck, or chest primary or metastasis causing Horner syndrome or partial third nerve palsy)
- ☐ Social history: smoker? (possible apical lung cancer causing Horner syndrome)
- ☐ If patient over 50: symptoms of giant cell arteritis (GCA)?
- ☐ System review questions: hemifacial, neck, or arm pain? (possible ICA dissection causing Horner syndrome)

Examination

- ☐ Visual acuity.
- ☐ Visual field defect to confrontation? (possible pituitary tumor causing partial third)
- ☐ Limitation of eye movements (especially elevation)? (possible myasthenia, or tumor/aneurysm causing partial third nerve palsy)
- ☐ Pupils
  - ☐ Is there anisocoria?
  - ☐ Smaller, normally reactive pupil on side of ptosis: possible Horner syndrome.
  - ☐ Larger, poorly reactive pupil on side of ptosis: possible partial third nerve palsy.
  - ☐ Relative afferent pupillary defect (RAPD)? (possible orbital apex tumor causing partial third nerve palsy)

☐ Eyelids
  ☐ Measure skin crease height and levator function (high skin crease and good levator function with otherwise normal examination: possible aponeurotic ptosis).
  ☐ Does the ptosis worsen on 2 minutes' sustained upgaze? (possible myasthenia; do ice test)
  ☐ Is there a Cogan lid twitch? (possible myasthenia) (Video 11.1)
  ☐ Increase in ptosis on manual elevation of contralateral eyelid (possible myasthenia) (Video 11.2).
  ☐ Remember to check the strength of eyelid closure (strength of orbicularis oculi) in all patients with ptosis (possible myasthenia, myotonic dystrophy, chronic progressive external ophthalmoplegia [CPEO]).
☐ Orbits: proptosis, injection, chemosis?
☐ Corneal and facial sensation to light touch: decreased sensation on side of ptosis? (possible cavernous sinus tumor)
☐ Orbicularis and facial muscle power (possible myasthenia or myopathy, if weak).
☐ If possible Horner syndrome:
  ☐ Examine the neck. Are there any lumps? (neck tumor)
  ☐ Examine the hands. Is there finger abduction or adduction weakness? (cervical spinal cord or lung apex C8/T1 lesion)
  ☐ Spoon test for facial sweating (see p. 296).
☐ If patient over 50: palpate temporal arteries
☐ Perimetry if field defect to confrontation, decreased vision, RAPD, diplopia, or motility defect
☐ Full neurologic examination if the patient has fatigable ptosis, diplopia, or orbicularis or facial weakness; are there any signs of systemic muscle weakness or fatigability to support a diagnosis of myasthenia?

Management Flowchart

PTOSIS

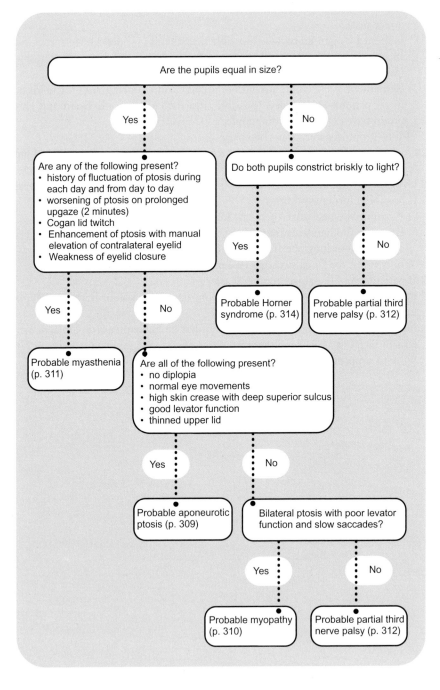

Aponeurotic Ptosis

CAUSE

- age-related dehiscence or disinsertion of the connective tissue aponeurosis connecting the levator muscle to the upper eyelid

DEMOGRAPHIC

- middle-aged or elderly patients

SYMPTOMS

- constant drooping of one or both upper lids
- no symptoms of myasthenia: no diplopia, no limb fatigability, no major change in the ptosis during the day or from day to day (note: some patients with aponeurotic ptosis do notice a slight worsening of the ptosis at night, due to fatigue of compensatory frontalis overaction)

SIGNS

- high skin crease (more than 7 mm from lid margin)
- high, deep superior sulcus
- thinned upper eyelid skin
- normal levator function (Fig. 11.1)
- no anisocoria
- no signs of myasthenia
    - no worsening of the ptosis on continuous upgaze for 2 minutes (i.e., no clinical fatigability)
    - no orbicularis weakness

INVESTIGATIONS

- none required

TREATMENT

- if the patient is significantly troubled: ptosis surgery

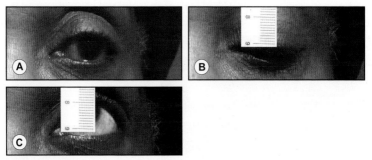

Fig. 11.1 (A) Left aponeurotic ptosis. The left upper lid has a high skin crease. Left upper lid levator function (B, C) is intact.

CAUTION

- Occasionally, patients have both an aponeurotic ptosis and ptosis of another (new) cause (e.g., myasthenia or partial third nerve palsy). Hence, finding a high skin crease and a thinned upper lid is not an absolute guarantee that a second disease process is not present.

Ptosis Due to Levator Myopathy

CAUSES

- mitochondrial myopathy, e.g., that leading to CPEO
- oculopharyngeal dystrophy
- myotonic dystrophy

DEMOGRAPHIC

- adults of all ages

SYMPTOMS

- Very slowly progressive bilateral ptosis.
- The patient may or may not also notice diplopia.
- In oculopharyngeal dystrophy: problems swallowing and change in voice.

SIGNS

- bilateral upper lid ptosis with poor levator function (Fig. 11.2)
- plus in some cases one or more of:
    - globally reduced eye movements (external ophthalmoplegia)
    - weakness of eyelid closure
    - weakness of other facial muscles

INVESTIGATIONS

- Genetic tests are possible on blood, but if these are negative then genetic tests, histology, and histochemical tests on a muscle biopsy specimen are more sensitive.

TREATMENT

- No specific treatment is possible for the genetic conditions.
- Ptosis surgery must be approached very cautiously in these patients as, if they also have weak orbicularis function (i.e., can't close the eyes properly), they have a high risk of postoperative corneal exposure problems.

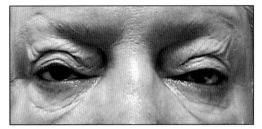

Fig. 11.2 Bilateral ptosis in chronic progressive external ophthalmoplegia (CPEO) secondary to mitochondrial myopathy.

Ptosis Due to Myasthenia Gravis

(See p. 212.)

DEMOGRAPHIC

- adults of all ages

SYMPTOMS AND SIGNS

- The hallmarks of myasthenic ptosis are:
  - Variability: the patient reports (or you observe) that the ptosis changes during each day (often being worse at night) and from day to day ("good days and bad days").
  - Fatigability (Fig. 11.3A and B):
    - Measure the ptosis in primary position.
    - Then ask the patient to keep their head still but to look far upward at a target on the ceiling continuously for 2 minutes.
    - Then remeasure the ptosis; an increase in the ptosis of 2 mm or more is suspicious for myasthenia.
  - A positive ice test (see p. 216) is also strongly suggestive of myasthenia (see Fig. 11.3C–E) as is improvement in ptosis after intramuscular injection of Prostigmin (neostigmine) (Fig. 11.4).
  - There may or may not also be a history of diplopia: myasthenic diplopia often has the same variability on history, and clinical fatigability, as the ptosis.
  - Myasthenia does not cause anisocoria: any patient with ptosis and anisocoria should be suspected of having Horner syndrome or partial third nerve palsy.

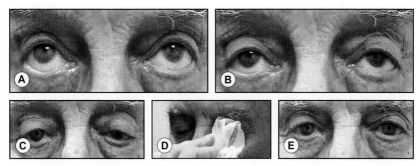

Fig. 11.3 This 63-year-old man complained of bilateral ptosis that was worse at night and varied from day to day. Testing clinical fatigability of the ptosis: (**A**) upper lid position immediately after the patient was asked to look upward to a point on the ceiling, (**B**) lid position after 2 minutes of sustained upgaze, demonstrating that the ptosis was clinically fatigable. Also note that the patient cannot sustain the amount of upgaze either. The ice test: (**C**) eyelid position with the patient looking straight ahead, immediately before ice application, (**D**) the patient closes his eyes and an ice pack is applied to the left eye for 2 minutes, (**D**) eyelid position immediately after ice pack removal, demonstrating an improvement in the left ptosis. The combination of definite clinical fatigability of the ptosis and positive ice test result enabled a clinical diagnosis of myasthenia.

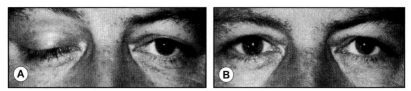

Fig. 11.4   Myasthenic ptosis (**A**) before and (**B**) after prostigmin (neostigmine) test.

INVESTIGATIONS AND TREATMENT

- See p. 216.

Ptosis Due to Partial Third Nerve Palsy

(See p. 219.)

CAUTION

- Partial third nerve palsies can be very subtle and very difficult to diagnose.
- Not all patients with early partial third nerve palsies report diplopia.
- Not all early compressive partial third nerve palsies have an enlarged pupil.
- It is, however, rare for a partial third nerve palsy to present with ptosis but entirely normal ocular motility and normal pupils.

CAUSES

- compressive
  - aneurysm (most often at internal carotid-posterior communicating artery junction; less often, basilar apex, posterior cerebral, superior cerebellar)
  - pituitary tumor (including acute-onset unilateral or bilateral partial third nerve palsy from pituitary apoplexy)
  - cavernous sinus or sphenoid wing meningioma
- ischemic
  - GCA
  - diabetes, hypertension, atherosclerosis

DEMOGRAPHIC

- adults of any age

SYMPTOMS AND SIGNS

- Ptosis may be mild, moderate, or severe.
- If anisocoria is present, the pupil on the side of the ptosis is larger and sluggishly reactive to light.
- If the patient has diplopia, it may be horizontal, vertical, or oblique, and the patient may have an exotropia, hypertropia, hypotropia, or oblique deviation on testing.

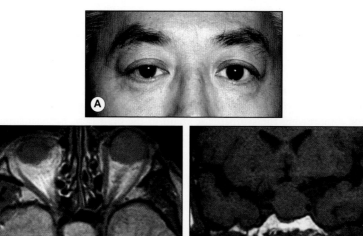

Fig. 11.5   **(A)** This 54-year-old man was referred by his optometrist "for treatment of right apo-neurotic ptosis." The patient complained of slowly progressive right upper lid drooping with no other ophthalmic symptoms. Pupils were of equal size in each eye and briskly reactive to light. Although the patient denied diplopia, eye movement testing revealed slightly limited elevation of the right eye with diplopia in upgaze. Perimetry showed bilateral upper temporal defects; magnetic resonance imaging revealed a pituitary tumor compressing and invading both cavernous sinuses (**B, C**). The ptosis was due to a compressive partial right third nerve palsy.

- A trap is that sometimes only the superior division of the third nerve is affected by a compressive lesion: in this case, the patient may only report diplopia when looking upward or if you ask them to look up (i.e., they may not have diplopia in primary position) (Fig. 11.5).
  - You must check for an ipsilateral hypotropia in upgaze, as this may be the only eye movement abnormality.

INVESTIGATIONS

- Urgent magnetic resonance imaging (MRI) plus magnetic resonance angiography (MRA) (or MRI plus computed tomographic angiography [CTA]) is mandatory for all suspected partial third nerve palsies (whether the pupils are normal or abnormal) because of the risk of aneurysm (see Chapter 6).

TREATMENT

- Treat the underlying cause.
- If ptosis persists and is stable more than 12 months after the cause has been treated, ptosis surgery can be contemplated.

Ptosis Due to Horner Syndrome

(See p. 292.)

CAUSES

- ICA dissection
- tumor compressing the sympathetic chain in the brainstem, cervical spinal cord, lung apex, neck, base of skull, or cavernous sinus
- cervical spondylosis
- brainstem stroke
- presumed ischemia due to atherosclerosis
- congenital

DEMOGRAPHIC

- any age

SYMPTOMS AND SIGNS

- Upper eyelid ptosis is usually only mild (and may be very subtle and difficult to detect).
- Upside-down ptosis of ipsilateral lower eyelid usually present (i.e., the lower eyelid is also weak due to reduced function of Muller's muscle, so it is higher than the lid on the opposite side).
- If a patient with Horner syndrome also has diplopia, a cavernous sinus lesion is likely (causing a sympathetic plexus lesion plus also a partial third or sixth nerve palsy).
- If heterochromia (different iris color) is present, the Horner is probably very long-standing or congenital.
- Pupils: in Horner syndrome, the following will be present:
  - Miosis (smaller pupil) on the side of the ptosis.
  - Both pupils constrict briskly to light.
  - The pupil on the side of the ptosis will show dilation lag when the room lights are switched off (it will take longer to dilate than the other pupil).
  - The amount of anisocoria will increase in the dark compared with in the light.
- A history of recent neck trauma (including "whiplash" injury, chiropractic manipulation, recent roller-coaster ride), neck or face pain, transient monocular visual loss, or other neurologic symptoms is suspicious for ICA dissection.
- If a neck tumor is the cause, it can sometimes be identified on palpation.
- Weakness of finger adduction suggests a lesion of the lower cervical spinal cord or brachial plexus.

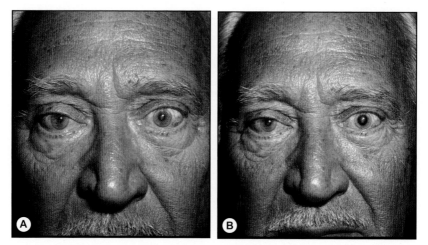

Fig. 11.6   Unilateral ptosis and anisocoria due to Horner syndrome. This 76-year-old man noticed drooping of his right upper eyelid. (**A**) There is moderate right ptosis. Note that the right pupil is slightly smaller than the left. (**B**) 10% cocaine test showed increased anisocoria after cocaine administration. The right pupil dilates minimally, the left pupil dilates markedly. A right Horner syndrome was diagnosed. The patient, a heavy smoker, was found to have a right apical lung tumor.

PHARMACOLOGIC TESTING

- to confirm the diagnosis of Horner syndrome: cocaine or apraclonidine test (p. 293) (Fig. 11.6)
- to localize the lesion causing Horner syndrome: hydroxyamphetamine or dilute phenylephrine test (p. 296)

INVESTIGATIONS

- Horner syndrome can be caused by a lesion anywhere in the head, neck, or upper chest, including tumor and ICA dissection.
- Therefore, unless there is very good evidence that the Horner syndrome is very long-standing or congenital, the patient requires cervical spine films and MRI of the head, neck, and upper thorax, looking specifically for a lesion of the sympathetic chain and MRA of the extracranial ICA, looking for dissection.

TREATMENT

- If ptosis persists and is stable more than 12 months after the cause has been treated, ptosis surgery can be contemplated.

Facial Weakness or Spasm

Introduction

FACIAL WEAKNESS

- Facial weakness can be due to disease of the:
  - facial muscles
  - neuromuscular junction
  - seventh nerve
  - brain
- Patients with facial weakness frequently present to ophthalmologists with symptoms of corneal exposure. The role of the ophthalmologist is twofold:
  - Ensure that the cause of the weakness has been established and, if possible, treated.
  - Protect the eye from complications such as corneal ulceration, while maintaining good vision and cosmesis.
- All patients with facial weakness must have their corneal sensation assessed. The combination of loss of sensation and loss of eyelid closure places the affected eye at great risk of potentially blinding complications. In addition, the finding of reduced corneal or facial sensation is of diagnostic importance.
- The most common cause of facial weakness is a unilateral lesion of the facial (seventh cranial) nerve. Rarer causes include myotonic dystrophy and other myopathies, myasthenia gravis, and brainstem or cortical disease.
- It is essential to resist the temptation to call all facial palsies "Bell's palsy." Although this is the most common diagnosis, it should be considered a diagnosis of exclusion. In view of the other possible diagnoses, all patients with new-onset facial nerve weakness should also be assessed by an otolaryngologist or neurologist.

INVOLUNTARY FACIAL MOVEMENTS

- Involuntary spasm of the orbicularis or other facial muscles can be due to disease of the:
  - seventh nerve
  - brain

- Patients with involuntary facial movements frequently present to ophthalmologists, particularly if the movements are centered on, or include, the orbicularis oculi muscles. The three most common patterns of abnormal movement are:
  - fine contractions of the eyelid muscle: orbicularis oculi myokymia
  - bilateral, usually forceful closure of eyes: blepharospasm
  - unilateral contractions of facial muscles: hemifacial spasm
- Many patients are concerned that their movement disorder is a marker of either serious neurologic disease or psychiatric illness. Part of the ophthalmologist's role is to reassure such patients that this is not usually the case. Once the disorder has been characterized, and investigations organized for the few patients who may have an underlying neurologic disorder, the main aims of the ophthalmologist are to identify any ocular disease that might be exacerbating the condition and (if necessary) to provide or organize appropriate treatment.

Examination Checklist

FACIAL WEAKNESS OR SPASM

Have you asked about, and looked for, all the following key features?

History

- ☐ The weakness or spasm
  - ☐ When did it start?
  - ☐ Speed of onset?
  - ☐ Development over time?
  - ☐ Variation through the day or from day to day?
  - ☐ Getting better or worse or staying the same?
- ☐ Other ophthalmic symptoms: diplopia, blurred vision?
- ☐ Other neurologic symptoms?
  - ☐ Deafness, tinnitus, or vertigo? (eighth plus seventh nerve palsy: high risk of cerebello-pontine angle [CPA] tumor, e.g., vestibular schwannoma)
  - ☐ In patients with facial spasm: is there spasm elsewhere in the body?
  - ☐ Numbness (particularly of same side of face), weakness, loss of balance?
- ☐ Previous medical and surgical history: cancer?
- ☐ If patient over 50: symptoms of giant cell arteritis (GCA)?
- ☐ System review questions.

Examination

- ☐ Visual acuity.
- ☐ Visual field defect to confrontation?
- ☐ Limitation of eye movements: sixth plus seventh nerve palsy: high risk of CPA tumor, e.g., vestibular schwannoma.
- ☐ Pupils: is there anisocoria?
- ☐ Eyelids: ptosis?
- ☐ Corneal and facial sensation to light touch: fifth plus seventh nerve palsy: high risk of CPA tumor, e.g., vestibular schwannoma.

☐ Orbicularis and facial muscle power: in the case of spasm, is there weakness as well as spasm?

☐ Hearing (to finger rub).

☐ If patient over 50: palpate temporal arteries.

☐ Perimetry if field defect to confrontation, decreased vision, relative afferent pupillary defect (RAPD), diplopia, or motility defect.

☐ Full neurologic examination if:

    ☐ The patient has a seventh nerve palsy that has not yet been fully investigated.

    ☐ The patient has unilateral facial spasm that has not yet been fully investigated.

Facial Weakness

FACIAL NERVE PALSY

Causes

- damage to the facial nucleus or fascicle
  - pontine infarction
  - demyelination
  - infiltration by tumor
- compression of the peripheral nerve
  - acoustic neuroma (schwannoma of the eighth cranial nerve)
  - other CPA or skull base tumors
  - parotid tumor
- inflammation of the peripheral nerve
  - viral infection (e.g., varicella zoster infection: Ramsay-Hunt syndrome)
  - infectious mastoiditis
  - sarcoidosis
- trauma (including surgical)
- idiopathic: "Bell's palsy"

Symptoms and Signs (Figs 12.1 and 12.2, Video 12.1)

Ophthalmic

- sore and/or watering eye
- blurred vision (corneal exposure)
- incomplete eyelid closure
- lower lid paralytic ectropion
- punctate epithelial loss of cornea
- reduced tear film (if nerve supply to lacrimal gland affected) or epiphora (failure of the lacrimal pump)

Other Symptoms of Facial Nerve Dysfunction

- problems with speech and eating/drinking
- drooping of the outer angle of the mouth
- inability to purse lips or "puff out" cheeks
- altered taste

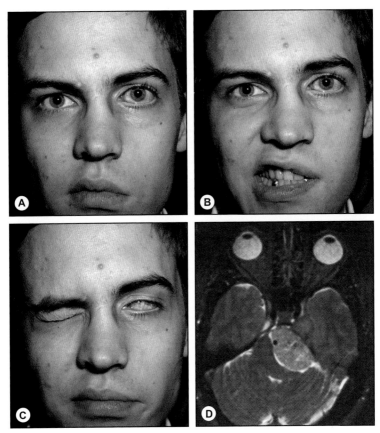

Fig. 12.1   This 24-year-old man was referred to his ophthalmologist "for treatment of left Bell's palsy." The patient complained of 6 months of left facial weakness and admitted on specific questioning to having a 10-month history of left deafness and tinnitus as well as numbness and tingling of the left side of the face. (**A**) The patient has marked left facial weakness. Note that the left eye is more open than the right due to left lower lid paralytic ectropion. (**B**) The patient cannot raise the lower portion of the left side of the face. (**C**) The patient cannot close the left eye tightly, nor can he lower the left brow. (**D**) Magnetic resonance imaging revealed a large meningioma in the left cerebellopontine angle.

Possible Localizing Symptoms and Signs

- loss of facial sensation: suggests a CPA lesion
- ipsilateral horizontal gaze palsy: pontine lesion
- double vision (horizontal; sixth cranial nerve palsy): suggests a pontine or a CPA lesion
- loss of hearing: suggests a CPA lesion
- vesicles in the external acoustic meatus: Ramsay-Hunt syndrome
- parotid lump

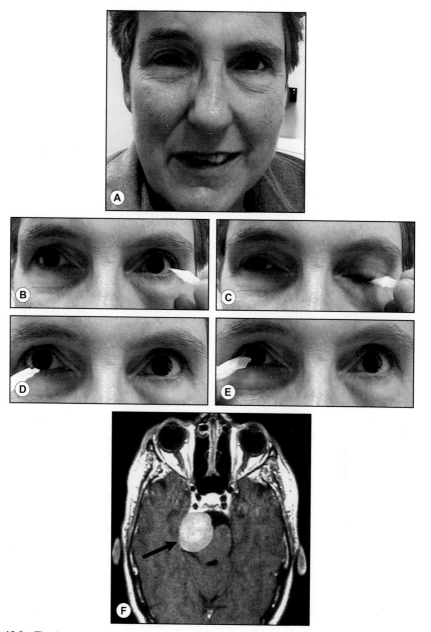

Fig. 12.2 The importance of testing corneal sensation in patients with facial weakness. This 44-year-old woman was referred by her doctor with right "Bell's palsy." (**A**) Examination revealed right-sided facial weakness. Corneal sensation testing revealed normal left corneal sensation (note reflex closure of eyelid) (**B**, **C**) but absent right corneal sensation (**D**, **E**). Abnormal corneal or facial sensation raises suspicion of a cerebellopontine angle tumor compressing both the fifth and seventh nerves, so magnetic resonance imaging was performed that revealed a large right-sided tumor (**F**) found at surgery to be a trigeminal schwannoma.

Differential Diagnosis

- "upper motor neuron" facial weakness due to contralateral cortical tumor or stroke (this usually spares the upper facial muscles)
- facial myopathy, typically bilateral and slowly progressive
- myasthenia gravis: other signs of this condition are usually present

Investigations

- assessment by otolaryngologist or neurologist
- magnetic resonance imaging (MRI) with detailed views of the course of the facial nerve

Ophthalmic Complications

- Exposure keratopathy and corneal ulceration: the risk of this is greatly increased if one or more of the following are present:
  - Severe orbicularis weakness.
  - Reduced corneal sensation.
  - Poor Bell phenomenon (the eyeball does not roll upwards on attempted forced closure of the eye).

Ophthalmic Treatment

- Regular review is required, especially if corneal sensation is reduced.
- Patients should be advised to seek immediate ophthalmic attention if their eye becomes unusually painful, red, or sticky.
- Lubricants.
  - Various drops, gels, and ointments are available.
  - The regimen is best guided by patient preference: some patients prefer to use drops frequently to maintain good vision, while others prefer to use ointments less frequently even though the ointment tends to reduce vision.
  - The patient must ensure that the lubricant covers the cornea.
- Eyelid taping at night.
  - Many patients sleep with their affected eye partially open.
  - A single piece of tape from the upper to the lower eyelid is an effective method of preventing this (should be placed horizontally not vertically).
- Tarsorrhaphy.
  - Not all patients require a tarsorrhaphy, and disfiguring lateral tarsorrhaphies should be avoided if possible.
  - Urgent temporary tarsorrhaphy (mattress suture on bolsters) if there are severe or worsening signs of exposure, if patient is very debilitated or has no caregiver who can help use lubricants, or if there is both corneal exposure and loss of corneal sensation.
- Other oculoplastic procedures.
  - Lateral canthal sling and medial canthoplasty for lower lid ectropion.
  - Insertion of upper eyelid gold weight: usually reserved for chronic facial palsies.

Involuntary Facial Movements

ORBICULARIS OCULI MYOKYMIA

Causes

- spontaneous repetitive firing of an orbicularis oculi motor unit
- usually idiopathic; may be precipitated by fatigue, stress, or excessive caffeine consumption
- very rarely, a presenting sign of multiple sclerosis (MS) or a compressive brainstem lesion

Demographic

- usually young adults

Symptoms and Signs

- Always monocular.
- Twitching or flickering of part of the orbicularis oculi muscle, most commonly affecting the lower lid.
- Occasionally forceful enough to cause oscillopsia.
- Contractions may last for several hours and recur over a period of weeks or months.
- Rarely, may progress to blepharospasm, hemifacial spasm, or a more generalized facial myokymia with facial weakness.

Investigations

- neuroimaging if persistent (more than 3 months) or spreads to involve other facial muscles

Treatment

- Usually resolves spontaneously.
- Avoid precipitating factors.
- Botulinum toxin injection into the affected part of the muscle is occasionally required for persistent cases.

BLEPHAROSPASM

Causes

- idiopathic: "essential blepharospasm"
- rarely associated with irritating or painful ocular diseases such as blepharitis, entropion, tear deficiency, corneal disease, or iritis ("reflex blepharospasm")
- associated with neurodegenerative diseases such as Parkinson disease or progressive supranuclear palsy (PSP) ("atypical blepharospasm" or apraxia of eyelid opening: see later)

Demographics

- middle-aged or elderly
- female predominance

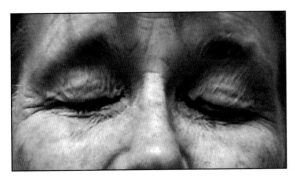

Fig. 12.3 Idiopathic blepharospasm.

Symptoms and Signs (Fig. 12.3, Video 12.2)

- Always binocular, although may begin as monocular eyelid myokymia.
- Patients typically present with a long history of either an increased blink rate or frequent, involuntary, forceful eyelid closure, causing embarrassment and, in severe cases, temporary blindness.
- Many complain of irritation similar to that caused by tear deficiency or blepharitis even if there are no signs of these conditions.
- The spasms usually involve the whole of both orbicularis oculi muscles, causing characteristic lowering of the eyebrows. Occasionally, the contractions are confined to the preseptal portions of the muscles.
- Some patients progress to a more generalized facial dystonia: Meige syndrome.

Differential Diagnosis

- Apraxia of eyelid opening ("atypical blepharospasm")
  - Patients with this condition have difficulty initiating eyelid opening, resulting in prolonged periods of bilateral eyelid closure.
  - A combination of varying degrees of orbicularis oculi spasm and inhibition of levator function.
  - Electromyographic studies have shown that some have inappropriate persistence of pretarsal orbicularis oculi activity during attempted eyelid opening.
  - Almost always associated with neurodegenerative disorders such as Parkinson disease or PSP.

Investigations

- None are required.

Treatment

- Treat any potentially exacerbating ocular disease, e.g., dry eye or blepharitis.
- Botulinum toxin injections to the orbicularis oculi muscles are the most effective current treatment.
  - Patients should be aware that the aim of treatment is to control rather than cure their symptoms.
  - The amount of botulinum toxin used should be individualized.

- The sites of injection are individualized but generally include upper and lower eyelids, brows, and, in some cases, forehead.
- The dose is adjusted according to response but usually high dose is needed.
- Injections usually need to be repeated every 2–4 months.
- Side effects (requiring adjustment of dose or position and/or number of injection sites) are uncommon but include transient ptosis or diplopia due to spread of the toxin into the orbit. These resolve spontaneously as the effects of the toxin wear off.
- Some patients with apraxia of eyelid opening benefit from botulinum toxin injection depending on how much of their eyelid closure is spastic. Most need high doses of toxin injected frequently; others may benefit from so-called "ptosis crutches" and still others may benefit from surgery, such as a levator resection or a frontalis sling procedure.
- Oral treatment, including tetrabenazine, clonazepam, and baclofen, has occasionally proved beneficial, particularly for patients with Meige syndrome.
- Partial or complete orbicularis oculi myectomy should be reserved for blepharospasm patients with severe symptoms that fail to respond to other forms of treatment.

HEMIFACIAL SPASM

Causes

- compression of the facial nerve in the CPA
  - usually by an intracranial artery or vein (sometimes more than one)
  - rarely by a tumor or aneurysm (1 in 200)
- idiopathic

Demographics

- most commonly middle-aged but can occur in childhood

Symptoms and Signs (Fig. 12.4, Video 12.3)

- Typically, patients progress over a period of months to years from mild twitching around one eye to repetitive synchronous spasm of all the facial muscles on the affected side.
- Most develop ipsilateral facial weakness with chronicity.
- Many have evidence of seventh nerve aberrant regeneration.

Investigations

- MRI of the brain with high-resolution views of the facial nerve and CPA

Treatment

- Posterior fossa surgery.
  - Microvascular decompression is curative in up to 90% of cases when vascular compression is present.
  - Potential complications include facial nerve palsy, ipsilateral hearing loss, and stroke.

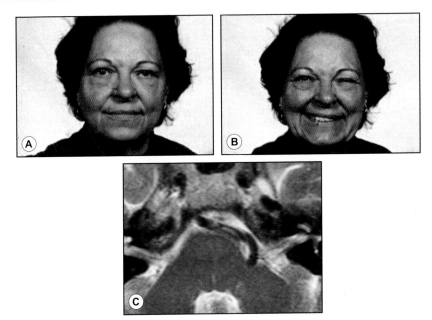

Fig. 12.4 Left hemifacial spasm. (**A**) Between spasms, the patient has a relatively normal appearance. (**B**) When the spasms occur, the left eyelid closes and the left lower face draws upward. (**C**) The patient underwent a magnetic resonance imaging that shows a tortuous basilar artery compressing the left seventh nerve at its exit from the brainstem.

- Botulinum toxin injections.
  - Provide reasonably effective control for many patients.
  - The treatment regimen is similar to that for blepharospasm.
  - Effects usually last 3–6 months or longer.
  - Additional injections may be given to lower facial muscles, but the orbicularis oris should be avoided because of the risk of causing problems with eating and drinking.
- Surgical destruction of the facial nerve has a high complication rate and should be avoided.

ABERRANT REGENERATION OF THE FACIAL NERVE

Causes

- previous facial nerve palsy
- rarely, as a primary phenomenon from a slow-growing tumor compressing or infiltrating the facial nerve

Demographic

- most commonly middle-aged but can occur in childhood

Symptoms and Signs

- Beginning several months after an acute facial palsy, patients develop involuntary closure of the eyelid on the side of the palsy when they move their mouth in certain directions, and their lower face twitches or pulls upward on the side of the palsy when they close the eye on that side.

Investigations

- none required assuming the facial nerve palsy was investigated

Treatment

- Botulinum toxin injections
  - Provide reasonably effective control for many patients.
  - The treatment regimen is similar to that for hemifacial spasm.

Unexplained Eye Pain, Orbital Pain, or Headache

Introduction

Headache or facial pain can both be due to disease in the:

- eye
- orbit
- fifth nerve
- meninges
- skull base
- paranasal sinuses
- internal carotid artery (ICA)
- neck

Headache and facial pain are common symptoms with multiple causes. The 2018 International Classification of Headache Disorders recognizes 70 primary and over 250 secondary headache types and subtypes, and 45 causes of cranial neuralgias and central causes of facial pain. Some patients will present to eye care professionals either because they have pain in or around the eye or because they have other ophthalmic symptoms or signs.

When presented with a patient whose principal symptom is headache or facial pain, the eye care professional has the responsibility to:

- Recognize and treat ophthalmic causes of headache and facial pain.
- Recognize ophthalmic symptoms and signs of an intracranial or systemic cause of headache or facial pain.

- Recognize common "benign" headache patterns with ophthalmic features.
- Know when to refer other patients for further investigation.

Examination Checklist

UNEXPLAINED EYE PAIN OR HEADACHE

Have you asked about, and looked for, all the following key features?

History

- ☐ The pain or headache
  - ☐ Where is it?
  - ☐ When did it start?
  - ☐ Speed of onset?
  - ☐ Development over time?
  - ☐ Triggers?
  - ☐ Getting better or worse or staying the same?
- ☐ Other neurologic symptoms?
  - ☐ Symptoms of raised intracranial pressure, e.g., nausea, vomiting, pulsatile tinnitus?
  - ☐ Symptoms of migraine, e.g., visual disturbance preceding headache, nausea, Photophobia?
  - ☐ Numbness, weakness, loss of balance?
  - ☐ Deafness, tinnitus, or vertigo? (possible cerebello-pontine angle [CPA] tumor)
  - ☐ Neck or arm pain: possible ICA dissection.
- ☐ Other ophthalmic symptoms: diplopia, blurred vision, redness, or swelling?
- ☐ Previous medical and surgical history: cancer?
- ☐ If patient over 50: symptoms of giant cell arteritis (GCA)?
- ☐ System review questions.

Examination

- ☐ Visual acuity.
- ☐ Refraction: undercorrected hypermetropia, overcorrected myopia, or presbyopia?
- ☐ Visual field defect to confrontation?
- ☐ Limitation of eye movements: sixth nerve palsy plus persistent orbital or hemifacial pain: high risk of skull base or cavernous sinus tumor.
- ☐ Pupils
  - ☐ Is there anisocoria?
  - ☐ Small pupil with ipsilateral pain: possible Horner syndrome due to tumor or ICA dissection.
  - ☐ Large pupil with ipsilateral pain: possible partial third nerve palsy due to aneurysm or tumor.
- ☐ Eyelids and adjacent skin
  - ☐ Ptosis: possible Horner syndrome or partial third nerve palsy.
  - ☐ Rashes: herpes zoster ophthalmicus.

☐ Corneal and facial sensation to light touch: if reduced: increased risk of compressive tumor.

☐ Orbicularis and facial muscle power: seventh nerve palsy plus persistent orbital or hemifacial pain: high risk of CPA tumor.

☐ Slit-lamp
    ☐ Conjunctiva, sclera: chemosis, injection?
    ☐ Anterior chamber: depth, cells, flare?
    ☐ Intraocular pressure (IOP)?
    ☐ Gonioscopy.
    ☐ Vitreous: cells?
    ☐ Disc: swelling, hemorrhages, pallor?

☐ If patient over 50: palpate temporal arteries.

☐ Perimetry if field defect to confrontation, decreased vision, relative afferent pupillary defect (RAPD), diplopia, or motility defect.

☐ Full neurologic examination if persistent headache or pain of unknown cause.

Ophthalmic Causes of Headache or Facial Pain

Most ophthalmic causes of headache or facial pain are easily diagnosed by their characteristic features, for example, the sharp "surface" pain of a corneal abrasion or the aching pain and photophobia of acute iritis. The following may be missed if not specifically considered.

HEADACHE DUE TO ANGLE-CLOSURE GLAUCOMA

- Typically severe pain in or around the affected eye.
- Usually associated with loss of vision, haloes around lights, and a red eye.
- Occasionally, patients experience recurrent episodes that resolve spontaneously with milder or no associated symptoms. Therefore, it is essential that all patients with atypical eye or facial pain are gonioscoped.

HEADACHE DUE TO HERPES ZOSTER OPHTHALMICUS

- Burning or aching, frequently severe pain in the distribution of the ophthalmic division of the trigeminal nerve.
- Often associated with hyperesthesia and/or numbness in the same area.
- Pain may precede the emergence of the vesicular rash by up to 1 week.
- If this diagnosis is suspected, the patient should be monitored closely and appropriate antiviral treatment started at the first signs of a rash or ocular inflammation. If no rash appears within 1 week, alternative diagnoses should be considered.

HEADACHE DUE TO REFRACTIVE ERROR

- Recurrent mild frontal and/or ocular headache.
- Normally absent on awakening.
- Precipitated or aggravated by prolonged visual tasks (e.g., reading for patients with presbyopia).
- Always remits with visual rest.
- Headaches are often attributed to refractive error; genuine cases are rare but rapidly respond to the use of appropriate glasses.

HEADACHE DUE TO HETEROPHORIA OR HETEROTROPIA

- Recurrent nonpulsatile mild to moderate frontal headache.
- Caused by significant heterophoria (close to or at limit of fusion range) or intermittent heterotropia.
- Patients often also complain of intermittent blurred vision or diplopia and difficulty adjusting focus.
- Usually absent upon awakening but worsens throughout the day.

Ophthalmic Symptoms and Signs of an Intracranial or Systemic Cause of Headache or Facial Pain

Intracranial causes of headache or facial pain include tumors, inflammation, or infection of the meninges, skull base, or paranasal sinuses and arterial dissection or aneurysm.

In general, headaches or facial pain due to an intracranial or systemic cause are of recent (and sometimes sudden) onset. Ophthalmic symptoms and signs may include:
- optic disc swelling (usually bilateral) with (usually) normal vision: raised intracranial pressure
- optic disc swelling (usually unilateral) with (usually) severe loss of vision: GCA
- single or multiple cranial neuropathies affecting third to sixth nerves: compression, infiltration, or inflammation
- anisocoria (Horner syndrome or third cranial nerve palsy)

Important disorders to consider include the following:

GIANT CELL ARTERITIS (GCA)

(See p. 85.)
- The headache of GCA may be "temporal," but is often bifrontal or diffuse.
  - Although headaches are common in elderly patients, most patients with GCA recognize a "new" type of, or unusually severe, headache.
  - However, some patients with GCA have no headache at all.
- Patients may also complain of ear, neck, jaw, or tongue pain.
- GCA may present with eye or orbital pain due to ocular ischemic syndrome (with or without headache).
  - This pain may worsen on standing up and improve on lying down.

- One or more of the following visual symptoms may also be present:
  - transient blurred vision (including "amaurosis fugax")
  - persisting blurred vision
  - transient diplopia (with a normal motility examination)
  - persisting diplopia (due to third, fourth, or sixth nerve palsy, orbital ischemic syndrome, or stroke)

RAISED INTRACRANIAL PRESSURE

- The headache is typically diffuse and constant (nonpulsatile). It is usually present on waking and aggravated by coughing, straining, or lying down.
- Disc swelling is usually bilateral (see p. 155).
- Unilateral or bilateral sixth cranial nerve palsies may be present ("false localizing sign").
- There may also be localizing signs of the cause of the raised intracranial pressure.
- Management is urgent neuroimaging (magnetic resonance imaging [MRI] and magnetic resonance venography [MRV] or computed tomographic [CT] scanning and CT venography [CTV]) looking for a space-occupying lesion or sinus thrombosis.
- Patients with papilledema require treatment of the underlying cause and regular monitoring of visual function (see p. 159).

PITUITARY APOPLEXY

- Sudden hemorrhagic infarction and expansion of the pituitary, usually associated with a pre-existing pituitary adenoma.
- The headache is typically severe and of sudden onset. It may be retro-orbital, frontal, or diffuse.
- Patients may have a reduced level of consciousness.
- Ophthalmic signs may include monocular or binocular visual loss, ptosis, and ophthalmoplegia.
- Patients require immediate admission for imaging, endocrine assessment (they frequently require urgent corticosteroid replacement), stabilization, and consideration of neurosurgical decompression.

INTERNAL CAROTID ARTERY (ICA) DISSECTION

ICA dissection should be considered in the differential diagnosis of all unilateral headache or facial pain, particularly if associated with Horner syndrome.

Causes

- spontaneous: associated with Marfan syndrome, fibromuscular dysplasia, etc.
- secondary to head or neck trauma, including "whiplash" or chiropractic manipulation

Symptoms and Signs

- Sudden onset of unilateral moderate to severe throbbing or aching pain, localized to the orbital, periorbital, or frontal region.
- The pain may be isolated or associated with:
  - Anisocoria: the most common associated symptom, due to disruption of the perivascular sympathetic supply.
  - Visual loss: ischemic optic neuropathy or retinal artery occlusion.
  - Oculomotor cranial neuropathies.

Investigations

- Neuroimaging: initially, MRI and MR angiography (MRA) or CT angiography (CTA) of the neck, possibly followed by catheter angiography.

Treatment

- Treatment remains somewhat controversial but usually consists of anticoagulation with heparin followed by warfarin for 6 months.

TRIGEMINAL NEURALGIA

Causes (Fig. 13.1)

- Secondary trigeminal neuralgia: MRI shows compression of the fifth nerve or one of its branches by tumor, aneurysm, or ectatic arterial loop; rarely due to multiple sclerosis (MS).
- Idiopathic trigeminal neuralgia: MRI shows no cause.

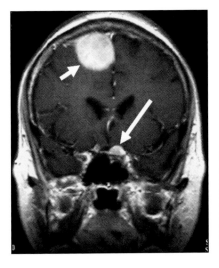

Fig. 13.1 This patient was diagnosed by her local doctor as having "trigeminal neuralgia"; after a further 2 years of severe persistent left facial pain, brain magnetic resonance imaging revealed a small left clinoidal meningioma *(long arrow)* to be the likely cause of her pain. A larger but asymptomatic hemispheric meningioma *(short arrow)* was incidentally identified as well.

Symptoms

- Persistent or recurrent unilateral facial or periocular pain.
- Pain may be constant and aching or transient, "electric shock-like."
- Sometimes, also symptoms of "pins and needles" or "ants crawling under the skin" in one or more of the trigeminal distributions.
- Pain triggered by innocuous stimuli in the trigeminal distribution (e.g., applying makeup, cold air, light touch).

Signs

- Finding one or more of the following ipsilateral to the pain increases the chance of a compressive or infiltrative tumor:
  - decreased corneal or facial sensation
  - ptosis or anisocoria (partial third nerve palsy or sympathetic lesion)
  - sixth, seventh, or eighth nerve palsy (CPA lesion)

Investigations

- All patients with unexplained, persistent, severe unilateral facial pain require MRI neuroimaging to exclude a serious cause for the trigeminal symptoms. The MRI requested should be a high-resolution scan with contrast, focused on the course of the fifth nerve.

Treatment

- secondary trigeminal neuralgia: treat the causative lesion
- primary trigeminal neuralgia
  - medical treatment: tricyclic antidepressants, carbamazepine, other drugs
  - surgical treatment: radiofrequency or surgical ablation of the trigeminal ganglion; decompression of the trigeminal nerve in the subarachnoid space; retrogasserian glycerol injection

Common "Benign" Headache Patterns With Ophthalmic Features

The characteristic feature of these conditions is that they are recurrent. Patients usually give a clear history of multiple episodes, sometimes over many years. Provided that there are no atypical features in the history and that examination (between episodes) is normal, no investigations are required. However, treatment can be difficult and most patients should probably be referred to a specialist.

MIGRAINE

CLINICAL DIAGNOSTIC CRITERIA FOR MIGRAINE

A. At least five attacks fulfilling B–D
B. Headache attacks lasting 4–72 hours (untreated or unsuccessfully treated)
C. Headache has at least two of the following four characteristics
  1. unilateral location
  2. pulsating quality
  3. moderate or severe pain intensity
  4. aggravation by or causing avoidance of routine physical activity (e.g., walking, climbing stairs)
D. During headache, at least one of the following:
  1. nausea and/or vomiting
  2. photophobia and/or phonophobia
E. Not better accounted for by another ICHD-3 diagnosis

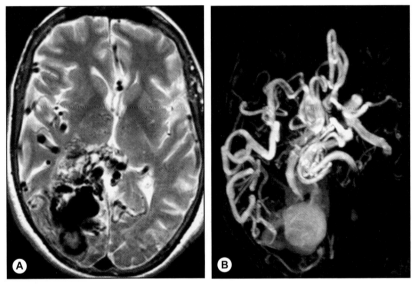

Fig. 13.2 This patient began having "migraines" with blurred vision at age 45. Perimetry revealed a left homonymous visual field defect, so magnetic resonance imaging (MRI) was performed, revealing a large right occipital arteriovenous malformation, which had been triggering visual seizures. (**A**) MRI. (**B**) Magnetic resonance angiography.

- All ages; frequently positive family history.
- Headaches are usually unilateral (but may be bilateral, especially in childhood), pulsating and of moderate or severe intensity.
- Associated with nausea and/or photophobia and phonophobia.
- An episode may last from a few hours to 3 days.
- Patients may present to eye care professionals either because their pain is localized to the periocular region or because they have associated visual aura (see p. 188) or, much more rarely, diplopia.
- Caution: many patients call all headaches "migraines." Don't believe it is "migraine" just because the patient tells you it is (Fig. 13.2)!

TRIGEMINAL AUTONOMIC CEPHALALGIAS (TACs)

- These are primary unilateral headaches in the territory of the trigeminal nerve associated with autonomic signs on the same side (e.g., tearing, ptosis, and miosis).
- TACs include cluster headache, paroxysmal hemicrania, short-lasting unilateral neuralgiform headache attacks with conjunctival injection and tearing (SUNCTs), short-lasting unilateral neuralgiform headache attacks with cranial autonomic symptoms (SUNAs), and long-lasting autonomic symptoms with hemicrania (LASHs).
- TAC sufferers, and their doctors, may be convinced that they have an "eye problem," because:
  - Excrutiating pain can be experienced in the eye or orbit.
  - There is often accompanying eye redness, tearing, or ptosis.
- TACs can be differentiated by length and frequency of recurrence of the headaches.
- Patients with TACs should be referred to a neurologist for management.

When to Refer Other Patients for Further Investigation

- The majority of headaches have no serious underlying cause, so routine investigation of patients with headaches should be avoided. However, isolated headaches may be the only presenting sign of serious intracranial pathology.
- Therefore, any patient presenting with a sudden or recent-onset new headache or facial pain should not be ignored, particularly if the pain is severe, if it is unlike any headache that they have suffered before and/or if it awakens the patient from sleep.
- We would recommend that such patients be promptly referred to a neurologist for further assessment.

Neuro-ophthalmic History Checklist

- ☐ age, occupation, marital status
- ☐ presenting complaint
- ☐ other ophthalmic symptoms
- ☐ previous ophthalmic history
- ☐ previous medical history
- ☐ medications and allergies
- ☐ previous surgical history
- ☐ family history
- ☐ social and occupational history
- ☐ if patient over 50: ask specifically for symptoms of giant cell arteritis (GCA) if history of transient or persistent blurred vision, transient or persistent diplopia, or headache
- ☐ system review questions
  - ☐ "head to toe": specific questions to detect previously undiagnosed systemic disease.

Neuro-ophthalmic Examination Checklist

- ☐ visual acuity
- ☐ color acuity
- ☐ visual fields to confrontation
- ☐ eye movements
  - ☐ fixation holding (is there nystagmus?)
  - ☐ primary position deviation (observation, cover test)
  - ☐ smooth pursuit (range of eye movements)
  - ☐ saccades (horizontal, vertical)
  - ☐ others types of eye movement only if required (see Chapter 6).
- ☐ pupils
  - ☐ record size of each in mm
  - ☐ do both constrict briskly to light?
  - ☐ is a relative afferent pupillary defect (RAPD) present on the "swinging light test?"
- ☐ lids—ptosis or lid retraction?
- ☐ orbits—proptosis, enophthalmos, injection, chemosis?
- ☐ corneal and facial sensation to light touch
- ☐ orbicularis and facial muscle power
- ☐ if patient over 50: palpate the temporal arteries for pulsatility and tenderness

- ☐ **perimetry (if required) before dilating drops**
- ☐ **slit-lamp examination**
- ☐ **plus if required:**
  - ☐ blood pressure
  - ☐ full neurologic examination
  - ☐ full systemic examination.

Miller, N. R., Subramanian, P. S., & Patel, V. R. (2020). *Walsh and Hoyt's Clinical Neuro-Ophthalmology: The Essentials* (4th edn). Wolters Kluwer, 2020. Philadelphia, PA.

The perfect "step up" from *The Neuro-ophthalmology Survival Guide*: an excellent resource for those wanting more detailed information about specific neuro-ophthalmic conditions. Summarizes key information from the "full" Walsh and Hoyt volumes.

Miller, N. R., & Newman, N. J. (eds.). (2005). *Walsh and Hoyt's Clinical Neuro-Ophthalmology* (6th edn), 3 vols. Lippincott Williams and Wilkins. Philadelphia, PA.

The ultimate reference text for neuro-ophthalmologists. Contains detailed descriptions on all common and rare neuro-ophthalmic diseases.

Lyons, C., & Lambert, S. (2022). *Taylor and Hoyt's Pediatric Ophthalmology and Strabismus* (6th edn). Elsevier. Amsterdam.

Contains excellent chapters on childhood strabismus and pediatric neuro-ophthalmic disorders.

Biousse, V., & Newman, N. J. (2020). *Neuro-Ophthalmology Illustrated* (3rd edn). Thieme. Stuttgart.

A lavishly illustrated text, written by two of the premier neuro-ophthalmologists in the world today, covers the diagnosis and treatment of neuro-ophthalmological disorders in detail. It includes more than 900 full-color images, line drawings, and charts that help readers understand these complex conditions.

Liu, G. T., Volpe, N. J., & Galetta, S. L. (2018). *Liu, Volpe and Galetta's Neuro-Ophthalmology: Diagnosis and Management* (3rd edn). Elsevier. Amsterdam.

An excellent guide to neuro-ophthalmic diagnosis and management.

Somlai, J., & Kovacs, T. (eds.). (2016). *Neuro-Ophthalmology*. Springer. New York, NY.

Edited by two prominent Hungarian neuro-ophthalmologists with chapters written by over 50 contributors, this is one of the most comprehensive texts on the market today.

Page numbers followed by "*b*" indicate boxes, "*f*" indicate figures, and "*t*" indicate tables.